Atlas
of Cardiothoracic
Surgery

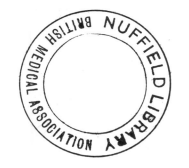

Atlas
of Cardiothoracic
Surgery

L. HENRY EDMUNDS, JR., M.D.
W. M. Measey Professor and Chief of Cardiothoracic Surgery
University of Pennsylvania
Philadelphia, Pennsylvania

WILLIAM I. NORWOOD, M.D., Ph.D.
Professor and Chief of Cardiovascular Surgery
Children's Hospital of Philadelphia
Philadelphia, Pennsylvania

DAVID W. LOW, M.D.
Assistant Professor of Surgery
Division of Plastic Surgery
Hospital of the University of Pennsylvania
Philadelphia, Pennsylvania

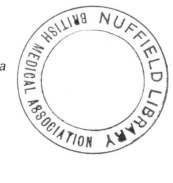
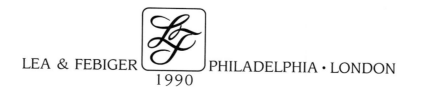
LEA & FEBIGER   PHILADELPHIA · LONDON
1990

Lᴇᴀ & Fᴇʙɪɢᴇʀ
600 Washington Square
Philadelphia, PA   19106-4198
U.S.A.
(215)922-1330

Lᴇᴀ & Fᴇʙɪɢᴇʀ (UK) Lᴛᴅ.
145a Croydon Road
Beckenham, Kent BR3 3RB
U.K.

Library of Congress Cataloging in Publication Data

Edmunds, L. Henry.
    Atlas of cardiothoracic surgery: L. Henry Edmunds, Jr.,
    William
  I. Norwood, David W. Low.
        p.   cm.
    Includes index.
    ISBN 0-8121-1224-5
    1. Heart—Surgery—Atlases.   2. Chest—Surgery—
    Atlases.
  1. Norwood, William I.   II. Low, David W.   III. Title.
    [DNLM: 1. Heart Surgery—atlases.   2. Thoracic Sur-
    gery—atlases.
  WG 17 E24a]
  RD597.E36   1989
  617.4'12'00222—dc20
  DNLM/DLC
  for Library of Congress   89-12294
                                                        CIP

PRINTED IN THE UNITED STATES OF AMERICA

Print number: 5 4 3 2 1

DEDICATION

To the teachers for whom we were students,
To the students for whom we are teachers.

Preface

THIS ATLAS is designed for practicing surgeons, residents, and students interested in contemporary cardiothoracic surgery. The illustrations and descriptions are presented in stepwise fashion to indicate the sequence of tasks and the anatomic relationships that appear. No attempt is made to discuss indications, results, or complications; these important tasks are better left to standard texts, scientific journals, and postgraduate training.

We have made a deliberate effort to make the atlas reasonably comprehensive and to cover those operations assigned to "thoracic surgery" by the American Board of Thoracic Surgery and the Residency Review Committee. However, no surgical atlas is truly comprehensive; it is not possible to include new modifications and variations of procedures, and it is not practical to include rarely used but sometimes valuable old techniques. We have tried to provide readers with a wide range of sound methods and efficient operations which have proved safe and effective in our hands. We hope that the atlas provides fundamental information for students who are learning operations and tune-ups for experienced surgeons when performing uncommon procedures.

Surgical operations are not commodities; each operation is unique. Patients vary, diseases vary, and decisions are made on the basis of knowledge, experience, and judgment. This book was seven years in the making as Dr. Low combined drawing with residencies in general and plastic surgery. During this time, we updated some procedures and learned new modifications from colleagues which are not in this book. Cardiothoracic surgery is not static, but fundamentals of operative conduct change more slowly than technical innovations.

For the most part, we were taught the operations that are described and illustrated. As we practiced, we made efforts to improve the safety, efficiency, and effectiveness of our surgery, and to develop new procedures. The operations taught to us are not the ones we taught to our students. We belong to a continuum of educators in cardiothoracic surgery, and this book portrays a moment in this continuum. Hopefully, these collective efforts benefit patients.

The authors thank Mary Wittrock, Claire Beckmann, and Myra Monahan for their secretarial skills, and Dr. W. Clark Hargrove, III, who described the WPW operation. We also thank C. C. F. "Kit" Spahr, Jr. and Raymond R. Kersey of Lea & Febiger for their patience and support.

Philadelphia, Pennsylvania

L. HENRY EDMUNDS, JR., M.D.
WILLIAM I. NORWOOD, M.D., PH.D.
DAVID W. LOW, M.D.

Contents

Section 1

Incisions

Median Sternotomy with Variations

MEDIAN STERNOTOMY

① Median sternotomy is the most rapid and least painful access to the anterior mediastinum, pericardium, and heart. The incision transects the sternum midway between the costal sternal articulations from the sternal notch to the xiphoid process.

② The skin incision begins just below the sternal notch and ends 1 to 2 cm below the tip of the xiphoid. The periosteum of the midline of the sternum is incised with the cautery. Fibrous bands between the two clavicular heads are divided.

③ The sternum is divided in the midline with either an oscillating or Stryker saw. Periosteal bleeding points are cauterized; bone wax is often used to control bleeding from the marrow. The innominate vein, ascending aorta, and right ventricle are vascular structures that can be injured during this incision. The two edges of the sternum are held apart with a Finochietto retractor or a variation of this instrument. Incision of fibrous bands overlying the strap muscles in the neck and a centimeter or two of the midline abdominal fascia facilitates wide retraction.

④ For closure, the two edges of the sternum are usually approximated with No. 6 stainless steel wire passed around or through the bone. The wire is twisted to firmly approximate the two edges. A combination of simple or mattress wire sutures is used. Usually two simple wire sutures are placed superiorly in the manubrium and upper body. Two mattress sutures are used in the midbody; one or two simple sutures are used in the lower body. Rarely, if the sternum is osteoporotic and friable, Teflon felt pledgets are used as illustrated to reduce the likelihood of the wire cutting through bone and costal cartilage. No. 5 polyester sutures tied with 5 or 6 knots may be used instead of wire to further reduce the likelihood of cutting through.

⑤ Soft tissues are approximated with one layer of running No. 1 absorbable suture followed by a subcutaneous running suture. Either a subcuticular suture of 4-0 absorbable suture or skin clips are used to close the skin.

After open heart surgery, the mediastinum is drained by two large bore (No. 36 Fr) chest tubes. One angled chest tube is inserted between the diaphragmatic pericardium and inferior wall of the heart and the other straight tube is placed on the anterior surface of the heart. Both are brought out through stab wounds in the anterior abdominal wall below the xiphoid.

CERVICAL COLLAR INCISION WITH PARTIAL STERNOTOMY

⑥ The thyroid gland and cervical trachea can be adequately exposed by adding a cervical collar incision to a partial upper median sternotomy. The sternotomy incision need only extend downward to the manubrium to allow access to the anterior structures at the root of the neck. Strap muscles can be incised or retracted as required.

RIGHT PARACLAVICULAR EXTENSION

⑦ The proximal subclavian vessels at the root of the neck, including the distal innominate on the right, can be exposed by combining a full or partial median sternotomy with a right or left paraclavicular or collar incision. Anterior cervical strap muscles are divided or retracted; the sternal insertion of the sternocleidomastoid muscle is also divided.

STERNOCLEIDOMASTOID EXTENSION

⑧ The cervical esophagus and contents in the carotid sheath can be exposed by extending the median sternotomy incision upward along the anterior border of the right or left sternocleidomastoid muscles. This incision can be extended to expose the larynx and hypopharynx and can be used for some operations on the cervical trachea. The carotid bifurcation is easily exposed through this extension.

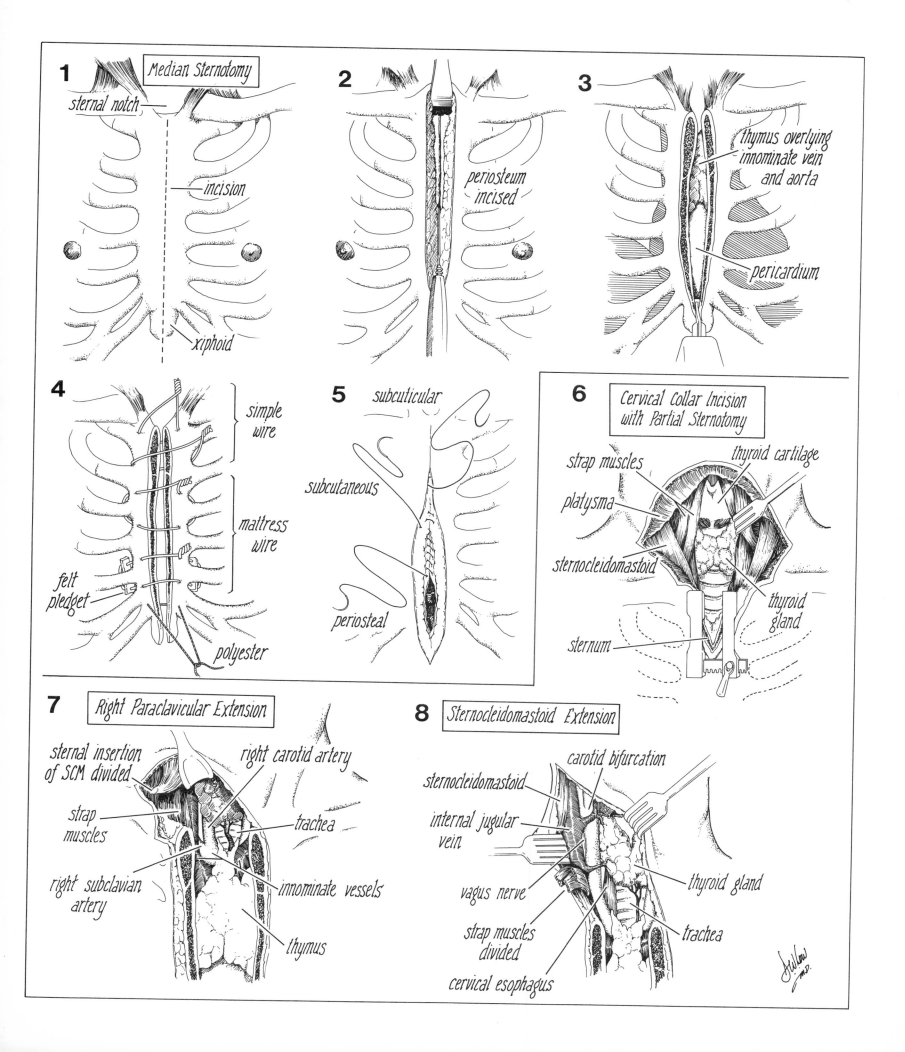

Median Sternotomy with Variations   *(Continued)*

THORACIC EXTENSIONS

⑨ To expose the aortic arch and proximal great vessels, a median sternotomy with left sternocleidomastoid extension can be combined with an extension into the left anterior third or fourth interspace. This allows lateral and outward reflection of the left anterior chest wall and good access to the ascending aorta, the arch, and the proximal portion of the descending thoracic aorta.

⑩ Exposure can be obtained by spreading ribs with a large retractor to allow the anterior chest wall and clavicle to move cephalad and outward. The two edges of the incised sternum are separated to expose the ascending aorta through this incision.

⑪ To expose the entire trachea from cricoid to carina, either a right collar incision or an incision along the right anterior border of the sternocleidomastoid muscle is combined with a partial upper sternotomy and right anterolateral thoracotomy. Usually, lower tracheal lesions can be satisfactorily exposed through a posterolateral thoracotomy; however, the more extended incision is needed to expose the entire trachea. The sternotomy incision is carried only to the third or fourth interspace, where it connects with the anterolateral thoracotomy.

⑫ These extended anterolateral thoracotomy incisions, which essentially displace the entire superior portion of the anterior chest wall, are easily closed if ribs are *not* resected. Adjacent ribs are stabilized with absorbable No. 1 suture pericostal ligatures and the sternum is closed with wire or heavy No. 5 polyester sutures as usual. Absorbable running sutures are used for soft tissues and skin.

REPEAT STERNOTOMY

Repeat median sternotomy must be done carefully to avoid incision of the innominate vein, ascending aorta, aortocoronary saphenous vein grafts, crossing right internal mammary artery-coronary graft, or anterior right ventricle. Until the heart and mediastinal structures are separated from the undersurface of the anterior chest wall, retraction of the incised sternal edges may tear any of these vascular structures. Closure of the pericardium during the previous operation does not ensure easy access the second or third time.

In all patients who have repeat midline sternotomy, both groins should be prepped into the surgical field and perfusion lines to the heart-lung machine should be made available for immediate partial cardiopulmonary bypass. Some surgeons routinely cut down over the common femoral artery and vein before beginning the sternotomy. Others locate the groin incision by palpating the femoral pulse, but do not expose the vessels or make the incision unless bleeding occurs.

⑬ After the sternum is exposed and previously placed sternal wires are removed, the outer table of the sternum is cut from notch to xiphoid with an oscillating saw. Following this, the inner table is cut carefully so that the saw does not penetrate below the underside of the sternum.

⑭ After the bone is cut, the two edges of the sternum separate slightly. With scissors or knife, the scar tissue between the underside of the sternal edges and deeper soft tissues is divided. The knife or scissors is held firmly against the underside of the sternum to avoid injury to the right ventricle, coronary grafts, aorta, or innominate vein.

⑮ As the space develops on both sides, the sternal edges can be elevated with bone hooks to facilitate incision of the scar tissue from the underside of the sternum and adjacent chest wall.

⑯ Alternatively, the xiphoid may be dissected out after the sternum is exposed. With the xiphoid elevated, the scar tissue between the underside of the intact sternum and heart (or pericardium) is cut with scissors bit by bit until a tunnel is developed from xiphoid to sternal notch.

⑰ With the closed scissors beneath the sternum, the bone is divided with an oscillating or Stryker saw. The two edges of the sternum and chest wall are dissected away as described above. This method risks injury if the tips of the scissors stray from the underside of the sternum but avoids injury that may occur from the oscillating saw if the heart lies against the sternum.

If significant bleeding occurs from injury to a major vascular compartment, a full dose of heparin is given immediately (3 mg per kg). After 2 minutes, the pump suckers of the heart-lung machine are used to aspirate field blood. No attempt should be made to separate the sternal edges until an arterial cannula is in place. The femoral artery is rapidly cannulated and shed blood is returned to the patient by way of the heart-lung machine. With this ability to return shed blood, the surgeon must dissect the heart away from the underside of the sternum and chest wall despite the bleeding to avoid enlarging the site of injury. As soon as possible, partial bypass is begun by cannulating the right atrium, right ventricle, or pulmonary artery; or by having an assistant cannulate the femoral vein.

The heart must be dissected out within the pericardium completely. This is recommended for all patients who require cold cardioplegia to achieve reliable and uniform myocardial preservation. If the patient has had one or both internal mammary arteries anastomosed to coronary vessels, great care must be taken to discover these pedicles to avoid injuring them. One method is to locate the distal coronary vessel downstream to the anastomosis and to dissect proximally until the anastomosis is located. The mammary pedicle is carefully dissected proximally until enough mobility is obtained to permit the planned operation. Particular care must be taken to separate the manubrium and upper anterior ribs from the mediastinal structures when mammary arteries have been used as grafts.

Entrance into either pleural space, if it has not been previously entered, permits rapid defibrillation of the heart if necessary before the heart is dissected out.

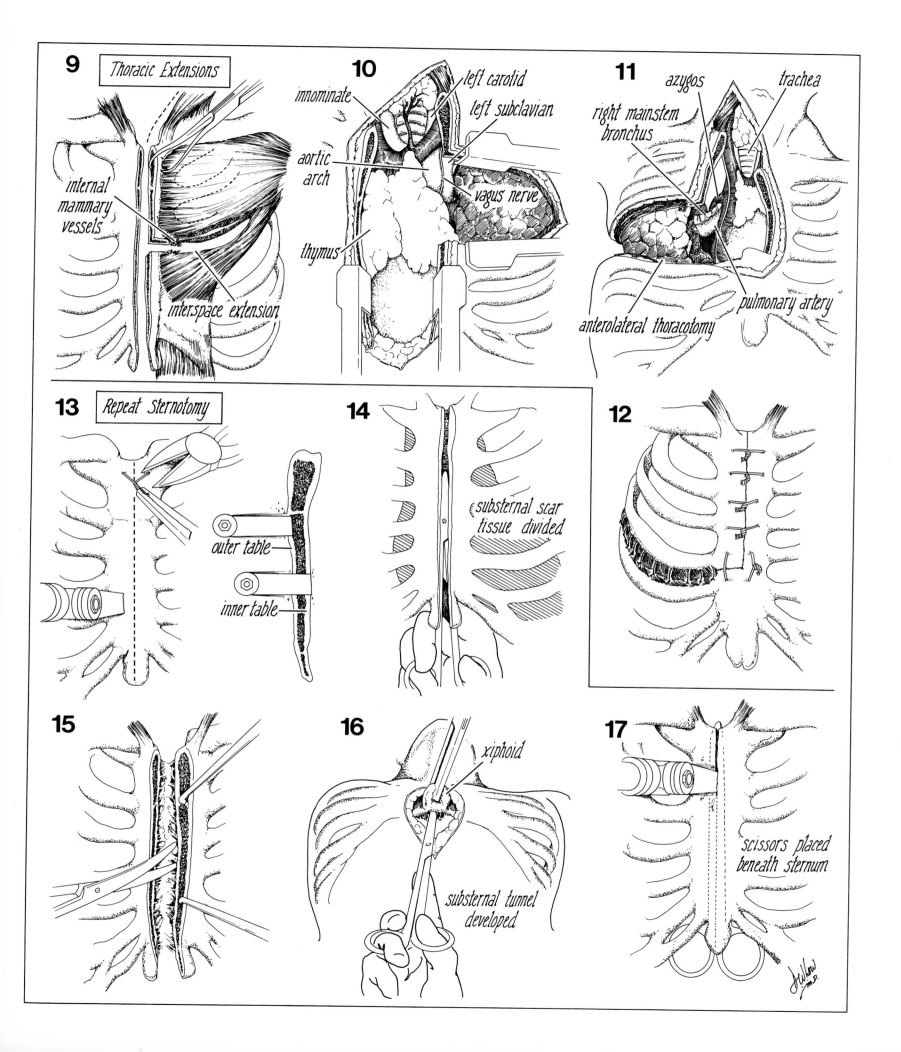

Thoracotomy with Variations

ANTERIOR THORACOTOMY

(18) An anterior thoracotomy incision is defined by the lateral edge of the sternum and anterior border of the latissimus dorsi. It can be made anywhere between the second and sixth ribs. For mediastinotomy, a short 3- to 4-inch incision and resection of the medial segment of the third rib provide adequate exposure of the anterior and middle mediastinum for node biopsy. A longer incision enters the ipsilateral pleural cavity and exposes the anterior pulmonary hilar structures. An anterior thoracotomy over the left fourth, fifth, or sixth rib exposes the anterior pericardium and left ventricle. If the planned anterior thoracotomy incision is small, the patient may be supine with the ipsilateral arm along the side. If a longer incision is planned, sandbags beneath the hip and shoulder should be used to rotate the patient 20 to 30 degrees toward the opposite side. The ipsilateral arm is suspended across the clavicle, neck, and face, or placed on a special arm board.

Usually a segment of rib is resected to enhance exposure. If wide exposure is needed, no rib is resected. Instead the anterior chest wall is elevated by entering the fourth or fifth intercostal space and incising the anterior costal cartilages of two to four ribs cephalad to the intercostal incision.

Usually a segment of rib is excised. The periosteum is incised longitudinally and elevated off the rib. The internal artery mammary artery and vein are identified in the intercostal space and either protected or ligated or clipped. The rib segment is cut and removed. The mediastinum and/or hemithorax is entered by incising the periosteum beneath the excised rib. If the rib is retained, the cephalad edge of the incised periosteum is reflected off the rib and the pleural cavity is entered through the intercostal space by incising the posterior periosteum beneath the rib.

Anterior thoracotomy incisions are closed by reapproximating adjacent structures. Incised cartilages are reattached to the sternum by single mattress sutures of polyester or wire. Usually it is possible to suture the intervening intercostal muscles to the sternal periosteum. When a rib is removed, adjacent intercostal muscles are closed by interrupted single or mattress sutures. Without rib resection, the reflected periosteum and attached intercostal muscles are folded over the rib and sutured to the intercostal muscle of the interspace below. The more superficial pectoralis minor, pectoralis major, and serratus anterior muscles are usually reapproximated with running 0 or No. 1 absorbable sutures.

MEDIASTINOTOMY

(19) For mediastinotomy, a short transverse incision is made over the anterior border of the third rib. A right mediastinotomy is illustrated. The internal mammary vascular pedicle is divided and the right pleura is gently pushed laterally to develop a plane between the right lobe of thymus, superior cava — right atrial junction and pericardium medially and the hilium of the lung laterally. Nodes may be found deep in the wound along the trachea.

(20) In men, longer anterior incisions may be made over the designated third, fourth, or fifth rib and extended laterally as exposure requires. In women, a submammary skin incision is made whenever possible. The breast is elevated. The pectoralis major muscle and interdigitations of the serratus over the designated rib are incised. The pectoralis minor muscle is divided.

(21) A convenient method of entering the chest with excision of a segment of rib is illustrated. The periosteum over the selected rib is incised longitudinally. The periosteum is elevated off the entire rib with a raspatory. The two ends are cut with shears and trimmed of any sharp spicules. The chest is entered by incising the posterior periosteum. Resection of a rib produces somewhat wider exposure and reduces the likelihood of adjacent rib fracture when the retractor is opened widely. Closure is achieved by approximating the adjacent intercostal muscles with interrupted single or mattress sutures.

(22) When a rib is not excised, the intercostal muscles between ribs can be incised directly. A modification, however, reduces bleeding and facilitates closure. The periosteum of the rib below (caudad to) the selected intercostal space is incised longitudinally with a cautery. With a raspatory, the cephalad margin is elevated and peeled from the rib to expose the posterior periosteum beneath the rib. The incision is made in the posterior periosteum to enter the pleural space.

LATERAL THORACOTOMY

(23) The patient is placed in the lateral position with the ipsilateral arm draped anteriorly and protected. A roll is placed on the opposite axilla to prevent brachial nerve injury. The upward leg is extended; the downward leg is flexed. Operation is usually facilitated by prior placement of a divided endotracheal tube so that the lung can be independently ventilated.

(24) The incision can be made over ribs 3 to 8 between the costochondral junction anteriorly and the auscultatory triangle (space between the borders of the trapezius and posterior latissumus dorsi inferiorly and rhomboids and posterior border of the scapula above).

(25) The latissimus dorsi, serratus anterior, and part of the pectoralis major muscles are divided over the selected rib. The rhomboids and trapezius muscles are reflected off the rib and retracted posteriorly. The rib can be excised or retained. If it is retained, the intercostal space can be incised. Closure of a direct intercostal incision with a retained rib is more difficult.

(26) When the incision is held open by a retractor, the scapula should be rotated and held anteriorly.

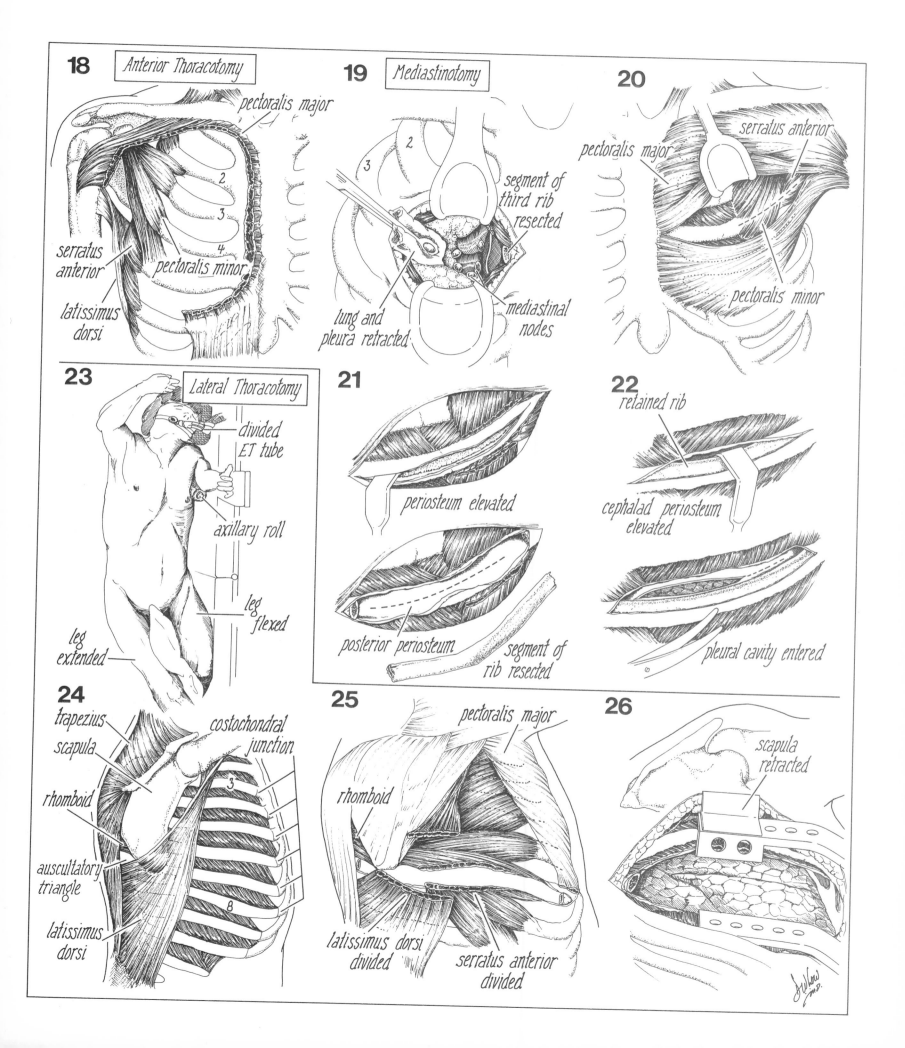

18 Anterior Thoracotomy

pectoralis major

2
3
4

serratus anterior

pectoralis minor

latissimus dorsi

19 Mediastinotomy

2
3

segment of third rib resected

lung and pleura retracted

mediastinal nodes

20

pectoralis major

serratus anterior

pectoralis minor

23 Lateral Thoracotomy

divided ET tube

axillary roll

leg flexed

leg extended

21

periosteum elevated

posterior periosteum

segment of rib resected

22 retained rib

cephalad periosteum elevated

pleural cavity entered

24

trapezius

scapula

rhomboid

auscultatory triangle

latissimus dorsi

costochondral junction

3

8

25

pectoralis major

rhomboid

latissimus dorsi divided

serratus anterior divided

26

scapula retracted

Thoracotomy with Variations *(Continued)*

POSTEROLATERAL THORACOTOMY

(27) This incision is similar to lateral thoracotomy but extends posteriorly and requires division of the rhomboid muscles. Anteriorly, the skin incision is parallel and over the fourth, fifth, or sixth rib from costochondral junction to auscultatory triangle. This skin incision should be made at least 2 cm below the tip of scapula to avoid overlying the tip. The incision curves around the scapular tip midway between the posterior border of the scapula and spine and may extend cephalad to the root of the neck if resection of the first, second, or third ribs is planned. The trapezius muscle must be cut if exposure of the posterior portion of high ribs is required; for incisions in the fourth or fifth interspaces, the trapezius muscle can usually be retracted or only partially incised.

(28) With lateral and posterolateral thoracotomy incisions, ribs are counted by entering the auscultatory triangle just posterior to the scapula and palpating the posterior portions of the ribs. The first rib, which has a small arc, is palpated cephalad and deep (medial) to the more easily palpated second rib.

(29) Once overlying muscles are divided or retracted, either a segmental rib can be resected or the chest may be entered through an intercostal space. In adults, exposure is better and closure is easier if a segmental rib is resected. In children and young adults, ribs are more easily separated and resection of a rib is not necessary for exposure.

(30) Thoracotomy incisions are usually closed with chest tube drainage. A straight tube placed through a lateral stab wound (so that the patient does not lie on the tube) is positioned so that the end is near the apex of the chest to remove air if the lung is incised. A low posteriorly angled tube is used to remove blood and fluid.

(31) Thoracotomy incisions are closed with absorbable sutures, although permanent sutures may also be used. If the rib is *not* resected, four or five heavy (No. 1) absorbable sutures are passed around the stripped rib and the one above to approximate the two. The intercostal muscles and periosteum are sutured over the stripped rib with continuous No. 1 absorbable suture to place the stripped periosteum against the rib. Sutures pass through the intercostal muscle and periosteum above and over the rib into the intercostal muscles below the stripped rib. Thereafter, the divided muscles are reapproximated with No. 1 or 0 absorbable sutures. For very thick muscles, two rows of sutures are used—one in the posterior muscle fascia and the other in the anterior fascia.

(32) When the rib is removed, the two edges of divided periosteum and attached intercostal muscles are approximated with interrupted No. 1 simple or mattress sutures. These are tied when the adjacent ribs are held together by a rib approximater. Continuous sutures are used to approximate the divided muscles, subcutaneous tissues and skin.

Before the chest is closed, intercostal nerves above and below the incision are injected with a long-lasting local anesthetic by means of a thin (No. 22) needle to reduce postoperative pain. After the needle tip enters the parietal pleura near the nerve, the plunger is pulled back to ensure that blood is not withdrawn and 0.5 to 2 ml are injected. Usually two nerves above and below the excised rib are injected.

AXILLARY THORACOTOMY

(33) A high, small incision between the latissimus dorsi posteriorly and pectoralis major anteriorly can be used to reach the apex of the lung and chest cavity. A segment of the lateral third rib should be removed, but the two large muscles can be retracted and need not be cut. This incision can be used to oversew apical blebs and is also the preferred approach to resect cervical and first ribs in patients with the thoracic outlet syndrome.

BILATERAL SUBMAMMARY THORACOTOMY

(34) This infrequently used incision consists of bilateral anterior thoracotomies with horizontal transection of the sternum. The skin incision is made over the xiphoid and beneath the breasts. Usually the fourth or occasionally the right fourth and left third interspaces are entered after the pectoralis major and minor and digitations of the serratus anterior muscles are divided. The internal mammary artery and vein are located in the selected interspaces and ligated and divided before the sternum is transected horizontally or obliquely.

This incision may be selected to expose the ascending and proximal descending aorta and can be used for intracardiac operations. The incision is closed by reapproximating the sternum with two wire sutures and the usual closure of the anterior thoracotomies.

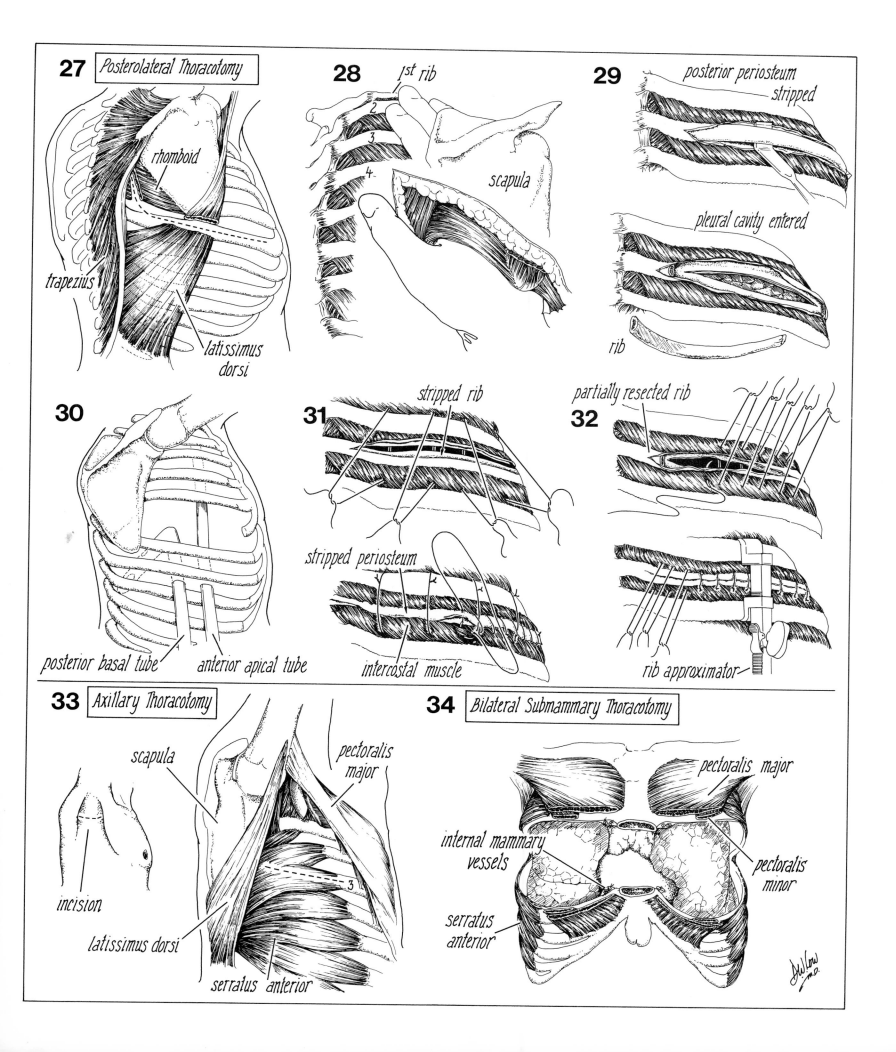

27 Posterolateral Thoracotomy

rhomboid

trapezius

latissimus dorsi

28 1st rib

scapula

29 posterior periosteum stripped

pleural cavity entered

rib

30 posterior basal tube anterior apical tube

31 stripped rib

stripped periosteum

intercostal muscle

32 partially resected rib

rib approximator

33 Axillary Thoracotomy

scapula

pectoralis major

incision

latissimus dorsi

serratus anterior

34 Bilateral Submammary Thoracotomy

pectoralis major

internal mammary vessels

serratus anterior

pectoralis minor

DOUBLE THORACOTOMY

(35) For aneurysms of the descending thoracic aorta, a single long posterolateral skin incision is made over the fifth rib. The pectoralis, serratus anterior, and latissimus dorsi muscles are divided over the fifth rib. The rhomboids and anterior border of the trapezius muscle are divided posteriorly. The skin, scapula, and muscle flap are elevated and the fourth or even third rib is resected. A long skin incision allows the high ribs to be reached. This incision exposes the proximal descending thoracic aorta.

To expose the distal descending thoracic aorta, the seventh or eight rib is resected. The overlying latissimus is sometimes elevated as a flap but more often is divided over the selected rib. The rib is excised. When the retractor is transferred to the lower chest wall incision, the distal descending thoracic aorta is satisfactorily exposed.

LEFT THORACOTOMY WITH DIAPHRAGMATIC INCISION

The overhanging costochondral margins impair exposure of the upper abdomen and retroperitoneum by abdominal incisions. Thoracoabdominal incisions are designed to expose the upper abdomen and lower mediastinum, and because of the location of the liver are almost always made on the left side. These incisions are used to expose the lower esophagus and upper stomach, the left diaphragm, and the thoracoabdominal aorta.

(36) A low lateral thoracotomy with resection of the left seventh or eighth rib combined with an incision in the left diaphragm produces excellent exposure of the esophageal hiatus, lower third of the esophagus, and lower abdomen. Transection of the costal margin, which causes considerable postoperative pain, is avoided.

The patient is positioned for a lateral thoracotomy and both the chest and upper abdomen are prepped. A generous thoracotomy incision is made over the seventh or eighth rib from the costal margin anteriorly to near the anterior border of the sacrospinalis muscles posteriorly. The rib is excised, but the costal margin is not broken. After retraction of the left lung, the esophageal hiatus at the diaphragm is located.

(37) For most operations, exposure requires an incision in the diaphragm that reaches the esophageal hiatus. This incision is made radially from the esophageal hiatus to the posterior chest wall and then anteriorly near the attachment of the diaphragm to the chest wall in an effort to preserve the function of the phrenic nerve. Although the circumferential incision is longer, it provides excellent exposure to the stomach and upper abdomen, and with retraction even the duodenum can be reached.

Cut edges of the diaphragm should be reapproximated with heavy (No. 1 or 0) permanent mattress sutures. The diaphragm and esophageal hiatus are reconstructed first. If the diaphragm is thin and friable, Teflon felt pledgets may be used with the mattress sutures.

STANDARD THORACOABDOMINAL INCISION

(38) The standard thoracoabdominal incision divides the costal margin and is usually carried across the left rectus abdominis to the midline. The patient is usually rotated about 30 degrees posteriorly to facilitate the abdominal incision. The incision starts over the seventh or eighth ribs posteriorly and is carried anteriorly across the costal margin and across the transverse abdominis and rectus abdominis muscles.

(39) After the chest and peritoneum are entered, the intervening diaphragm is cut either radially to the esophageal or aortic hiatus or circumferentially as described above. This incision gives somewhat better exposure of the abdomen but is considerably longer and more painful than the combined thoracotomy-diaphragmatic incision.

(40) Closure of this incision requires approximation of the cut costal margin. Removal of a small (1 cm) segment of cartilage facilitates approximation of the two ends with one or more heavy single or mattress sutures. The abdominal part of the incision can be closed with interrupted or running sutures layer by layer. The thoracotomy part of the incision is closed, usually with one chest tube for drainage in a standard fashion.

EXPOSURE OF THORACOABDOMINAL AORTA

(41) A similar incision can be used to expose the lower chest and upper posterior mediastinum and is excellent for operations on the thoracoabdominal aorta. The patient is either positioned for a straight lateral thoracotomy or rotated slightly posteriorly. The incision is placed over the eighth or ninth rib and carried past the rib end onto the abdominal wall. The rib can be excised and the abdominal wall muscles are carefully transected down to but not into the peritoneum. The plane between the posterior wall of the transverse abdominus muscle and the peritoneum is developed and, with gentle dissection, the peritoneum and its contents are pushed anteriorly. The diaphragm is incised about one inch from its attachment to the body wall, around laterally.

(42) Further dissection provides excellent exposure of the lower descending thoracic aorta, the thoracoabdominal aorta, and the left kidney. Development of the plane outside the peritoneum facilitates retraction and exposure.

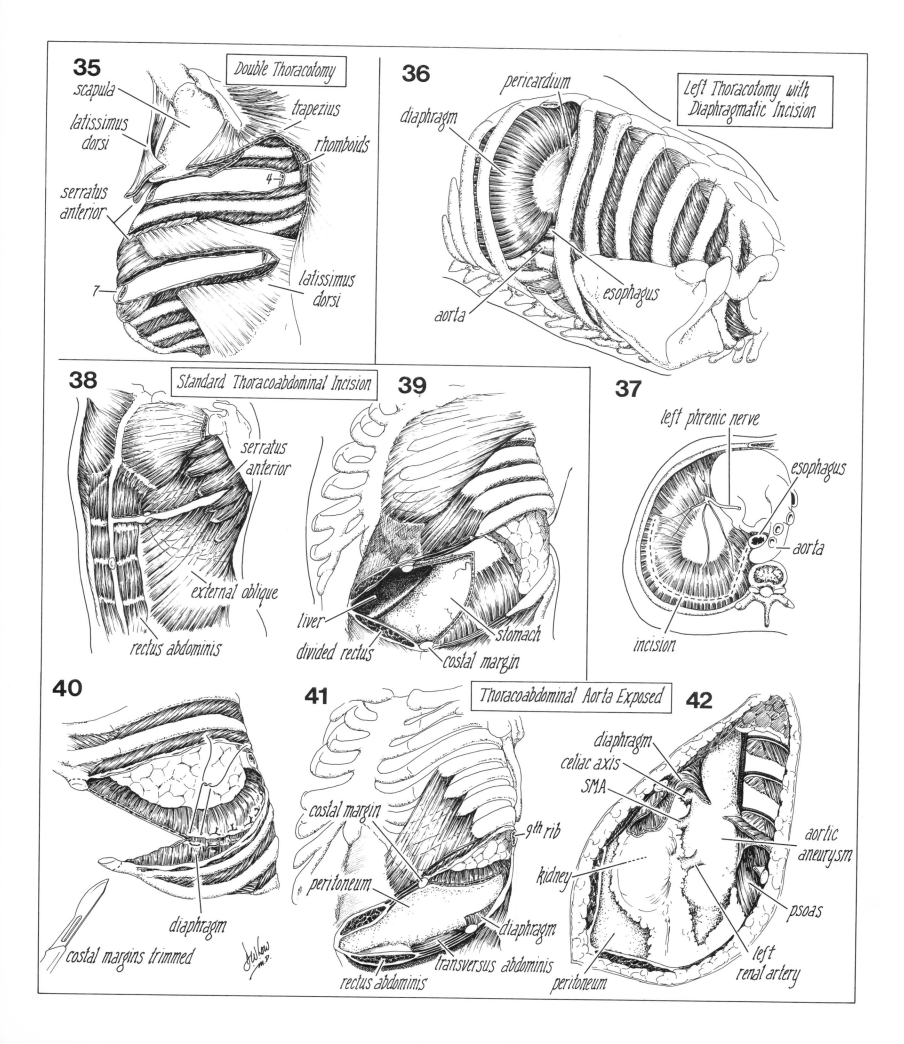

35 — Double Thoracotomy

scapula
latissimus dorsi
serratus anterior
7
trapezius
rhomboids
4
latissimus dorsi

36 — Left Thoracotomy with Diaphragmatic Incision

diaphragm
pericardium
aorta
esophagus

38 — Standard Thoracoabdominal Incision

serratus anterior
external oblique
rectus abdominis

39

liver
divided rectus
stomach
costal margin

37

left phrenic nerve
esophagus
aorta
incision

40

diaphragm
costal margins trimmed

41 — Thoracoabdominal Aorta Exposed

costal margin
peritoneum
rectus abdominis
9th rib
diaphragm
transversus abdominis

42

diaphragm
celiac axis
SMA
kidney
aortic aneurysm
psoas
left renal artery
peritoneum

Section 2

Acquired Heart Disease

Epicardial Pacemaker

Occasional patients require epicardial pacemaker leads. These are most easily placed during median sternotomy for intracardiac surgery or myocardial revascularization.

MEDIAN STERNOTOMY

① With the heart exposed and after the intracardiac repair and/or revascularization is complete, "sutureless," corkscrew, ventricular pacemaker leads may be placed in left ventricular muscle. Usually two leads are placed: one in the bare area of the apex just to the left of the distal left anterior descending coronary artery, and the other along the obtuse margin away from a marginal vessel at approximately mid-ventricle. "Sutureless" electrodes are twisted into the myocardium by 3.5 turns and eventually heal into place by epicardial scarring into the porous cloth washer.

② Plunge ventricular epicardial electrodes are sutured onto the epicardial surface with two sutures after the electrode is buried into a small hole made with a No. 11 scalpel blade. A "fish-hook" electrode may also be used for the ventricle, but a mattress suture should be used in addition to the "barb" to keep the electrode from backing out.

③ Permanent atrial epicardial leads are sutured directly to the right atrium near the base of the right atrial appendage with two 4-0 monofilament sutures tied over Teflon felt pledgets to reduce bleeding.

④ Permanent epicardial pacemaker leads are passed into the subcutaneous tissue of the left (usually) or right upper abdomen by blunt dissection. A space between the costal attachment of the diaphragm and rib is made with a Crile clamp. The clamp is passed beneath the costal margin anterior to the abdominal musculature into the subcutaneous tissue of the upper abdominal wall. A 3 cm transverse incision is made 5 to 8 cm below the costal margin over the lateral border of the rectus muscle in the upper abdomen. The incision is deepened down to the abdominal muscles. By blunt dissection, a small pocket is made between the abdominal wall muscles and the subcutaneous tissue. Through this incision, a Crafoord or DeBakey clamp can be passed beneath the costal margin into this precordial space. The electrode leads are grasped and passed into the pocket where the leads are coiled. Placement of the permanent leads should be well lateral of chest tubes and temporary pacing wires. Despite placement of permanent leads, temporary pacing wires are used during the immediate postoperative period to permit rapid control of heart rate.

⑤ After closure of the chest, the permanent leads may be attached to the pacemaker generator. The pacemaker should be programmed at the lowest rate so as not to interfere with a temporary pacemaker. The generator is placed in the abdominal subcutaneous pocket after connection to the permanent epicardial leads with the writing surface up in contact with the subcutaneous tissue.

LEFT ANTERIOR THORACOTOMY

⑥ When epicardial electrodes are prescribed as an independent procedure, a left anterior thoracotomy incision is used. A 10 to 15 cm incision over the fifth rib is made with the patient intubated and under general anesthesia. A segment of rib is resected and the mediastinum, pericardium, and usually the left pleural space are opened by incising the posterior periosteum.

⑦ The pericardium is grasped with forceps and opened 6 to 8 cm. Traction sutures on the edges facilitate exposure. The left anterior descending coronary artery is located. Two ventricular sites lateral to the coronary vessel are located.

⑧ Either the sutureless coil or a sutured plunge electrode is placed in the most cephalad site first. The second electrode is placed near the ventricular apex.

⑨ A transverse incision is made over the lateral border of the left rectus muscle 5 to 8 cm below the costal margin. If necessary, a generator can be placed in the right upper quadrant. A subcutaneous pocket is made for the pacemaker generator and all bleeding is controlled by cautery or ligature. With the pocket made, a Crafoord or DeBakey clamp is blindly passed beneath the costal margin into the mediastinum. First one and then the second electrode are pulled into the subcutaneous pocket and connected to the pacemaker generator. Excess length is generally coiled, partially in the chest and partially in the subcutaneous pocket. A small No. 28F angled catheter is inserted into the left chest for drainage of blood and fluid. The pericardium is loosely closed with two or three interrupted sutures. Both wounds are closed with running absorbable sutures.

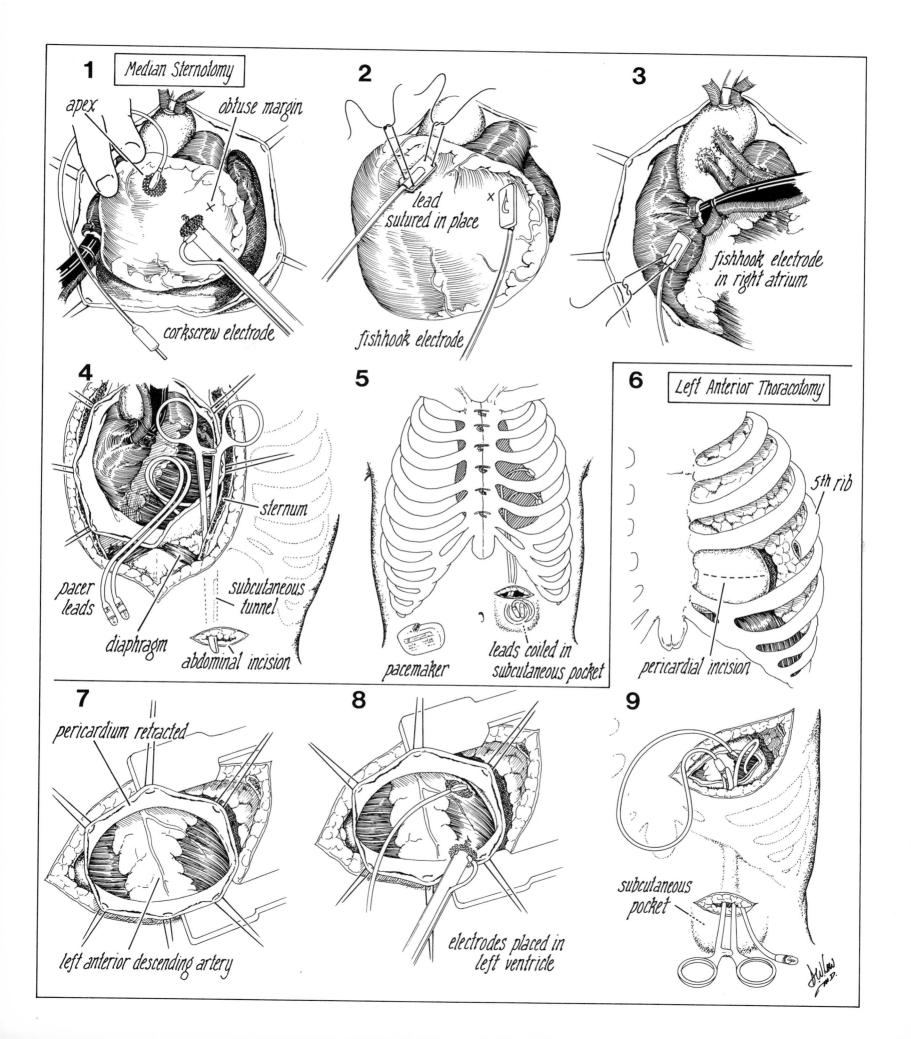

1 Median Sternotomy
apex
obtuse margin
corkscrew electrode

2
lead sutured in place
fishhook electrode

3
fishhook electrode in right atrium

4
sternum
pacer leads
diaphragm
subcutaneous tunnel
abdominal incision

5
pacemaker
leads coiled in subcutaneous pocket

6 Left Anterior Thoracotomy
5th rib
pericardial incision

7
pericardium retracted
left anterior descending artery

8
electrodes placed in left ventricle

9
subcutaneous pocket

Automatic Internal Cardiac Defibrillator

This device is prescribed for selected patients at risk for spontaneous ventricular fibrillation or who have experienced ventricular tachycardia and remain at risk despite drug therapy.

(1) The heart is exposed through a median sternotomy incision or a small anterior left thoracotomy with resection of a segment of the fifth rib.

(2) Exposure through the left anterior thoracotomy incision is illustrated. The pericardium is incised and retracted to provide wide exposure of the heart. Adhesions are carefully taken down and any previously placed bypass grafts are protected.

(3) The posterior defibrillator patch is placed behind the heart next to the posterolateral surface of the left ventricle. Two or three sutures are used to anchor the patch to the myocardium.

(4) The anterior defibrillator patch is placed on the anterior surface of the right ventricle directly opposite the posterior patch. If the patient has had previous bypass grafts or has a functioning internal mammary arterial graft, the pericardium is not dissected away from the epicardium. Instead, the space between the pericardium and chest wall is dissected out so that the anterior defibrillator patch can be placed outside the pericardium over the right ventricle opposite the posterior patch. The position of the patches should allow most of the defibrillator current to pass through a large area of ventricular septum.

(5) Two corkscrew epicardial pacemaker leads are placed in the anterolateral portion of the left ventricle if a sternotomy incision is used, and near the apex if a left thoracotomy is used. The pacing and sensing thresholds of both leads are established by overdrive pacing and measurement of the electrocardiographic "R"-waves.

(6) A subcutaneous pocket for the generator is created in the left upper quadrant of the abdomen.

(7) With the defibrillator patches connected to an external defibrillator and the epicardial leads connected to an electrical stimulator, the heart is electrically fibrillated to determine the electrical energy required to defibrillate the heart. External defibrillator paddles and an external defibrillator must be available to administer an effective shock in case the shocks delivered by way of the internal patches fail. The defibrillation threshold is tested beginning at 10 to 15 joules. An acceptable defibrillation threshold is between 10 and 25 joules. The threshold for ventricular fibrillation is first tested; afterward the threshold for ventricular tachycardia is induced by programmed electric stimulation by means of the epicardial leads is determined. The effect of changing the direction of the current is also tested.

(8) The epicardial and internal defibrillator patch leads are connected to the AICD device. The leads are passed subcutaneously and beneath the costal margin from the sternotomy wound to the subcutaneous pocket. When they are connected, the generator is tested by first inducing ventricular fibrillation by means of temporary pacing wires placed on the heart and then by inducing ventricular tachycardia. If acceptable, the wounds are closed.

(9) If necessary, one or both epicardial leads may be replaced without thoracotomy by percutaneous insertion of ventricular pacemaker leads under fluoroscopy. A small incision beneath the clavicle is necessary to enable the lead or leads to be passed subcutaneously and connected to the AICD device.

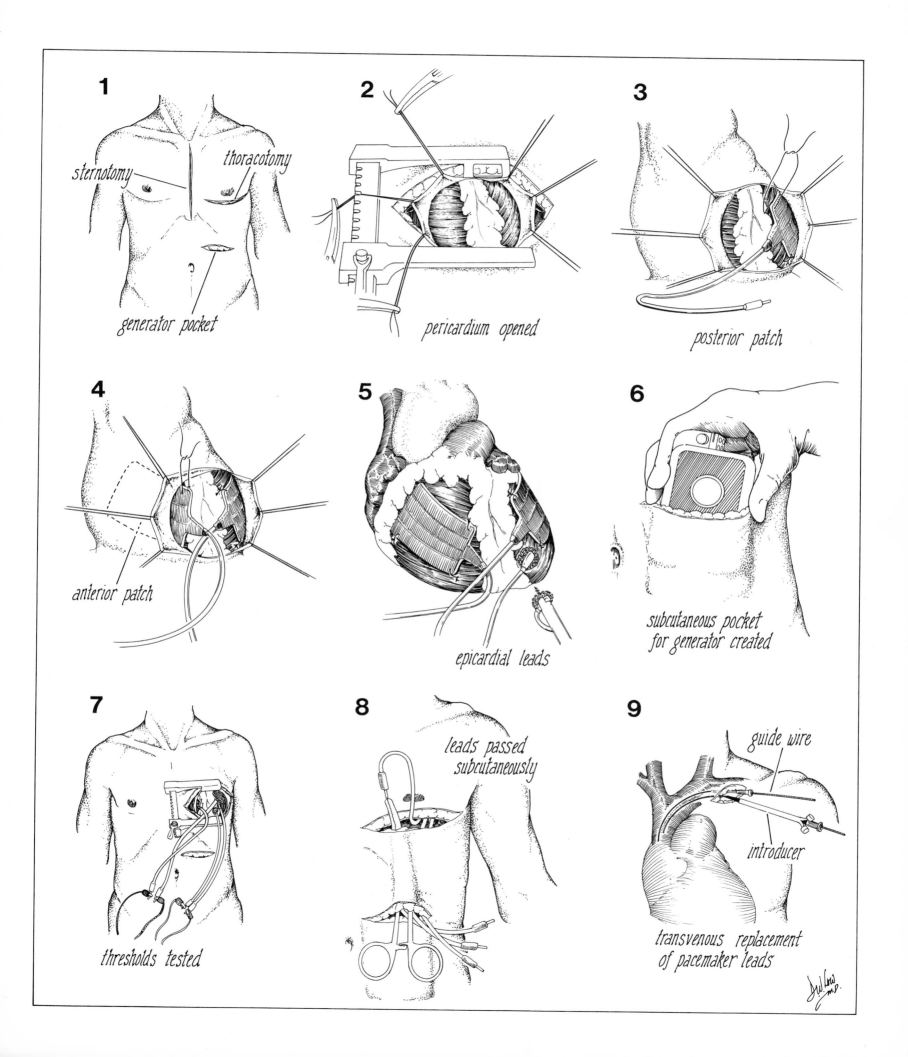

1 sternotomy · thoracotomy · generator pocket

2 pericardium opened

3 posterior patch

4 anterior patch

5 epicardial leads

6 subcutaneous pocket for generator created

7 thresholds tested

8 leads passed subcutaneously

9 guide wire · introducer · transvenous replacement of pacemaker leads

Pericardium

PERICARDIOCENTESIS

1 The subxiphoid approach is usually used to aspirate pericardial fluid. If a large effusion is present, a needle can be inserted through the left fourth or fifth intercostal spaces directly into the pericardium, but this route may lacerate a mammary vessel or the right atrium and therefore is not as commonly used as the subxiphoid location.

Local anesthesia is used; the electrocardiogram is monitored. Traditionally, the precordial lead of the electrocardiogram is attached to the aspirating needle with an alligator clip to detect a "current of injury" (negative deflection of the QRS complex) when the needle tip touches the heart, but this is rarely helpful. The bore of the needle is selected on the basis of the expected fluid; a 20 gauge needle is adequate for an effusion and a 16 gauge is better for blood or pus. A 12 to 18 cm long needle or catheter with a needle stylet is used. A needle is preferred because the catheter often kinks when the stylet is withdrawn.

The anesthetic weal is placed just to the left of the xiphoid tip about 2 to 3 cm below the costosternal angle. The needle is angled 45 degrees to the horizontal, vertical, and sagittal planes and directed toward the middle of the left scapula. The needle is slowly advanced beneath the left rib, through the attachment of the diaphragm into the pericardial space beneath the inferior border of the heart. Sometimes the tip of the needle can be felt to "pop" into the space at the same time as fluid starts to drip from the needle hub. The motion of the heart can be detected by bobbing of the needle; aspiration of blood that clots and has the same hematocrit as peripheral blood indicates that the tip is within the heart. Once pericardial fluid is obtained, a syringe and a three-way stopcock are added and the fluid is aspirated.

PERICARDIOTOMY

2 Suspected acute tamponade is best treated by pericardiotomy from the subxiphoid location. After injection of local anesthesia, a 5 to 6 cm vertical incision along the left border of the xiphoid is made through the rectus muscle and the posterior rectus fascia. The plane between the rectus and transversus thoracis muscle is dissected superiorly beneath the costal margin through the attachment of the diaphragm into the inferior margin of the pericardium. This approach is rapid and provides excellent drainage of the pericardial cavity, particularly if clotted blood or thick pus is present. The wound can be closed directly or around a large draining chest tube.

PERICARDIAL WINDOW

3 A "pericardial window" is occasionally prescribed as a palliative procedure for patients who have recurrent malignant pericardial effusions. The operation is designed to provide permanent drainage of the pericardial sac into the left hemithorax. A 10 to 12 cm incision is made over the anterior left fifth rib. A segment of the rib is excised and the pericardium and anterior surface of the heart are exposed by incising the posterior periosteum and parietal pleura.

4 The largest amount of pericardium that can be removed through this incision is excised. A wooden tongue blade between the heart and pericardium and a cautery with a bent blade facilitate the excision and reduce bleeding from the edges. Usually, most of the pericardium over the left ventricle anterior to the left phrenic nerve and most of the pericardium over the right ventricle can be removed. A chest tube is inserted through a stab wound into the left pleural space before the wound is closed.

PERICARDIECTOMY

Pericardiectomy can be performed through a median sternotomy, transverse sternotomy, or left anterior thoracotomy. A median sternotomy is usually preferred because postoperative pain is less and cannulation for bypass is easier if manipulation of the heart produces bleeding or unstable hemodynamics. The operation is usually prescribed for constrictive pericarditis and is designed to remove all of the thickened pericardium adherent to ventricular epicardium. Cardiopulmonary bypass is available on a standby basis.

5 The pleura and thymus are dissected from the anterior surface of the thickened pericardium when a median sternotomy is selected. The plane between the epicardium and thick pericardium is first established near the left lateral border of the heart away from the expected location of the left anterior descending coronary artery. A 3 to 5 cm vertical incision is gradually deepened with the scalpel until myocardial muscle is visible.

6 With the scalpel, a plane between myocardial muscle and the undersurface of the thick fibrous and occasionally calcified pericardium is gradually established.

7 The pericardium is painstakingly separated from the underlying myocardium, initially over the anterior left ventricle and apex. It is important to release the underlying myocardium from the overlying scar. Bleeding is controlled by fine figure-of-eight or mattress sutures, with or without small pledgets. The coronary vessels are carefully avoided. Arrhythmias can usually be controlled by careful retraction; occasionally drugs or even partial bypass are needed. To avoid pulmonary congestion, a good portion of the left ventricle is released before removing the constricting pericardium from the surface of the thin-walled right ventricle. Usually the pericardium over the left ventricle to the left phrenic nerve is excised first.

8 The inferior pericardium is removed next. This dissection requires establishing a plane between the diaphragm and thickened pericardium and between the epicardium and pericardium. The right ventricle can then be safely released. Pericardium is excised up to and beyond the right atrioventricular groove; however, it is not usually necessary to remove it from the right atrium and cavae if the dissection is difficult.

9 It is important to remove the thickened pericardium from the lateral left ventricle posterior to the left phrenic nerve. It is usually possible to gently retract the released anterior heart rightwards and continue the dissection around behind the phrenic nerve to the left pulmonary veins. When this is done, a triangular piece of pericardium is excised and only a 1 cm strip containing the left phrenic nerve is left.

After removal of the pericardium, all bleeding is carefully controlled with sutures before closure with drainage tubes in the anterior mediastinum and left hemithorax.

A left anterior thoracotomy facilitates removal of the pericardium posterior to the left phrenic nerve but complicates and sometimes precludes removal of part of the pericardium over the right ventricle and some of the inferior pericardium. Initiation of cardiopulmonary bypass, which usually is not necessary, and control of right ventricular bleeding are more difficult from a left thoracotomy.

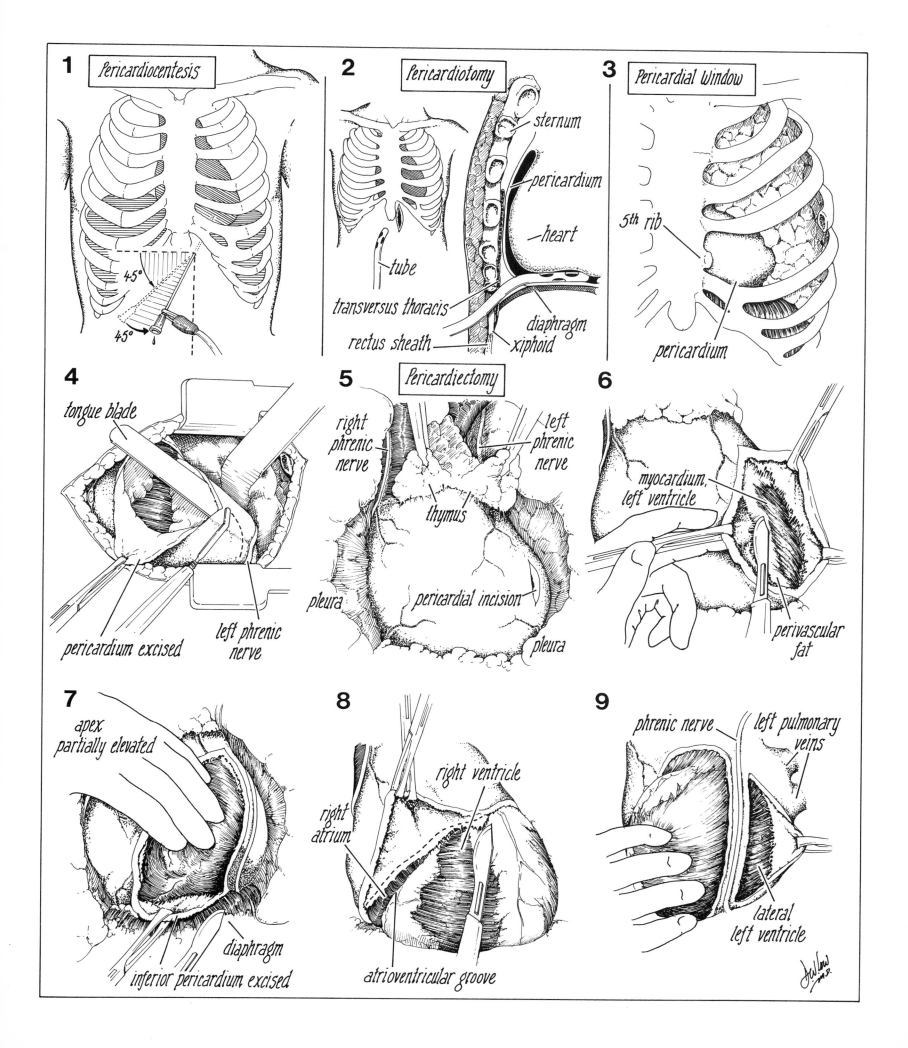

1 Pericardiocentesis

45°
45°

2 Pericardiotomy

sternum
pericardium
heart
tube
transversus thoracis
rectus sheath
diaphragm
xiphoid

3 Pericardial Window

5th rib
pericardium

4

tongue blade
pericardium excised
left phrenic nerve

5 Pericardiectomy

right phrenic nerve
left phrenic nerve
thymus
pleura
pericardial incision
pleura

6

myocardium, left ventricle
perivascular fat

7

apex partially elevated
diaphragm
inferior pericardium excised

8

right ventricle
right atrium
atrioventricular groove

9

phrenic nerve
left pulmonary veins
lateral left ventricle

Cannulation for Cardiopulmonary Bypass, Cold Cardioplegia, Air Maneuvers

For most open-heart operations, venous and arterial cannulas are inserted directly into the right atrium and ascending aorta from the median sternotomy incision. For special situations, however, other cannulation sites may be either advantageous or required. Basically, the arterial cannula can be inserted anywhere in the arterial system that is large enough to accommodate the entire cardiac output. Common alternative sites for arterial cannulas include the descending thoracic aorta and the common femoral, external iliac, and axillary arteries. Heparin should be given before any cannulas are inserted.

Flow is limited through peripherally placed venous catheters, but more than one can be used simultaneously. Whenever possible, the tip of a peripherally placed venous catheter should be advanced into the right atrium or the largest available vein. Common alternative sites of venous cannulas include the internal jugular vein (particularly the right), the common femoral and external iliac veins, the right ventricular outflow tract, and the main pulmonary artery.

AORTIC CANNULATION

1 The ascending aorta may be cannulated in various ways, and it is likely that no two surgeons use identical techniques. One good way is to place two concentric purse-string sutures of 2-0 polyester in the ascending aorta upstream but near the origin of the innominate artery and slightly toward the medial wall of the aorta. The area should be palpated to detect calcification or atherosclerotic plaque before the sutures are placed.

2 The full thickness of aortic wall is incised for about 4 mm with a No. 11 blade and covered with a finger as the blade is withdrawn. The hole beneath the finger can be enlarged with blunt metal dilators under the covering finger. The cannula is then easily slipped in with a twisting motion to reduce the chance of raising an internal flap.

3 The purse-string sutures are tightened and secured with clamped tourniquets. A heavy tie is placed around the cannula and one tourniquet to prevent dislodgement and the cannula is sutured to the skin edge to secure it further.

The same technique can be used with small modifications to cannulate other sites in the ascending or descending thoracic aorta. To cannulate an artery, the vessel must first be exposed. Both axillary and femoral arteries are easily exposed by incisions placed over them; the external iliac artery is usually exposed through a small oblique lower abdominal incision combined with retroperitoneal dissection.

4 Once the artery is exposed, a one-inch segment is isolated using appropriate bulldog clamps and suture-tourniquets. Either a transverse or a longitudinal incision can be used; both have advantages and disadvantages. After the arteriotomy is made, the artery is dilated with a hemostat or right-angled clamp. The beveled catheter (No. 16 to 24 Fr, depending on the size of the patient) is inserted and directed toward the heart. The umbilical tape used to encircle the artery cephalad to the arteriotomy is tied down over the cannula to prevent leakage. This tape can be bridled and tied again around the cannula to prevent dislodgement. After connection to the arterial line, the whole assembly is further secured to the skin by two or three heavy sutures.

After bypass, the securing sutures and tapes are cut. The cannula is withdrawn as the artery is occluded by an appropriate vascular clamp. Usually the arteriotomy can be closed by a single over-and-over continuous stitch of 5-0 monofilament suture. Occasionally separation of atherosclerotic intima from adventia occurs. This may be repaired by a running 5-0 monofilament, horizontal mattress suture followed by a continuous over-and-over stitch. If the arterial wall is torn up by the cannulation, repair using a vein patch (obtained from a segment of the nearby saphenous vein) may be necessary.

Because the patient has been heparinized, catheter thrombectomy of the distal vessel is usually not necessary.

RIGHT ATRIAL CANNULATION

5 For operations on the ascending aorta and aortic valve and for myocardial revascularization, a single large-bore cannula in the right atrium is sufficient. The cannula is inserted through a purse string suture (0 polyester) around the right atrial appendage or placed at a convenient spot in the right atrial wall. The tip is placed near the entrance of the inferior vena cava. A "two-stage" cannula with a narrow tip placed within the ostium of the inferior vena cava and with a second opening in the mid-right atrium often drains better when the heart is retracted upward. With a single right atrial catheter, some blood passes into the right ventricle and pulmonary artery through the lungs.

6 To further reduce pulmonary blood flow, both cavae may be cannulated through two separate purse-string sutures placed in the right atrium. The superior vena cava (SVC) is generally cannulated by way of the right atrial appendage, but may be cannulated directly through a purse-string suture in the caval wall. The inferior vena cava (IVC) is cannulated through a purse-string suture near the right atrial inferior vena cava junction. However, if a right atriotomy is not planned, the two purse-string sutures may be placed anywhere on the right atrial wall. Tapes or clamps placed around the caval cannulas within the inferior and superior cavae will divert all venous return into the heart-lung machine. Only blood from the coronary sinus enters the right atrium. Once the aorta is clamped and the heart is arrested, only small amounts of blood reach the right atrium from thebesian veins and by way of small coronary collaterals. However, cardioplegic solutions injected into the aortic root reach the right atrium from the coronary sinus.

Some surgeons prefer two venous cannulas for myocardial revascularization procedures; most use two caval cannulas for mitral valvular procedures.

PULMONARY ARTERY

7 Under special circumstances, the main pulmonary artery may be cannulated with a single large cannula passed through a purse-string suture in the outflow tract of the right ventricle and passed through the pulmonary valve. The pulmonary artery can be cannulated in this way when the mitral valve is exposed from a left thoracotomy. This site may also be used to decompress the left heart with a drainage catheter.

INTERNAL JUGULAR VEIN

8 The right internal jugular vein is the preferred site for peripheral cannulation. The vein is exposed through an oblique cervical incision over the anterior border of the sternocleidomastoid (a transverse incision can also be used). Only the anterior wall of the vein need be exposed; dissection of the vein and placement of encircling tapes are not necessary. The can-

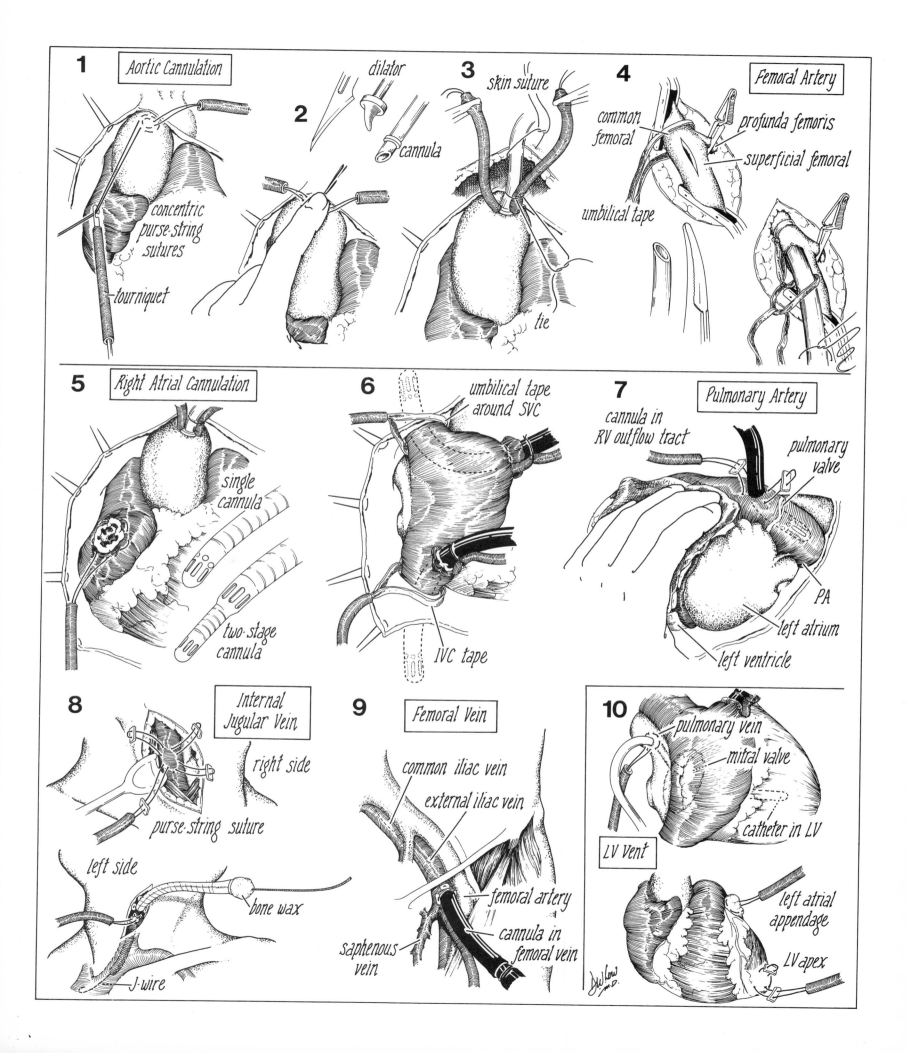

nula may be inserted and advanced into the right atrium through a purse-string suture of 3-0 monofilament suture buttressed with small Teflon felt pledgets. When the *left* internal jugular vein is used, a J-shaped guidewire is first passed through the innominate vein into the superior cava and right atrium. The venous cannula can be passed over the wire after a needle hole is made in the tip. Blood loss is prevented by a plug of bone wax in the opposite end which is cut off for connection to the venous line. Catheters up to 28 Fr can usually be passed into the right internal jugular vein of adults; however, flows exceeding 4 L/min can be achieved with an 18 Fr catheter if the catheter tip is in the right atrium.

FEMORAL VEIN

9 The common femoral vein is the most common site for insertion of peripheral venous catheters. After exposure of the vessel medial to the femoral artery, the cannula may be inserted through either a purse-string suture of a longitudinal venotomy made in a temporarily isolated segment of vein. The catheter is gently advanced toward the heart as far as it will go and may reach the lower inferior vena cava. In adults, the common femoral vein may accept catheters up to 24 Fr in diameter; however, smaller catheters (No. 20 Fr) are preferred because flow is partly related to the relative diameters of the catheter and surrounding vein. The external iliac vein, which is exposed as is the artery through a retroperitoneal incision, is seldom used.

LV VENT

10 During cardiopulmonary bypass, blood reaches the left atrium from bronchial arteries, thebesian veins, and the coronary system; and from around atrial and caval catheters. The left ventricle is therefore often vented to prevent distension. Usually the left ventricle is decompressed by means of a catheter (18 or 24 Fr), which is inserted through the junction of the right superior pulmonary veins and left atrium and is passed through the mitral valve. Alternatively, the left atrial appendage may be used to pass a left atrial venting catheter; however, cannulation of the left atrial appendage is more difficult through a median sternotomy than is cannulation of the right superior pulmonary vein–left atrial junction. Placement of a suction or venting catheter through a purse-string suture in the right ventricular outflow tract or preferably the main pulmonary artery is another convenient method to decompress the left ventricle and reduce the risk of air embolism. Lastly, the apex of the left ventricle, just to the left of the distal third of the left anterior descending coronary artery, may be used to place a No. 18 or 24 Ferguson venting catheter. For apical venting, a single No. 1 or 0 pledgeted mattress suture is first placed in the bare area of the ventricular apex, a stab wound is made, the catheter is inserted into the ventricular cavity away from valves or papillary muscles and the mattress suture is pulled up and placed in a tourniquet choke to maintain the catheter in place and to prevent air and blood leaks.

COLD CARDIOPLEGIA

Myocardial preservation and therefore postoperative function require avoidance of ischemic injury during periods when coronary blood flow is interrupted. Cold potassium cardioplegia has largely supplanted other methods of preventing ischemic myocardial damage. Although much debate continues over the merits of blood versus crystalloid solutions and the value of various additives, potassium (20 to 30 mEq/L) and cold (approximately 4° C) are the two essential constituents.

We administer blood or crystalloid cardioplegic solution by means of a No. 14 angiocatheter inserted into the aortic root during bypass immediately after the ascending aorta is clamped. The aorta is not clamped after bypass starts until the heart either fibrillates or is decompressed by insertion of a left atrial catheter. If the aortic valve is competent, 0.6 to 1 L of cold cardioplegic solution is infused at line pressures up to 180 mm/Hg into the aortic root to arrest the heart. At the same time, the

heart is bathed and entirely covered with cold saline slush at approximately 0 to 1° C. The heart must be kept flaccid during the infusion; if the ventricle becomes hard or distended, the infusion is stopped and an incision is made in the junction of the left atrial-right superior pulmonary vein to decompress the heart. When the heart is flaccid, the infusion is restarted and continued until the electrocardiographic tracing is flat.

Often myocardial septal temperature is monitored with a thermistor inserted near the left anterior descending coronary artery into the ventricular septum. Septal temperature is maintained below 18° C during the period of coronary ischemia.

If myocardial temperature is not monitored, cardioplegic solution (200 to 300 ml) is reinfused every 20 minutes and the heart is simultaneously bathed in cold saline slush. Although this ritual interrupts surgery for 2 to 3 minutes, it is usually possible to space the breaks for cardioplegic infusions so that steps in the operation are not inconvenienced. The interval between infusions is almost never extended beyond 20 minutes, but may be shorter if electrocardiographic activity reappears or myocardial temperature rises above 18° C, or if less time is convenient for the operative procedure.

The cardioplegic solution enters the perfusate from the coronary sinus. In patients with renal failure, repeat doses of cardioplegic solution contain only 5 to 10 mEq/L/L. For most patients, the 20 to 30 mEq/L concentration is used for repeat doses. Saline used to bathe the heart is aspirated into the cell saver system, from which packed red cells are recovered and returned to the perfusate.

The cardioplegic infusion system can also be used to vent the aortic root and left heart between infusions. The system drains by gravity into the venous reservoir. This method of venting may not always be adequate to fully decompress the heart during the period of arrest and should be supplemented by a stab incision in the left atrial-right superior pulmonary vein junction and insertion of a venting catheter if the heart becomes full.

AIR MANEUVERS

Open heart surgery exposes virtually every patient in whom the heart is opened to the risk of air embolism. For this reason, we have developed a series of steps to protect against this complication whenever the ascending aorta or left heart is opened, even if only a left atrial vent catheter is used during myocardial revascularization.

When the aorta is clamped and the heart arrested, sutured incisions in the left atrium, ventricle, and aorta are not tied until the heart is filled with blood. The patient is tilted head down and the anesthesiologist firmly inflates the lungs and holds the inspiration to drive blood from the lungs into the left heart. The atrial appendage is inverted and the ventricle is massaged and shaken to dislodge air. As air and blood leave the loose suture line, ventriculotomy sutures are tied. If necessary, the left ventricle is kept decompressed by means of a catheter in the left atrium or pulmonary artery. Left atrial suture lines are pulled up when all air is removed, but are usually not tied until after the aortic clamp is removed and the heart is reliably ejecting. For ascending aortic incisions, perfusion flow is reduced and the anterior surface of the ascending aorta is inverted somewhat to dislodge air through the bleeding suture line. The suture line is tied during this brief period of hypotension and a No. 19 needle is immediately inserted into the highest (most anterior) surface of the aorta. Sometimes suction is applied to the needle as perfusion is raised. Lung inflation is released as soon as the suture lines are tied or pulled up.

The heart is kept decompressed until effective contractions are re-established. When the heart begins to eject, a number 19 needle is reinserted into the ascending aorta to provide a place for air to exit. The needle can be placed on suction if there is a substantial likelihood of trapped air; usually just the needle hole is allowed to bleed.

The aortic needle is allowed to bleed until bypass is stopped and the heart is providing the entire circulation. Left atrial suture lines are tied at this time and the aortic needle hole is closed with a pledgeted mattress suture.

Excision of Atrial Myxoma

Excision of Atrial Myxoma

These uncommon tumors usually present in the left atrium but may rarely occur in the right atrium. The tumor is very friable and embolizes easily. It often attaches to the septum ovalis but may attach to any part of the atrium, including the atrioventricular valves and even part of the ventricle. Because of a high rate of recurrence, full-thickness excision of the atrial attachment with adequate margins must be performed.

CANNULATION FOR LEFT ATRIAL MYXOMA

(1) The heart is exposed through a midline sternotomy and the aorta is cannulated. A portion of the pericardium is cleared to provide material for a patch. With minimal or no manipulation of the heart, both cavae are cannulated through the right atrium near the caval junctions if the tumor is in the left atrium.

CANNULATION FOR RIGHT-ATRIAL MYXOMA

(2) If the tumor is large or in the right atrium, peripheral cannulation by way of the femoral or iliac veins below and internal jugular or superior cava (directly) above is recommended.

EXCISION, LEFT ATRIAL MYXOMA

(3) As soon as bypass begins, the heart is *electrically* fibrillated and the aorta is simultaneously clamped. A small incision is made in the left atrium at the junction of the right superior pulmonary vein to decompress the ventricle. Cold cardioplegic solution is then given, and tapes are placed around both cavae to develop a dry field in the right atrium.

(4) If the tumor is large, pericardial attachments surrounding both cavae should be divided to allow the lateral left atrial incision to extend behind both cavae to the inferior and superior left atrial walls. As this incision is made, the tumor usually bulges out and small pieces may break off if technique is rough.

(5) The atriotomy is widely extended both superiorly and inferiorly to expose the tumor and allow a clear view of the pedicle.

(6) If the pedicle is attached to the septum ovalis, the right atrium is opened by an incision parallel to the septum. Pressure on the right atrial surface of the septum everts the tumor through the left atrial incision and facilitates precise location of the pedicle. With the pedicle in full view, the first incision in the atrial septum is made.

(7) With Allis clamps used to retract septal edges, the entire full thickness of septum to which the pedicle is attached is excised with 0.5 to 1.0 cm margins. If possible, the lateral intra-atrial conduction tracts are preserved, but they are sacrificed if complete excision of the tumor pedicle cannot otherwise be achieved. The entire tumor and pedicle are removed. The atrium, valves, and ventricle are carefully inspected to ensure that no tumor emboli remain.

The defect in the interatrial septum is closed by a pericardial patch sewn in place with running 3-0 monofilament sutures. It is convenient to place the pericardial patch on a piece of wet cardboard to facilitate trimming. Three equidistant sutures are placed through patch and septal defect before the patch is lowered into the heart and the cardboard is removed.

(8) After repair of the septal defect or other site of pedicular attachment, the left atrium is closed with a running horizontal mattress suture (3-0 monofilament) followed by an over-and-over continuous suture. If the wall is thin and friable, Teflon felt strips may be used to strengthen the suture line. Before the left atrial suture line is tied down, air is carefully evacuated from the atrium, ventricle, and aortic root.

(9) The right atrial incision is closed similarly. Air is evacuated by releasing a caval tape and filling the right atrium with blood before the suture line is tied. Two temporary atrial and two ventricular pacemaker wires are placed for possible use during the early postoperative period.

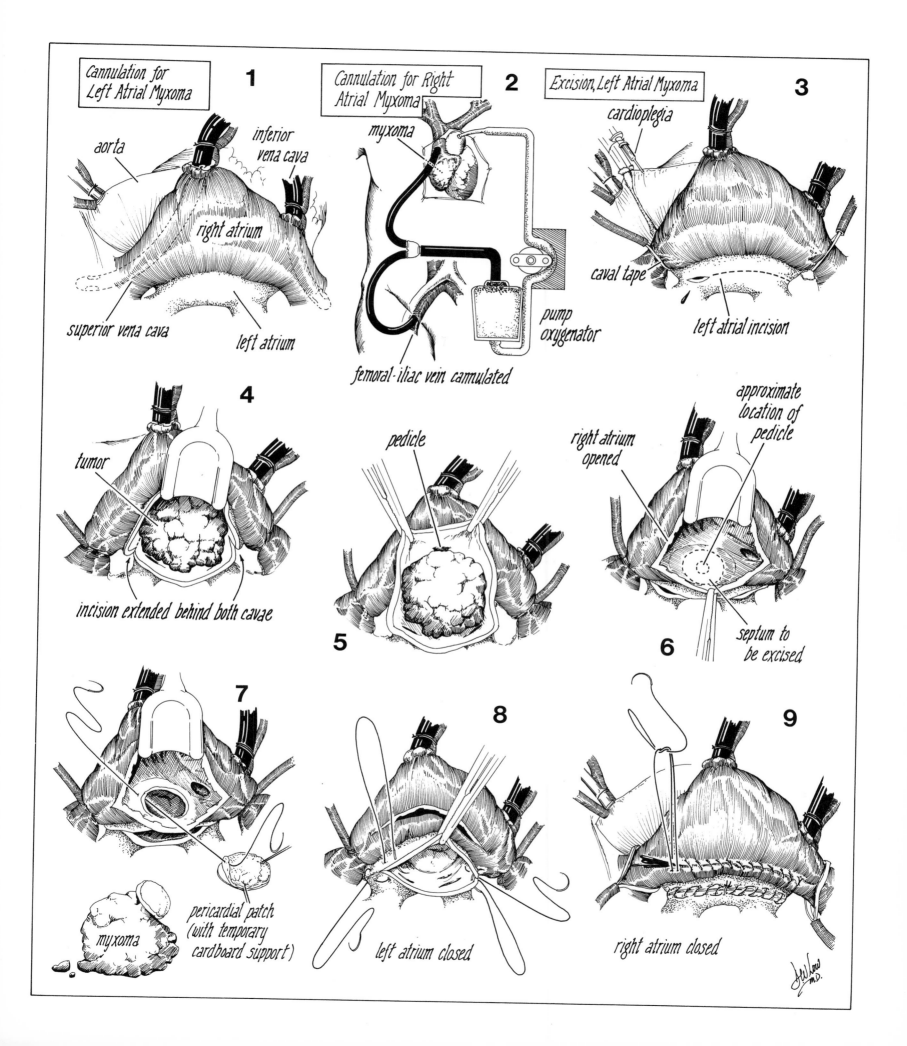

1 Cannulation for Left Atrial Myxoma

aorta
inferior vena cava
right atrium
superior vena cava
left atrium

2 Cannulation for Right Atrial Myxoma

myxoma
pump oxygenator
femoral-iliac vein cannulated

3 Excision, Left Atrial Myxoma

cardioplegia
caval tape
left atrial incision

4

tumor
incision extended behind both cavae

5

pedicle

6

right atrium opened
approximate location of pedicle
septum to be excised

7

myxoma
pericardial patch (with temporary cardboard support)

8

left atrium closed

9

right atrium closed

Tricuspid Valve

TRICUSPID VALVE COMMISSUROTOMY

Repair of the tricuspid valve is preferred to replacement whenever the prospect of a functionally satisfactory valve exists. Tricuspid stenosis, usually due to rheumatic fever, occurs less commonly than tricuspid insufficiency.

(1) To expose the tricuspid valve, both cavae are separately cannulated by means of purse-string sutures placed in the right atrium. The right atrial appendage is used for cannulation of the superior cava; a purse-string suture placed laterally and near the inferior vena cava-right atrial junction is preferred for cannulation of the inferior vena cava. Tapes are placed around both cavae to direct all caval blood flow into the cannulas. The aorta is crossclamped and the heart is arrested with cold cardiplegic solution to stop blood flow into the coronary sinus. The right atrium is opened posterior to the superior caval purse-string and atrioventricular groove and anterior to the inferior caval purse-string.

(2) Tricuspid stenosis usually results from fusion of the commissures with minimal chordal thickening and fusion. Leaflets may sometimes be fibrotic and thickened, but are nearly always pliable enough that a commissurotomy and valvuloplasty are possible. Often tricuspid stenosis is associated with some degree of tricuspid insufficiency.

The valve is carefully inspected and the position of the coronary sinus and presumed location of the A-V node and bundle of His are determined. The location of the fused commissure between the septal and anterior leaflets is found. This is aided by inspection of chordal attachments to the valve edges. The fused commissure is incised toward, but not completely to, the annulus. Care is taken to ensure that chordal attachments to the anterior leaflet are not injured or cut. If chordae are thickened and fused, they can be separated and debrided to improve the secondary orifice of the valve.

The postero-septal commissure is similarly located and partially incised; however, the fused commissure between the anterior and posterior leaflets is not incised for fear of producing free insufficiency. After partial incisions in the two fused commissures, saline is introduced through the enlarged opening to fill the right ventricle and test valve competence. Usually one or both of the commissural incisions can be extended to further enlarge the tricuspid opening without increasing the amount of incompetence. A bicuspid valve is produced. If leaflets do not coapt securely, a ring annuloplasty may be added to improve competence. A small amount of tricuspid regurgitation is acceptable and generally preferable to valve replacement.

SUTURE ANNULOPLASTY

(3) Tricuspid annuloplasty is the most common operation on the tricuspid valve in adults and is designed to correct tricuspid valve insufficiency. Two methods are currently used. Semicircular suture annuloplasty can be performed rapidly but is less secure than the Carpentier ring annuloplasty. Both operations are usually performed in conjunction with other valvular and/or revascularization procedures.

The tricuspid valve is carefully inspected for intrinsic disease of the leaflets and chordae. Occasionally, if a simple ruptured chordae is present, a wedge of leaflet containing the ruptured chorda is excised. The adjacent edges of the leaflet are sewn to each other with 5-0 monofilament interrupted mattress sutures. Most often, dilation of the annulus is responsible for the tricuspid insufficiency and leaflets and chordae are not diseased.

The semicircular suture annuloplasty, described by de Vega, consists of a single suture of No. 1 monofilament suture placed in the annulus of the anterior and posterior tricuspid leaflets only. The ends are buttressed with pledgets of Teflon felt. The suture, passed once through a pledget of felt (approximately 1 cm x 0.6 cm), begins in the annulus at the commissure between the septal and anterior leaflets of the tricuspid valve. The suture continues anteriorly in and out of the annulus around both anterior and posterior leaflets to the commissure between the septal and posterior leaflets, anterior to the coronary sinus. The suture is passed twice through a second Teflon pledget and then passes in and out of the annulus back to the starting point.

(4) The suture is passed through the original felt pledget.

(5) Alternatively, the running suture may be placed as an over-and-over continuous suture around the in-and-out suture to the starting point.

(6) The continuous suture is snugged up (using a nerve hook if necessary) and is tied to itself with either a tricuspid ring obturator in place or with two fingers of an assistant placed through the valve to the first knuckle. As the suture is drawn up, the tricuspid annulus is constricted. The knot is tied and atrium is closed. It is prudent to assess the degree of residual tricuspid insufficiency by injection of the right ventricle with a syringe of saline and by a finger inserted through the right atrial appendage shortly after bypass is stopped.

CARPENTIER RING

(7) The Carpentier ring annuloplasty utilizes a prosthetic ring held in place with interrupted pledgeted mattress sutures of No. 0 polyester. The annulus is sized with a tricuspid obturator, but if the annulus is dilated ring size is selected according to the patient's size - 28 for a small woman to 34 for a large man.

The pledgeted mattress sutures are placed in the annulus around the anterior and posterior leaflets with the pledget located on the atrial surface of the annulus. The opening of the ring is located along the annulus of the septal leaflet nearest the anterior commissure.

(8) The pledgets are placed on the ventricular side of the annulus along the septal leaflet, and sutures are carefully passed through a tiny rim of valve leaflet tissue and the annulus, but not through atrial tissue, to avoid injury to the bundle of His. When all sutures are placed, they are tied and the atrium is closed.

The proximity of sutures near the bundle of His may cause permanent or temporary atrioventricular conduction block. Some surgeons prefer to place sutures in the triscuspid annulus with the heart beating. We prefer the dry motionless heart, but carefully place sutures in a small rim of valve tissue and the annulus along the septal annulus, and do not include atrial tissue. Temporary atrial and ventricular pacing wires are recommended after triscuspid annuloplasty operations.

TRICUSPID VALVE REPLACEMENT

Prosthetic tricuspid valves are more prone to develop thrombi and presumably emboli than are left-sided prosthetic valves. Because pulmonary and right ventricular pressures are lower than aortic and left ventricular pressures, valvuloplasty is usually applicable unless substantial portions of the anterior and posterior leaflets are destroyed. Bioprosthetic valves are generally preferred over mechanical valves; coumadin anticoagulation is recommended postoperatively for both types of prosthesis.

(9) The destroyed valve is excised. If possible, chordal attachments to the septal leaflet and the entire septal leaflet are retained. The valve annulus is sized.

(10) Interrupted pledgeted 0-polyester mattress sutures are placed around the anterior and posterior portions of the annulus and through the sewing ring of the prosthesis as illustrated.

(11) Sutures along the septal leaflet are passed first through the retained leaflet (in such a way as to gather any redundant leaflet tissue into the stitch) and then carefully and superficially through the ventricular edge of the tricuspid annulus. These sutures avoid the AV node and bundle of His and thus avoid complete heart block when the valve is tied down.

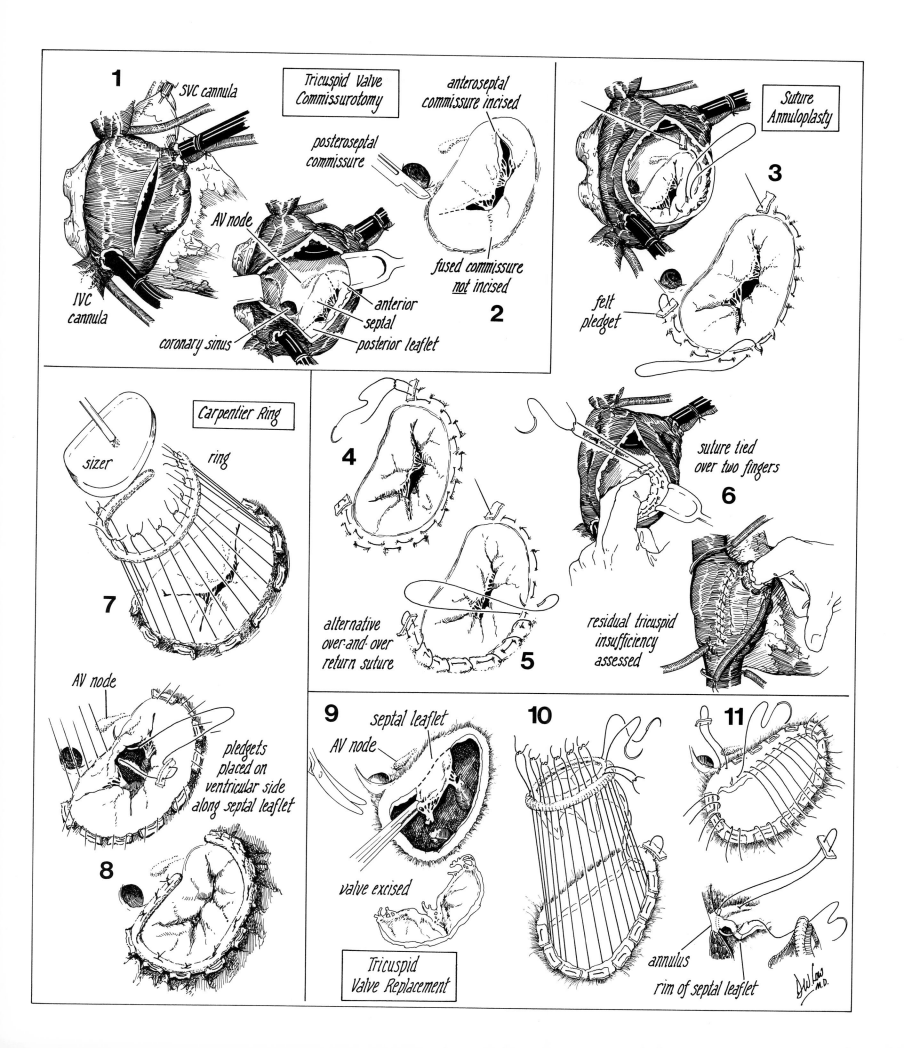

1 SVC cannula

IVC cannula

Tricuspid Valve Commissurotomy

anteroseptal commissure incised

posteroseptal commissure

AV node

coronary sinus

anterior
septal
posterior leaflet

fused commissure *not* incised

2

Suture Annuloplasty

3

felt pledget

Carpentier Ring

sizer   ring

7

AV node

pledgets placed on ventricular side along septal leaflet

8

4

alternative over-and-over return suture

5

suture tied over two fingers

6

residual tricuspid insufficiency assessed

9 septal leaflet
AV node

valve excised

10

11

annulus

rim of septal leaflet

Tricuspid Valve Replacement

J.W. Low M.D.

Mitral Valve Reconstruction

The high incidence of complications related to prosthetic valves has stimulated renewed efforts to reconstruct both stenotic and regurgitant mitral valves. Severely calcified valves or valves with shrunken, rigid anterior leaflets usually cannot be repaired.

The normal mitral valve has two leaflets with approximately the same surface area. The broad anterior leaflet subtends about 170 degrees of the mitral annulus and closes a disproportionate amount of the center of the orifice during ventricular systole. Part of the annulus of the anterior leaflet is in continuity with the aortic annulus and cannot be shortened. The longer but more narrow posterior (mural) leaflet subtends approximately 210 degrees of the mitral annulus and can function as an immobile buttress. The anterior leaflet, however, must be flexible and mobile for the valve to function and must coapt with the mural leaflet to close the orifice during systole. The anterior and posterior papillary muscles provide chordal attachments to both leaflets.

Good exposure in a dry, motionless operative field is required for mitral valve reconstruction. Traction sutures placed carefully in the annulus at each commissure improve exposure. Initial inspection of the valve should assess the width and potential mobility of the anterior leaflet and the degree and location of calcification.

STENOTIC VALVE

1 If the valve is stenotic, the fused commissures are incised first. This must be done carefully along the line of fusion and with inspection of the chordal attachments beneath the fused leaflets. In most patients, a small linear depression marks the line of fusion. As the leaflets are separated using a No. 15 scalpel, the chordal attachments to each free edge are checked. The incision is extended to or to within 1 or 2 mm of the valve annulus.

2 Thickened, fused chordae are trimmed and split to gain both length and mobility. Sometimes layers of fibrous tissue can be peeled off chordae and leaflets, revealing a strong, mobile, near-normal structure beneath. Chordal incisions can be extended 1 to 2 cm into the papillary muscles to gain length. Unnecessary chordae are excised.

3 Thickened, calcified, immobile leaflets can be debrided also. Patience is required as bits of fibrous tissue and calcium are peeled away from both surfaces of the leaflets. The anterior leaflet must be mobile for the valve to function properly.

RUPTURED CHORDAE

4 Degenerative mitral valve disease causes mitral insufficiency from dilatation of the annulus, redundant prolapsing leaflets, and one or more ruptured chordae. After careful inspection, a plan of repair is developed. Wedge-shaped portions of the leaflet attached to the ruptured chord may be resected. Leaflet edges are approximated with interrupted 5-0 monofilament mattress sutures buttressed with tiny pledgets of excised valve tissue. Larger trapezoid sections of leaflet tissue may be excised from the mural leaflet. If the anterior leaflet remains redundant, a triangular portion at each commissure can be removed and the free edge of the leaflet rotated and sutured to the annulus at the commissures. This effectively shortens both chordae and free edge.

REDUNDANT CHORDAE

5 Elongated redundant chordae may be plicated to prevent leaflet prolapse. The most popular method incises the tip of the papillary muscle and folds the excess chord into the incision. This technique risks infarction of part of the papillary muscle. Alternatively, elongated chordae may be plicated to the underside of the leaflet or to adjacent chordae.

ANNULAR RING

6 Many incompetent mitral valves require reduction of dilated annuli. We prefer the Carpentier ring, which both reduces the size of the annulus and elevates the mural annulus and leaflet to provide better apposition with the anterior leaflet. The annular ring is sized using an obturator, which measures the length of the anterior annulus between the two commissures. The broken ring is sutured in place with interrupted pledgeted mattress sutures passed around the ring and through the fabric. All sutures pass through the atrium and junction of valve leaflet and annulus so that the ring is securely anchored and does not compromise the valve orifice.

7 The ring may also be anchored with a running over-and-over suture of 2-0 monofilament. This technique is faster but does not produce as secure a fixation of the ring. Two or three continuous sutures are used; two or three interrupted sutures are added to prevent rotation of the ring.

8 After the valve is reconstructed, it must be tested for competence and lack of stenosis. If two fingers can be passed through the valve to the first knuckle, and if spaces between the chordae (secondary orifice) are sufficiently open, stenosis is relieved.

Valve competence is more difficult to assess. This is done by filling the ventricle with saline solution injected through a small catheter passed through the reconstructed valve. The leaflets should float together and prevent regurgitation at the free edges. When the surgeon is satisfied with the reconstruction, a No. 18 Foley catheter with a cut atrial hole is left to decompress the ventricle.

9 The left atrium is closed with a running horizontal mattress suture followed by an over-and-over stitch. Left atrial sutures are not tied until all air has been removed from the left ventricle, atrium, and aortic root, and until the heart is beating. After bypass is stopped, final evaluation of valve function is determined by finger palpation (through the untied atrial suture line) and by Doppler echocardiography using an esophageal probe. If the valve is not satisfactory, it is replaced.

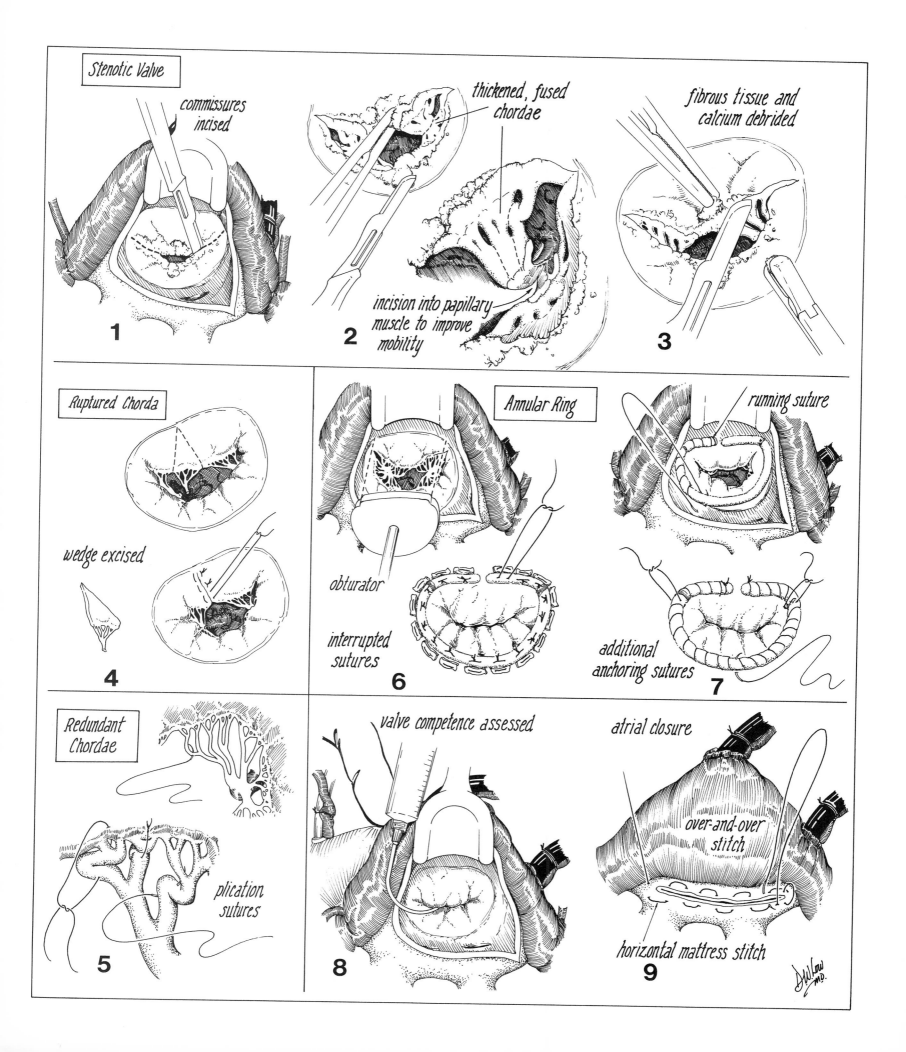

Stenotic Valve

1 commissures incised

2 thickened, fused chordae · incision into papillary muscle to improve mobility

3 fibrous tissue and calcium debrided

Ruptured Chorda

4 wedge excised

Annular Ring

6 obturator · interrupted sutures

7 running suture · additional anchoring sutures

Redundant Chordae

5 plication sutures

8 valve competence assessed

9 atrial closure · over-and-over stitch · horizontal mattress stitch

Mitral Valve Replacement

The mitral valve may be exposed through a median sternotomy or a right or left thoracotomy. Median sternotomy is the most common incision, is easy and familiar, and provides access to other valves and the coronary arteries. Right thoracotomy is available for special circumstances and is an alternative for patients who have had a previous median sternotomy. Exposure of the mitral valve from a left thoracotomy requires cannulation of the right ventricular outflow tract or pulmonary artery for venous access and cannulation of the left femoral, external iliac artery or descending thoracic aorta for arterial return.

RIGHT THORACOTOMY

1 For right thoracotomy, the patient is positioned with the right arm forward, a roll in the left axilla, and a sandbag along the spine. The shoulders and hips are rotated about 15 to 20 degrees posteriorly to provide access to the right groin (in case the femoral artery is cannulated) and anterior chest wall and sternum. Usually the left knee is flexed and the right leg extended and rotated slightly laterally.

2 A curvilinear submammary incision is made and extended posterior to the tip of the scapula. The fifth rib is excised. For better cephalad exposure, the costosternal junction of the fourth rib may be cut. The lung is retracted posteriorly; it is convenient to use a flap of pericardium hinged along the right phrenic nerve to help retract the lung from the operative field. Suture of the anterior edge of pericardium to the chest wall improves exposure and helps retract the heart toward the operator.

3 The ascending aorta can be cannulated in most patients. The right atrial appendage is retracted caudad and purse-string sutures are placed in the exposed ascending aorta well above the aortic valve. After the cannula is inserted, it is tied to the chest wall anteriorly to protect it. Both cava are cannulated from right atrial incisions made within purse string sutures. Caval tapes are not necessary unless the right atrium is entered. After bypass begins and the heart is arrested with cold cardioplegic solution, the mitral valve is exposed by means of an incision in the left atrium posterior to the interatrial groove. The incision extends slightly behind the inferior vena cava, which is mobilized by cutting the pericardial attachment. The mitral valve is directly ahead and does not require strong retraction of the right atrium and interatrial septum as required when a median sternotomy is used.

LEFT THORACOTOMY

4 A similar position is used to expose the mitral valve through a left thoracotomy. Only the hips are rotated posteriorly, however, to permit access to the left femoral artery for insertion of the arterial cannula; the shoulders remain perpendicular to the table with the left arm forward. The chest is opened through a posterolateral thoracotomy incision and the fifth rib is excised (the rib need not be excised in children, but its excision provides better exposure in adults). The lung is retracted posteriorly. The pericardium is opened wide to expose the left atrium and left pulmonary artery.

5 The main pulmonary artery can be cannulated through either an incision in the right ventricular outflow tract below the pulmonary artery or a purse-string suture placed near the origin of the left pulmonary artery as it begins its curve around the left main bronchus. Pericardial attachments must be incised to expose the thin-walled left pulmonary artery. If a right ventriculotomy is used, a small incision is made horizontally within a large mattress suture buttressed with Teflon felt pledgets. The epicardial incision is deepened into the chamber by a blunt instrument, and then the cannula is advanced into the main pulmonary artery. Retraction on the anterior pericardial edge helps to rotate the right ventricular outflow tract toward the surgeon. Usually the left femoral artery is used for the arterial cannula; less often the descending thoracic aorta is exposed by retracting the lung anteriorly. The ascending aorta is not available; therefore, cardiac arrest and cold cardioplegia cannot be used. Usually the heart fibrillates and remains in ventricular fibrillation while the mitral valve is exposed. Coronary vessels are perfused and fibrillation is maintained by moderate hypothermia.

6 After bypass starts, the mitral valve is exposed by an anterior incision in the left atrial wall which is roughly parallel to the atrioventricular groove. The mitral valve is anterior and the anterior wall of the left atrium must be retracted strongly for the valve to be seen.

MEDIAN STERNOTOMY: LEFT ATRIAL INCISION

7 Three different cardiotomy incisions may be used to expose the mitral valve from a median sternotomy incision. After the ascending aorta and both cavae are cannulated, the heart is mobilized by incising pericardial attachments along the right edge of the superior vena cava to and beyond the junction of the azygous vein, the attachments to the anterior wall of the right pulmonary veins and attachments to the inferior vena cava as it passes through the diaphragm. The space bounded by the inferior cava and inferior right pulmonary vein and left atrium and pericardium is opened. This allows the operator to rotate the patient's heart toward the patient's left and exposes the left atrium posterior to the interatrial groove. The atriotomy starts at the superior border of the right superior pulmonary vein as it enters the left atrium, continues caudad parallel to the interatrial septum, and curves posteriorly behind the inferior cava toward the mitral annulus.

LEFT AND RIGHT ATRIA INCISED

8 In patients with small left atria, the mitral valve may be better exposed through an incision in the interatrial septum. Tapes are placed around both caval cannulas to exclude venous return from the right atrium. An incision is made perpendicular to the left atriotomy in the anterolateral wall of the right atrium. The interatrial septum is incised across the fossa ovalis to expose the entire mitral annulus.

RIGHT ATRIUM AND SEPTUM INCISED

9 In patients with large left atria, the mitral valve may be exposed by opening the right atrium widely and incising the interatrial septum. The lateral wall of the left atrium is not incised. The septal incision is made primarily in the fossa ovalis but is extended slightly into the muscular septum superiorly and inferiorly. When the medial edge of the septum is retracted, the anterior mitral annulus appears just beneath the retractor.

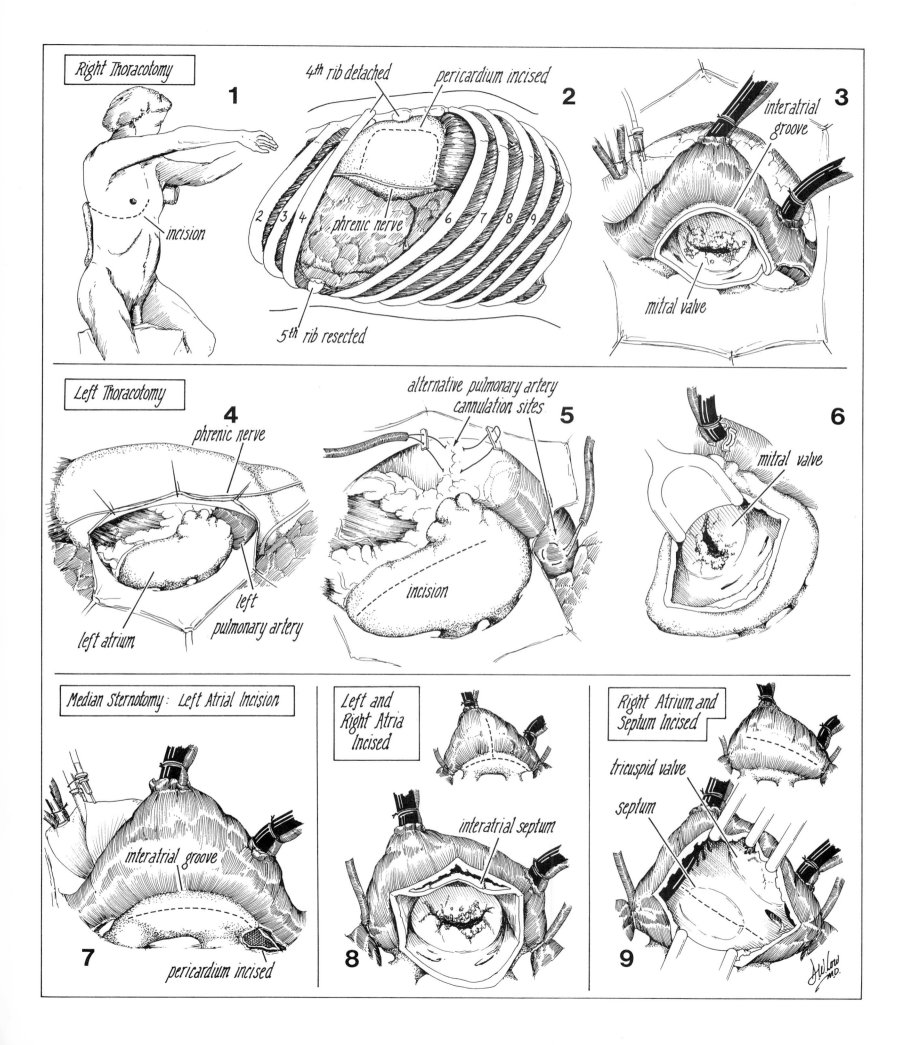

Right Thoracotomy — **1**

2 — 4th rib detached / pericardium incised / phrenic nerve / 5th rib resected / 2 3 4 6 7 8 9

3 — interatrial groove / mitral valve

Left Thoracotomy — **4** — phrenic nerve / left atrium / left pulmonary artery

5 — alternative pulmonary artery cannulation sites / incision

6 — mitral valve

Median Sternotomy: Left Atrial Incision — **7** — interatrial groove / pericardium incised

Left and Right Atria Incised — **8** — interatrial septum

Right Atrium and Septum Incised — **9** — tricuspid valve / septum

SUPERIOR APPROACH

(10) The mitral valve may also be exposed from the superior approach. The aorta must be clamped and the heart arrested to retract the ascending aorta medially and anteriorly. This exposes the superior wall of the left atrium from the base of the left atrial appendage to the edge of the superior cava. If the cava is dissected from the right pulmonary artery and retracted anteriorly, the incision may continue behind the cava toward the right superior pulmonary vein. This incision exposes the mitral valve, which is surprisingly close to the anterior edge of the atriotomy.

The aorta is usually clamped and the heart arrested when the mitral valve is replaced from a median sternotomy or right thoracotomy. Cardioplegia improves exposure by relaxing the ventricles and reducing pulmonary venous blood flow. The aorta is difficult to clamp from a left thoracotomy and is therefore not clamped. The ventricles may be electrically fibrillated while the valve is replaced.

MITRAL VALVE REPLACEMENT

(11) The exposed mitral valve must be excised carefully to avoid injury to the left ventricle, aortic valve, and adjacent structures. A 2 to 3 mm rim of leaflet is left attached to the annulus. The chordae remain attached to the leaflets and are transected at the tips of the papillary muscles. The papillary muscles are not excised. If calcium extends into the annulus, it must be carefully broken up and removed without injuring the annulus or ventricular endocardium.

(12) Many surgeons retain part of the diseased mitral valve in hope of reducing the incidence of postoperative ventricular rupture and improving postoperative ventricular function. If a bioprosthesis is inserted, only a wedge of the central anterior mitral leaflet need be removed to prevent impairment of blood flow through the prosthesis. If mechanical valves are used, more leaflet tissue must be removed. This can often be done by cutting deep wedges into the leaflets between major chordal attachments. Residual valvular tissue must not interfere with movement of the prosthetic valve mechanism and must not create an obstruction at the "secondary" or subannular valve orifice.

(13) Once the diseased valve is excised, the annulus is sized using the obturator supplied by the manufacturer of the prosthesis. If the left ventricular cavity is small and/or hypertrophied, a low profile prosthesis is preferred so that the prosthesis does not injure ventricular endocardium.

The prosthetic sewing ring can be sutured to the annulus in several ways. It is helpful to retract the valve annulus toward the operator by two or three traction sutures. Most often, Teflon-pledgeted mattress sutures of polyester are placed through the atrium near the annulus into the annular attachment to the ventricle. If the mural leaflet and a portion of the anterior leaflet are retained, the suture, which is passed from atrium through ventricular annulus, is passed through the leaflet near its attachment to the annulus before it is passed through the prosthetic sewing ring. It is important that the needles exit through the fibrotic annulus and not through the adjacent friable ventricular muscle. Needles are then passed from below upward through the prosthetic sewing ring. It is convenient to begin at the anterior commissure and proceed along the mural (posterior annulus) to the posterior commissure first.

(14) With the prosthesis held laterally, sutures in the anterior annulus are placed beginning at either commissure. Traction on newly placed sutures retracts the annulus into view for the next stitch. Usually 15 to 18 mattress sutures suffice to anchor the prosthesis in place. When these sutures are tied, the mitral annulus is everted into the sewing ring. This reduces the possibility that residual tissue can interfere with the valve mechanism. If pledgeted mattress sutures are passed from the ventricular annulus to the atrium so that the pledgets are positioned below the annulus, annular tissue may interfere with the mechanism of many mechanical valves.

(15) If the mitral annulus is fibrotic, thick, and firm, the prosthesis may be inserted with either simple interrupted sutures (no pledgets) or with one or two continuous sutures of 2-0 monofilament material. The annulus must be well exposed for the continuous suture. This double needle suture is conveniently started at the anterior commissure. After three or four over-and-over sutures, the prosthesis is placed into position. The mural (posterior) annulus is completed first, then the suture is continued around the anterior annulus. A hook is used to tighten all loops before the posthesis is tied into place.

In occasional patients, particularly those with prosthetic valve endocarditis, part of the mitral annulus is destroyed. Before the prosthetic valve is chosen, the annulus must be reconstructed and/or a means to anchor the prosthesis devised. The circumflex coronary artery lies in the atrioventricular groove along the posterior mitral annulus. The annulus that connects ventricle and atrium is very thin and may require carefully placed pledgeted mattress sutures to reconstruct or reinforce the atrioventricular junction. Care must be taken that these sutures do not tear the ventricular endocardium and the endocardial pledgets do not interfere with the mechanism of the prosthesis. If the septal portion of the annulus is destroyed, deep mattress sutures, which will probably cause third degree heart block, may be required.

(16) If the annulus adjacent to the aorta annulus is destroyed, the aorta can be opened and pledgeted mattress sutures passed from the sinus of Valsalva and aortic root to anchor the prosthesis. These sutures must be carefully placed to avoid injury or distortion of the aortic valve.

VENTRICULAR APPROACH

(17) Occasionally in patients with ventricular aneurysms, the mitral valve is replaced from the ventriculotomy. With the aorta clamped, exposure of mitral valve from the ventricle is not difficult through a large anterior or posterior ventriculotomy when the heart is rotated anteriorly. Pledgeted mattress sutures are usually used to anchor the valve with pledgets and knots placed on the ventricular side of the annulus.

EXCISION OF PROSTHETIC VALVE

(18) Excision of a prosthetic mitral valve is more difficult than excision of the native diseased valve. After the valve is exposed, it should be carefully inspected to determine the cause of failure and the presence of vegetations or thrombi. With a long-handled No.15 blade, the scar tissue over the sewing ring is incised around the entire circumference. A Kocher clamp is placed in the sewing ring near the posterior commissure and the valve is retracted superiorly and anteriorly. With the knife blade, sutures are cut and fibrous tissue adjacent to the sewing ring is delicately cut away along the edge of the sewing ring. The knife is directed toward the ventricular cavity at all times. When the knife enters the ventricle, the Kocher is replaced by a hook beneath the sewing ring. The plane between annulus and sewing ring is expanded until the valve is removed. With traction sutures to improve exposure, potentially obstructing tags of fibrous tissue or calcium are excised and the annulus is prepared for the new prosthesis. In infected patients, the annulus should be carefully inspected for abscesses and necrotic tissue, which are removed.

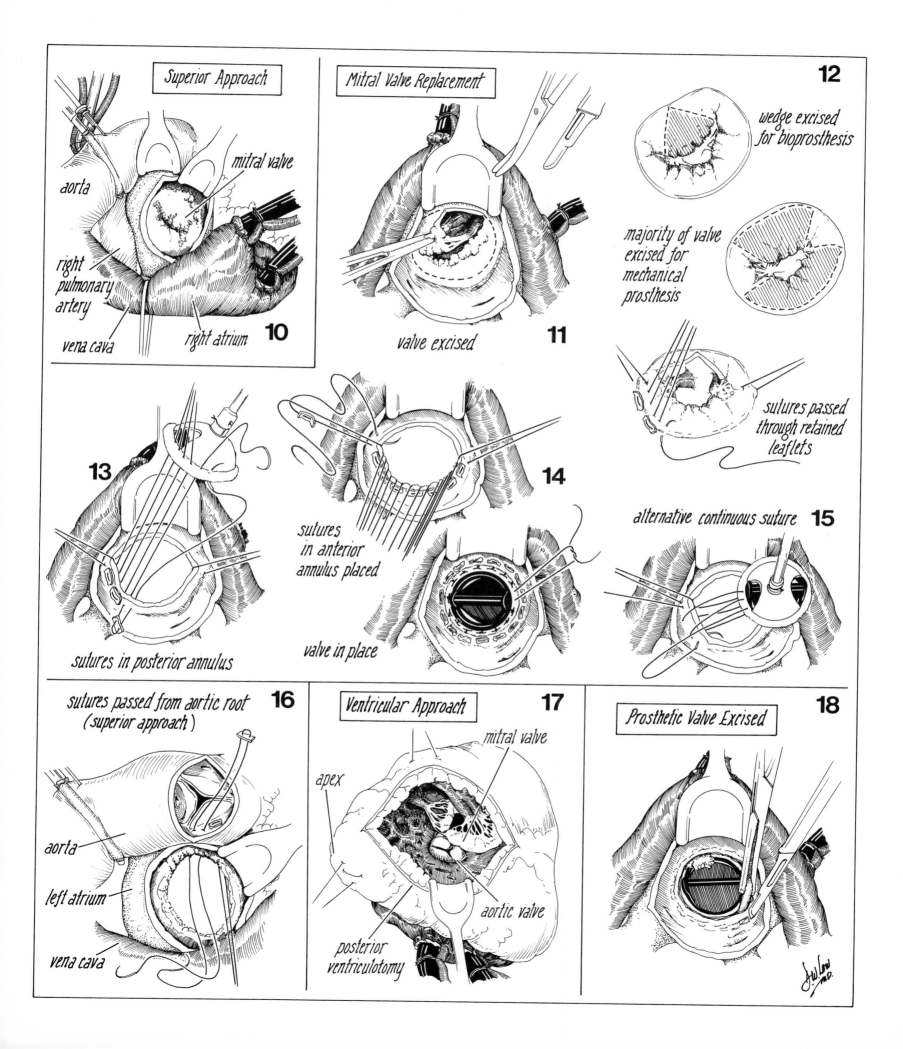

Superior Approach

aorta

mitral valve

right pulmonary artery

vena cava

right atrium

10

Mitral Valve Replacement

valve excised **11**

12

wedge excised for bioprosthesis

majority of valve excised for mechanical prosthesis

sutures passed through retained leaflets

13

sutures in posterior annulus

sutures in anterior annulus placed

valve in place **14**

alternative continuous suture **15**

sutures passed from aortic root (superior approach) **16**

aorta

left atrium

vena cava

Ventricular Approach **17**

apex

mitral valve

aortic valve

posterior ventriculotomy

Prosthetic Valve Excised **18**

Aortic Valve Replacement

A variety of satisfactory aortic valvular prostheses are available. Considerations with respect to the incidence of thromboembolism, need for warfarin anticoagulation, durability of prosthesis, hemodynamic characteristics of the valve, and the preferences of the surgeon and an informed patient determine the selection. The operation is frequently combined with other procedures such as mitral valve replacement and coronary artery bypass grafts.

(1) The heart is exposed through a midline sternotomy, and after heparin, the ascending aorta is cannulated just upstream to the origin of the innominate artery. A large bore, single or "two-stage" cannula is placed into the right atrium. On bypass, the patient is cooled to 28 to 32° C. A small incision is made in the left atrium near the junction with the right superior pulmonary vein. As the ascending aorta is clamped just upstream to the aortic cannula, a No. 18 Ferguson catheter is placed into the left atrium to decompress the heart. If aortic insufficiency is absent or minimal, the heart is arrested with direct injection of cold cardioplegic solution into the ascending aorta and simultaneous application of cold (4° C) saline to the surface of the heart.

(2) The ascending aorta is opened through an oblique or hockey-stick incision. If not previously arrested, the left and right coronary orifices are injected directly with cold potassium cardioplegic solution using soft silastic Spencer-Malette catheters placed directly into the coronary ostia. The coronary catheters may be perfused from a pump-controlled cardioplegic system or manually by using multiple syringe injections. If both coronary arteries are patent, both are perfused to achieve complete cardiac arrest. Reperfusion of the coronary arteries and reapplication of cold external saline are done every 20 to 25 minutes to prevent myocardial ischemic damage. Left ventricular septal temperature is often monitored, and either a cooling coil or sponge soaked in saline slush is placed in the pericardial well to maintain a low (<18° C) left ventricular temperature.

(3) The cephalad flap of aorta is tacked to the pericardium and traction sutures are placed at the top of each aortic commissure to improve exposure.

(4) The valve is inspected and excised. The excision usually begins at the least diseased commissure and carefully follows the annulus. If calcification is severe or granular, a small Hibbs sponge is placed through the opened valve into the left ventricle to trap potential emboli produced by the excision.

(5) After removal of the diseased valve, calcium is carefully debrided from the annulus with rongeur, knife, and forceps. Calcium extending onto the anterior leaflet of the mitral valve and onto the surface of the ventricular septum is removed carefully to avoid injury to the mitral leaflet and conduction system. Thorough calcium debridement should be carried out to ensure the maximum diameter of the annulus and secure anchorage of sutures. Often calcium chips can be "extruded" from the annulus without removing fibrous tissue.

In patients with acute bacterial endocarditis, small abscesses may be present in the aortic annulus. When encountered, these must be completely opened and all the necrotic material removed. Pledgeted sutures may be necessary to reconstruct the annulus and obliterate the abscess cavity before inserting the valve prosthesis.

(6) The valve annulus is sized using the valve sizer. If a bioprosthesis that requires rinsing is selected, sutures are placed in the annulus and pinned to the drapes surrounding the wound while the valve is prepared. If a mechanical prosthesis is selected, sutures are passed through the valve sewing ring immediately after placement of the annulus.

(7) Pledgeted 2-0 polyester mattress sutures are used to anchor aortic prostheses. With tilting disc valves, it is important to evert the aortic annulus away from the disc mechanism; therefore, sutures are passed through the aortic annulus from above downward and then through the sewing ring from below upward (in the direction of the blood flow).

(8) When tied down, these sutures evert the aortic annulus against the sewing ring and prevent tissue from interfering with valve closure.

Other surgeons prefer other suture techniques including simple, unpledgeted sutures, mattress sutures without pledgets, figure-of-eight sutures, pledgeted mattress sutures with pledgets placed on the ventricular side of the annulus, and running sutures. When running sutures are used, No. 0 or No. 1 monofilament suture material is preferred and at least three separate sutures are used. The over-and-over suture between annulus and sewing ring is placed with the prosthesis held 1 to 2 inches above the annulus. It is convenient to begin suture placement at the commissure between the left and right cusps and continue toward the surgeon along the annulus of the left coronary cusp. When all sutures are placed, the loops are pulled up (using a nerve hook), and the ends of the three sutures are tied to each other.

(9) The aorta is closed with a running horizontal mattress suture of 3-0 monofilament suture followed by an over-and-over suture. Usually a double-ended suture with a 4 x 6 mm Teflon felt pledget is placed at each end of the aortotomy. One end of each suture is used for the mattress sutures; the other is used for the over-and-over suture. When the aorta is very thin and/or friable, the sutures are passed through strips of Teflon felt (as illustrated).

Before releasing the aortic cross-clamp, all air is evacuated from the left atrium, ventricle, and aortic root. The patient is turned "head down" and the lungs are inflated while the aortic suture line remains open. The ventricular vent is occluded. Perfusion flow is reduced as the aortic clamp is released. The sutures are tied as blood under low pressure flows out of the aortotomy. In addition, a No. 19 needle is placed in the ascending aorta at its most anterior (highest) point to permit escape of air as the heart begins to contract and eject. Distension of the noncontracting or poorly contracting ventricle is prevented by reopening the left ventricular vent catheter.

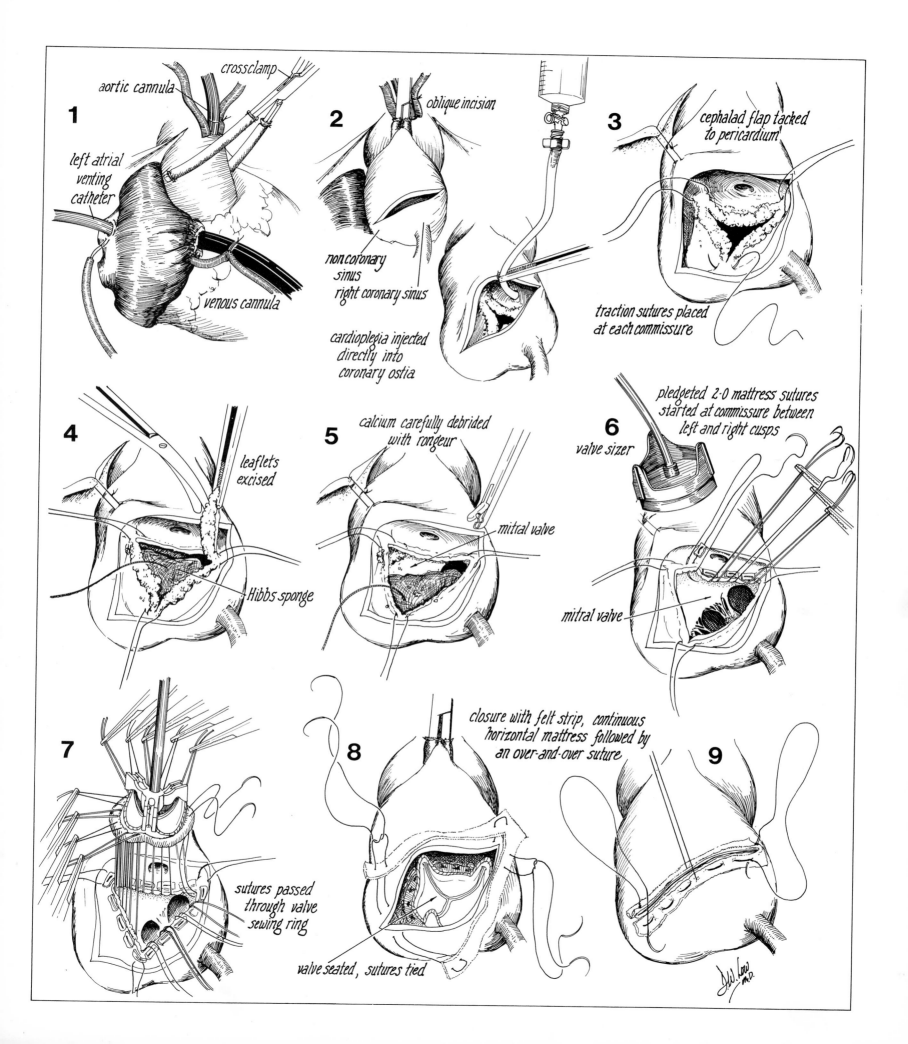

1 aortic cannula crossclamp left atrial venting catheter venous cannula

2 oblique incision non coronary sinus right coronary sinus cardioplegia injected directly into coronary ostia

3 cephalad flap tacked to pericardium traction sutures placed at each commissure

4 leaflets excised Hibbs sponge

5 calcium carefully debrided with rongeur mitral valve

6 pledgeted 2-0 mattress sutures started at commissure between left and right cusps valve sizer mitral valve

7 sutures passed through valve sewing ring

8 valve seated, sutures tied

9 closure with felt strip, continuous horizontal mattress followed by an over-and-over suture

D.W. Low M.D.

Insertion of Aortic Allograft Valve

Currently, aortic valve allografts are used in selected adolescent children and young adults. This valve does not require coumadin anticoagulation, and its durability in young patients far exceeds that of preserved xenografts (heterografts). The allografts are harvested by sterile or "clean" technique from brain-dead donors or within 12 hours from cadavers. The excised tissue includes the valve, ascending aorta, and a portion of the ventricular muscle and anterior mitral leaflet below the valve. The diameter of the graft is carefully measured and recorded. The graft is then immersed in a solution of nutrients and antibiotics at 4° C. After a series of cultures and solution changes, the graft is packaged in a vinyl envelope with nutrient solution and 10% dimethyl sulfoxide (DMSO). The packaged graft is frozen at a controlled rate of temperature change to −40° C to minimize cell destruction by crystallization. Packaged grafts are stored in a liquid nitrogen freezer at −150° C until use within 1 year. All cultures must be negative for at least 72 hours before the graft is available for use.

(1) The heart is exposed by means of midline sternotomy and the ascending aorta and right atrium are cannulated (single or two-stage venous cannula). Before bypass starts, the outside diameter of the aortic root is carefully measured. One or more grafts with diameters approximately 5 mm less are transferred in a liquid nitrogen cannister to the operating room. Bypass is started and the patient is cooled to 26° C. A 24 Fr catheter is inserted into the junction of the left superior pulmonary vein and left atrium and passed into the ventricle; after the heart fibrillates, the ascending aorta is clamped. The ascending aorta is opened by a hockey stick incision which extends down into the noncoronary sinus midway between the two commissures to a point approximately 4 or 5 mm from the aortic annulus. Cold cardioplegic solution is infused directly into both coronary sinuses and the heart is immersed in cold saline. Cardioplegia is renewed every 20 minutes, or sooner if myocardial septal temperature exceeds 18° C.

(2) The aortic valve is excised as close to the aortic wall and mitral annulus as possible. The rim of attached leaflets should be minimal and is debrided of all calcium. Three traction sutures of 2-0 polyester are placed in the aortic wall at the downstream attachments of the native valve commissures. These should be an equal distance apart. The valve annulus is sized using any commercial sizer. An allograft valve which is 2 to 3 mm smaller in diameter is selected and transferred to the first of three thawing solutions. The graft is thawed in nutrient solution containing DMSO until warmed above the freezing point. The DMSO is rinsed out in the next two solutions.

(3) While the heart is kept cool, the allograft is carefully trimmed. The excess ascending aorta beyond the downstream attachments of the commissures is removed. The allograft is mounted on the index finger of the left (or nondominant) hand and the excess ventricular septum and mitral leaflet is trimmed from the circumference of the graft. The base of the valve is trimmed back to leave 5 mm of tissue between the attachment of the cusps in the depths of the sinuses and the upstream end of the graft.

Excess aortic wall within the sinuses is trimmed. A 2 mm rim of aorta is left around the attachment of the leaflets to the allograft aortic wall at the commissures. This rim expands to 4 mm at the depths of the sinuses. The trimmed sinuses should be U-shaped, with three commissural "posts" about 4 mm wide.

(4) Three equidistant 4-0 double-needled monofilament sutures are placed approximately 5 mm upstream to the leaflet attachment line of the excised recipient valve. These sutures are placed midway between the excised commissures and upstream to the deepest part of the recipient's sinuses of Valsalva.

The allograft is rotated counterclockwise 120 degrees so that the residual septal musculature of the allograft opposes the mitral-aortic annulus of the recipient. The rotated valve is inverted into the left ventricle.

(5) The three previously placed monofilament sutures are passed through the base of the allograft opposite the deepest point of the allograft sinuses of Valsalva. These sutures are tied. The base of the allograft valve is sutured to the base of the recipient aorta and left ventricular outflow tract by a continuous over-and-over suture using the three tied sutures in turn. It is convenient to begin with the right coronary cusp suture.

(6) Suture bites for the upstream suture line should be substantial in both the allograft and aorta, and it is important to pass the needles from allograft base into the recipient aorta in the direction of future blood flow (that is, vertical rather than tangential sutures should be used). The sutures are tied to each other to complete the upstream suture line.

(7) Two of the three allograft commissural "posts" supporting the right cusp are everted and, with traction sutures, lined up with the previously placed traction sutures in the recipient aorta. The position of the coronary ostium is checked. The downstream suture line of the right cusp is made first.

(8) It is particularly important for proper function of the valve that the horseshoe-shaped, scalloped sinus of Valsalva be maintained. An over-and-over stitch of 4-0 monofilament suture is used. With traction on the commissural posts, the stitch starts at the depths of the sinus and proceeds up each post. The needle passes perpendicular to the cut edge of the allograft through either graft or recipient aorta first. The suture line makes a miniature horseshoe wherein the distance between the two downstream commissural attachments is slightly less than the chord length of the arc made by the suture line in the depths of the sinus. A V-shaped downstream sinus suture line would compromise the billow of the cusp and coaptation of the leaflets and cause valvular incompetence.

(9) After the right cusp is sutured, the third commissural post is everted. The two traction sutures of the commissure between the left and noncoronary cusps are lined up. The left cusp is attached next and the noncoronary cusp last. The sutures are tied to each other at the downstream apex of the three commissures. Traction sutures are removed. The aortotomy is closed without distortion of the aortic root. Two mm in the aortic wall are used and sutures are evenly spaced. A double row of over-and-over sutures of 4-0 monofilament suture material is used unless the aortic wall is very friable and requires a horizontal mattress stitch or interrupted mattress sutures with Teflon felt. Air maneuvers are carried out before the aortic clamp is released.

After rewarming is completed and bypass is stopped, left ventricular pressure is measured using a No. 20 spinal needle passed through the right ventricular wall and interventricular septum into the left ventricle. Simultaneous radial (or femoral) arterial and left ventricular pressures are recorded to detect any stenosis of the valve. The presence of a palpable "tap" in the aortic root and a normal aortic dicrotic notch and diastolic pressure confirm the absence of significant aortic insufficiency.

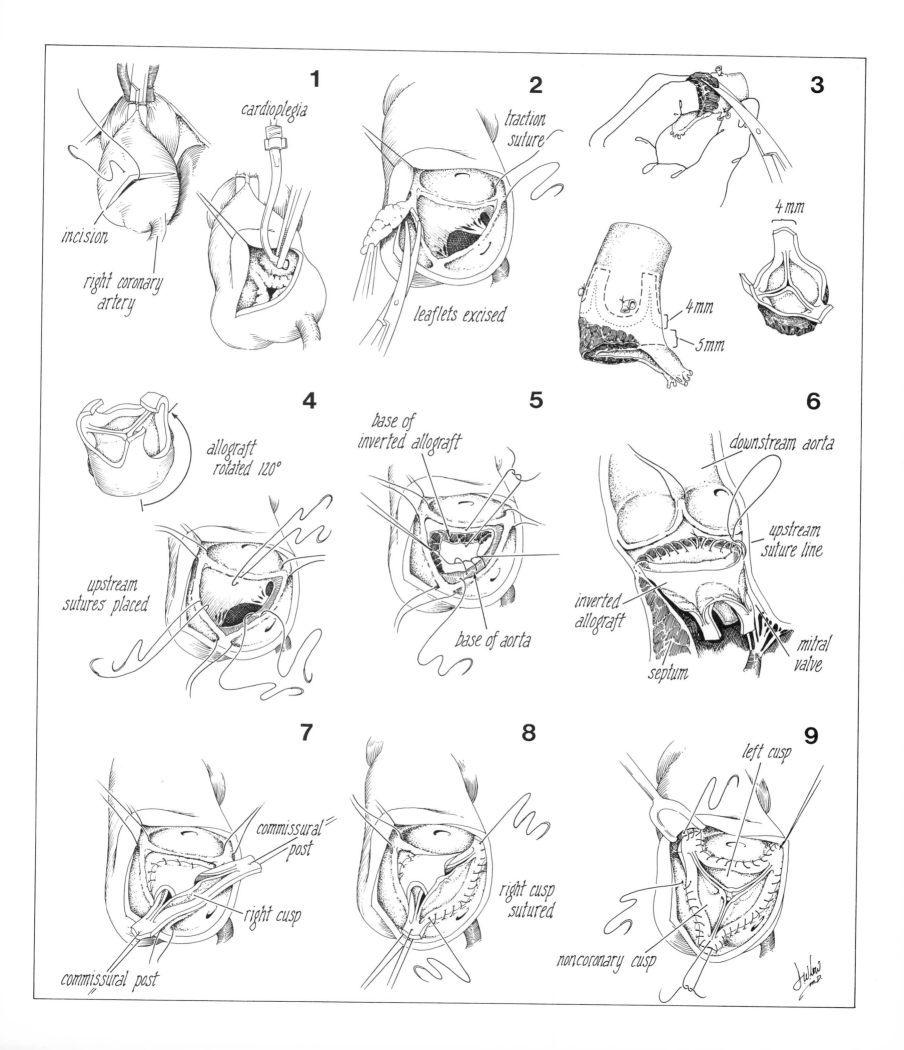

1

cardioplegia

incision

right coronary
artery

2

traction
suture

leaflets excised

3

4 mm

4 mm

5 mm

4

allograft
rotated 120°

upstream
sutures placed

5

base of
inverted allograft

base of aorta

6

downstream aorta

upstream
suture line

inverted
allograft

mitral
valve

septum

7

commissural
post

right cusp

commissural post

8

right cusp
sutured

9

left cusp

noncoronary cusp

Enlargement of the Aortic Annulus

The aortic annulus may be enlarged to accommodate a larger aortic valvular prosthesis in one of several ways. An incision across the annulus of the noncoronary cusp into the fibrous trigone can enlarge the circumference of the annulus 2 to 3 cm. A vertical incision across the annulus of the left coronary cusp will increase the circumference 1 to 2 cm. Further enlargement of the aortic annulus and left ventricular outflow tract is made possible by incision and patching of the aortic annulus and ventricular septum as described by Konno.

(1) The relevant anatomy of an incision across the noncoronary annulus is illustrated. The incision avoids the annulus of both atrioventricular valves and extends into the fibrous trigone of the heart.

(2) The aortotomy is continued vertically across the aorta annulus of the noncoronary cusp beyond the anterior mitral leaflet and anterior to the posterior commissure of the mitral valve.

(3) The incision extends to but not into muscle of the left ventricular outflow tract. The anterior leaflet of the mitral valve is not incised. A preclotted woven Dacron patch is carefully measured and cut to maximally widen the annulus and adjacent subannular and supra-annular aortic walls. Pericardium or polytetrafluoroethylene (PTFE or Teflon) may also be used. The patch is conveniently cut from a tubular prosthesis of the approximate desired diameter of the enlarged aortic root. Distances from the apex of the subannular incision to the annulus, between the two cut ends of the annulus, and from annulus to the cephalad apex of the aortotomy are measured and marked on the tubular prosthesis. If an oblique or hockey-stick incision was made in the supra-annular aorta, this prosthesis is measured and marked accordingly so that the resulting patch will not distort the aortic root.

(4) The subannular portion of the patch is sutured in place using a running 4-0 monofilament suture with or without a small Teflon pledget at the apex of the incision. The suture lines are carried about 1 cm across the aortic annulus into the aortic root and tied, but are not cut.

(5) The aortic prosthesis is selected and inserted as described elsewhere. The plane of the valve should not be altered, but should remain perpendicular to the flow-path from left ventricular outflow tract to aortic root. Sutures buttressed with Teflon felt pledgets are passed from outside in across the patch to anchor the valve sewing ring to the patch.

(6) After insertion of the valve, the aorta is closed by suturing the edges of the patch to the edges of the aorta with a continuous running suture.

(7) A second method of enlarging the annulus 1 to 1.5 cm involves an incision in the left coronary sinus of Valsalva. A vertical incision across the annulus of the left coronary cusp is extended for approximately 1 cm into the anterior leaflet of the mitral valve.

(8) When the edges of the cut annulus are separated (with traction sutures), a diamond-shaped defect in the posterior aorta and mitral leaflet develops.

(9) This defect is closed with a patch of pericardium or prosthetic material as illustrated. Before the patch is sutured to the aorta, pledgeted anchoring sutures for the aortic valvular prosthesis are placed so that the pledgets lie between the patch and left atrial wall.

(10) The aortotomy is closed. The prosthesis is inserted and sewn into the enlarged annulus.

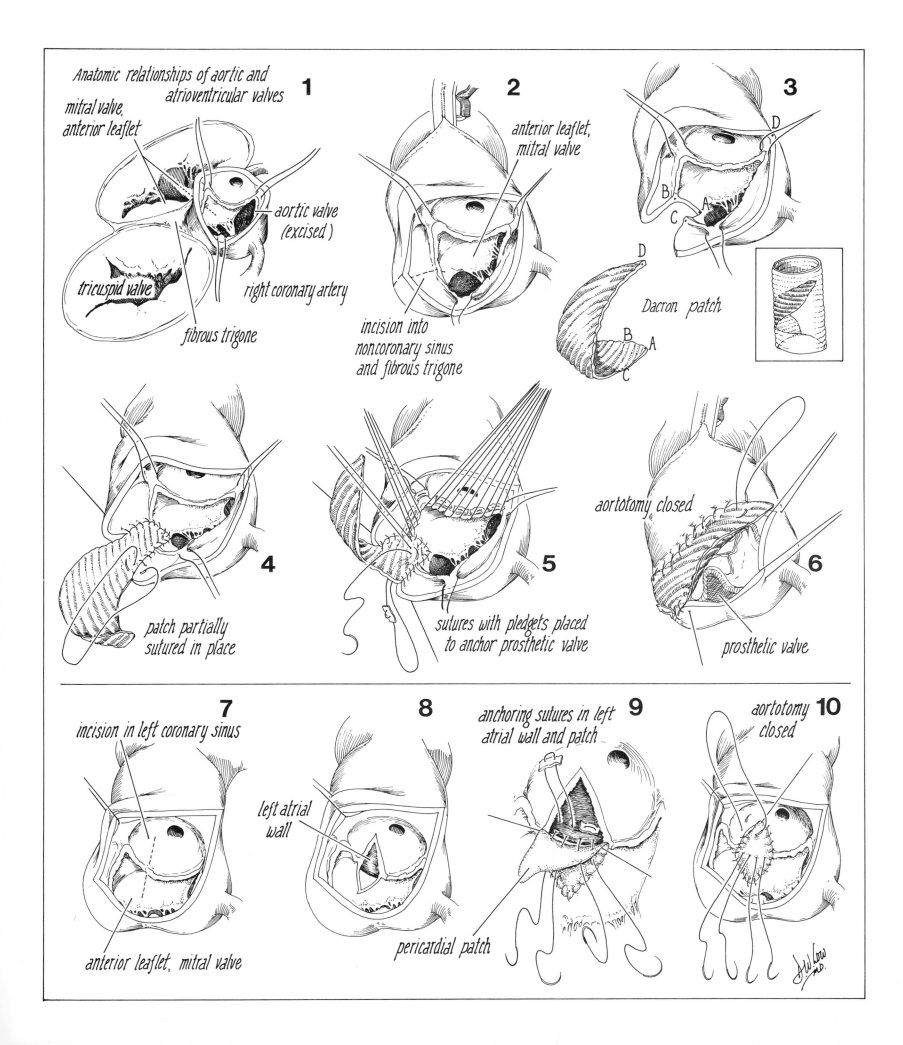

1 Anatomic relationships of aortic and atrioventricular valves

mitral valve, anterior leaflet

aortic valve (excised)

tricuspid valve

right coronary artery

fibrous trigone

2 anterior leaflet, mitral valve

incision into noncoronary sinus and fibrous trigone

3 Dacron patch

4 patch partially sutured in place

5 sutures with pledgets placed to anchor prosthetic valve

6 aortotomy closed

prosthetic valve

7 incision in left coronary sinus

anterior leaflet, mitral valve

8 left atrial wall

pericardial patch

9 anchoring sutures in left atrial wall and patch

10 aortotomy closed

11 The Konno method extends a vertical aortic incision into the anterior wall of the right ventricular outflow tract beneath the pulmonary valve (which is normally more cephalad than the aortic valve) and medial to the origin of the right coronary artery.

12 The aortic valve is excised. The aortic annulus and adjacent ventricular septum are incised 3 to 5 cm in line with the aortotomy. The incision in the septum does not transect the bundle of His.

13 The size of the aortic valvular prosthesis is chosen by placing the obturator in the annulus. Traction sutures are placed at both ends of the cut annulus.

14 A patch of woven Dacron is carefully measured and cut to cover the defect in the ventricular septum below the annulus and in the aortic wall above the annulus. With a double-ended 3-0 monofilament suture buttressed with a Teflon felt pledget, the apex of the patch is sutured to the apex of the septal incision.

15 The patch is sewn to the right ventricular surface of the septum. Generous bites of ventricular muscle (but usually not full thickness) are taken to securely anchor the patch to the muscle and separate the two ventricular cavities. Both ends are tied to single sutures placed between the patch and cut ends of the aortic annulus. These tied sutures are held and will be used later to sew the patch to the edges of the aortotomy.

16 The valve prosthesis is inserted with pledgeted 2-0 polyester mattress sutures. Sutures are passed through the Dacron patch with pledgets outside. The prosthesis must be securely anchored around its entire circumference to prevent paravalvular leak. The valve sutures are tied and cut.

17 A second patch of preclotted woven Dacron, pericardium, or other suitable prosthetic material, is cut to close the defect in the right ventricular outflow tract. A running 3-0 monofilament suture with a strip of Teflon felt is used to anchor this patch to the first patch at or slightly cephalad to the plane of the prosthesis. One of the retained sutures used to anchor the patch to the ventricular septum and cut edge of the annulus is used for this suture line. The suture is tied to its opposite at the other end of the Dacron patch.

18 The same suture is used to sew the patch to the cut edges of the right ventricular outflow tract. Usually full-thickness bites of ventricular muscle are taken. Air is evacuated from the right ventricle before this suture line is completed.

19 The aortotomy is closed using the retained 3-0 monofilament sutures used to tie the septal patch to the cut edges of the aortic annulus. Air is evacuated from the left heart and aortic root before this suture line is tied. Suture line leaks are closed with simple, pledgeted mattress or figure-of-eight sutures.

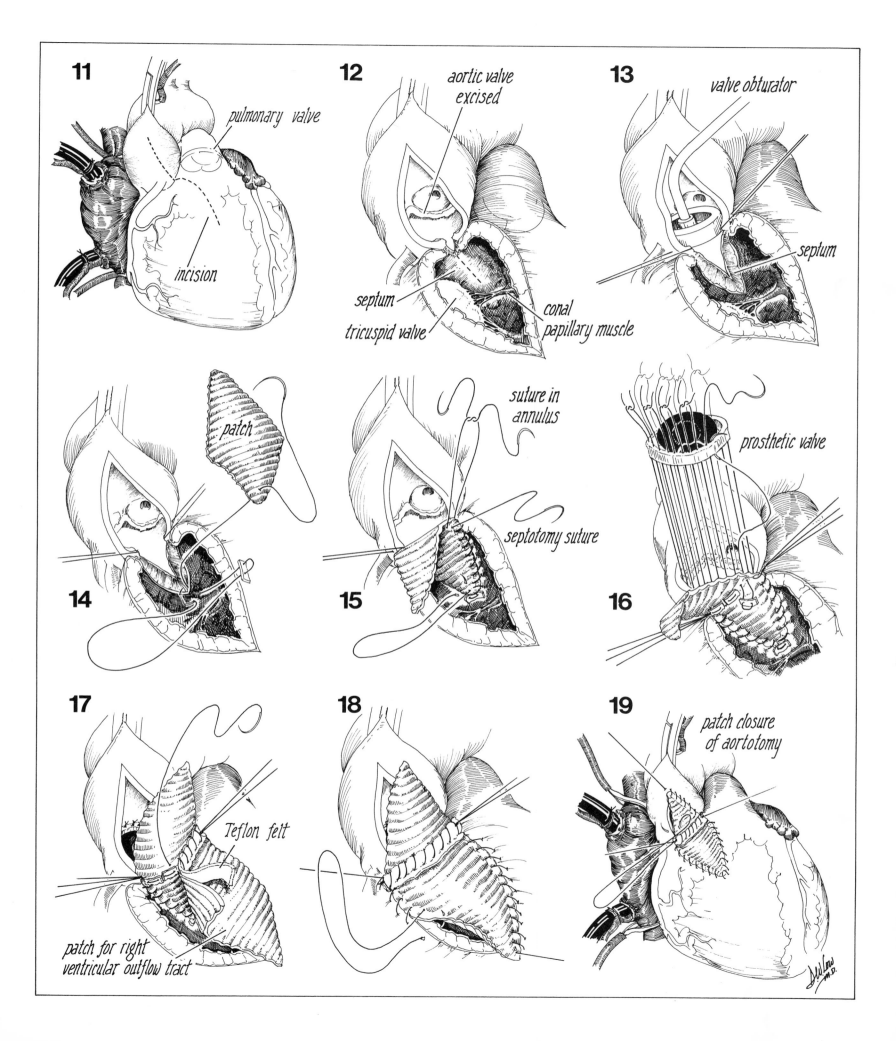

Left Ventricular-Aortic Conduit

This is an uncommon operation, useful in patients with severe calcific aortic stenosis associated with extensive calcification of the ascending aorta.

1 The midline sternotomy incision is extended inferiorly to just above the umbilicus. The abdomen and chest are opened. A femoral artery is prepared for cannulation and a purse-string suture is placed in the right atrium.

2 The left lobe of the liver is retracted toward the patient's right after the triangular ligament is incised. The upper abdominal esophagus and gastroesophageal junction are retracted to the patient's left. A 4 cm segment of the abdominal aorta upstream to the celiac artery is exposed as it passes through the diaphragm.

3 A side-biting vascular clamp is placed on the exposed segment. The aorta is opened longitudinally with knife and scissors.

4 A preclotted, commercially available, valved conduit is sutured end-to-side to the aortotomy. A porcine valve is preferred in adults, and the surgeon must be sure that the direction of the valve is correct. The valve is positioned so that it is nearer the aorta than the left ventricular apex. The anastomosis is made with continuous 3 or 4-0 monofilament nonabsorbable suture.

5 Heparin is given and the patient is cannulated for bypass. A catheter is inserted through the junction of the right superior pulmonary vein and left atrium into the left atrium. Because the ascending aorta cannot be clamped safely, the heart is electrically fibrillated after cardiopulmonary bypass is started. The patient is cooled to 28° C. The apex of the left ventricle is lifted to expose the bare area lateral to the left anterior descending coronary artery and inferior to any large diagonal branches. The area of diaphragm directly adjacent to the left ventricular apex (and exit site of the conduit) is marked by a stitch.

6 An ordinary laboratory cork borer of appropriate size is used to cut a circular hole in the apex of the left ventricular. The hole should be inferior to the papillary muscle of the mitral valve and should not injure the ventricular septum. The core of excised myocardium is removed.

7 The cuffed ventricular end of the conduit is sutured to the ventricular wall with interrupted pledgeted mattress sutures of 0 gauge polyester material. The sutures are passed outside in around the circumference of the ventriculotomy and through the sewing ring of the conduit. All sutures are placed before any are tied.

Before tying the final sutures, all air is expressed from the left ventricle by stopping the left atrial vent and lifting the apex of the heart during a gentle Valsalva maneuver.

The interrupted suture line is reinforced with a continuous suture of 2-0 monofilament material to ensure complete hemostasis.

8 A small portion of diaphragm is excised with cautery at the previously marked site. The ventricular portion of the conduit is brought through the diaphragmatic hole as the heart is replaced in the pericardium. Rewarming may begin and the heart is defibrillated at this time. The two ends of the conduit are trimmed at a convenient place for anastomosis.

9 The trimmed ends of woven Dacron are anastomosed with a 3-0 monofilament continuous suture. Before this is tied, air is expressed out of both ends of the conduit. When clamps are removed, tacking sutures are placed between conduit and diaphragm to prevent herniation of abdominal contents.

When rewarming is completed, bypass is discontinued and cannulas are removed. The abdomen is not drained. Routine mediastinal drains are placed in the chest. The incision is closed with continous sutures.

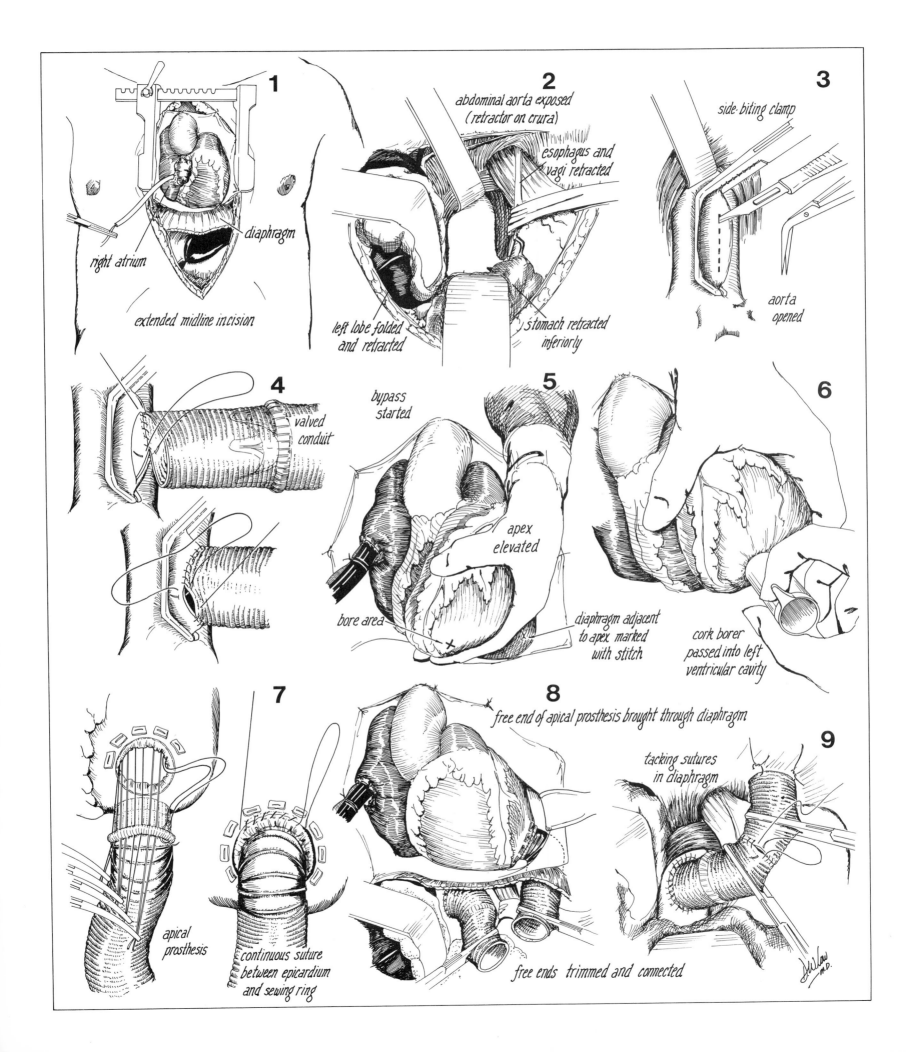

1
right atrium
diaphragm
extended midline incision

2
abdominal aorta exposed
(retractor on crura)
esophagus and
vagi retracted
left lobe folded
and retracted
stomach retracted
inferiorly

3
side-biting clamp
aorta
opened

4
valved
conduit

5
bypass
started
apex
elevated
bore area
diaphragm adjacent
to apex marked
with stitch

6
cork borer
passed into left
ventricular cavity

7
apical
prosthesis
continuous suture
between epicardium
and sewing ring

8
free end of apical prosthesis brought through diaphragm
free ends trimmed and connected

9
tacking sutures
in diaphragm

Simultaneous Replacement Aortic Prosthesis and Mitral Valve

The operation illustrated and described here is for a patient with a defective aortic valvular prosthesis. Reoperation is carried out through a median sternotomy.

1 The aorta, cavae, and entire heart are dissected free of all adhesions to ensure uniform and adequate cooling during cardioplegia and to facilitate exposure. After heparin, the ascending aorta is cannulated and *both* cavae are cannulated separately by means of purse-string sutures in the right atrium near the atrial-caval junctions. The patient is cooled to 26 to 28° C on bypass. A small incision is made in the left atrium at its junction with the right superior pulmonary vein to decompress the heart. As the ascending aorta is clamped, the heart is emptied by inserting a suction catheter into the left atrium and/or left ventricle.

2 The dissection of the aortic root should be completed to expose the previous downstream suture line. The aorta is opened through the previous incision or one nearby to expose the malfunctioning or infected prosthesis. Cold cardioplegic solution is injected directly into both coronary ostia through Spencer-Malette catheters, and the heart is submerged in cold saline to obtain cardiac arrest.

3 The valve is carefully inspected and any friable, loose material is removed. Cultures are obtained. The prosthesis is removed by incising the scar tissue covering the sewing ring circumferentially around the entire valve. A sharp hook is driven into the sewing ring adjacent to the noncoronary sinus of Valsalva. With a No. 15 scalpel blade (several changes will be needed), the plane between the outer portion of the sewing ring and the valve annulus is identified and deepened until the knife slips into the left ventricular outflow tract beneath the sewing ring. The knife is angled toward the center of the outflow tract away from the fibrous trigone and anterior mitral leaflet at all times. The surgeon works around the circumference of the prosthesis and carefully separates the sewing ring and annulus by sharp dissection as different sections of the sewing ring are retracted in turn.

After the valve is removed, the annulus, outflow tract, and aortic root are carefully inspected for abscesses, injuries, potential embolic material, or strands of scar tissue that may interfere with the new prosthesis. Abscesses are thoroughly debrided of necrotic material and obliterated if possible by approximating adjacent wall. Any tears, incisions, or abscesses that detach the annulus from the aorta or left ventricular outflow tract are repaired before the annulus is sized. If the mitral valve is beyond repair and replacement prescribed before the valve is exposed, chordal attachments to the anterior leaflet of the mitral valve are conveniently cut by way of the aortic root after the aortic prosthesis is removed.

5 The small incision in the left atrium is enlarged posterior to the interatrial septum to expose the diseased mitral valve. This valve is excised as described previously.

6 The mitral prosthesis is sized, selected, and sutured to the mitral annulus before the aortic prosthesis is inserted.

7 The left atriotomy is closed, preferably with two running sutures before the aortic valve is inserted. A Foley catheter is placed across the mitral prosthesis to prevent valve closure and to aspirate the left ventricle before the atrial suture line is completed. The atrial sutures are not tied at this time.

8 The aortic prosthesis is inserted, usually with pledgeted interrupted 2-0 polyester mattress sutures passed firmly through the annulus and adjacent scar. Coronary ostia are checked to ensure that the new prosthesis does not interfere with coronary blood flow. The prosthesis is placed as closely as possible against the scarred annulus.

9 The aortotomy is closed with a double suture line of 3-0 monofilament with or without strips of Teflon felt. Before this suture line is tied, all air is carefully and thoroughly removed from the heart and ascending aorta. After removal of the aortic clamp, cardiac contractions are restarted. The catheter across the mitral prosthesis is not removed until strong reliable cardiac contractions return. The left atrial sutures are not tied until bypass is stopped and it is clear that the heart can maintain an adequate circulation. During this period, the atrial sutures are held firmly to prevent bleeding and entrance of air into the left atrium.

During the period of aortic crossclamping, cold blood or crystalloid cardioplegic solution is injected into both coronary ostia and the heart is bathed in cold saline every 20 minutes to prevent myocardial ischemia. Septal temperature is often monitored; a cooling pad is often used.

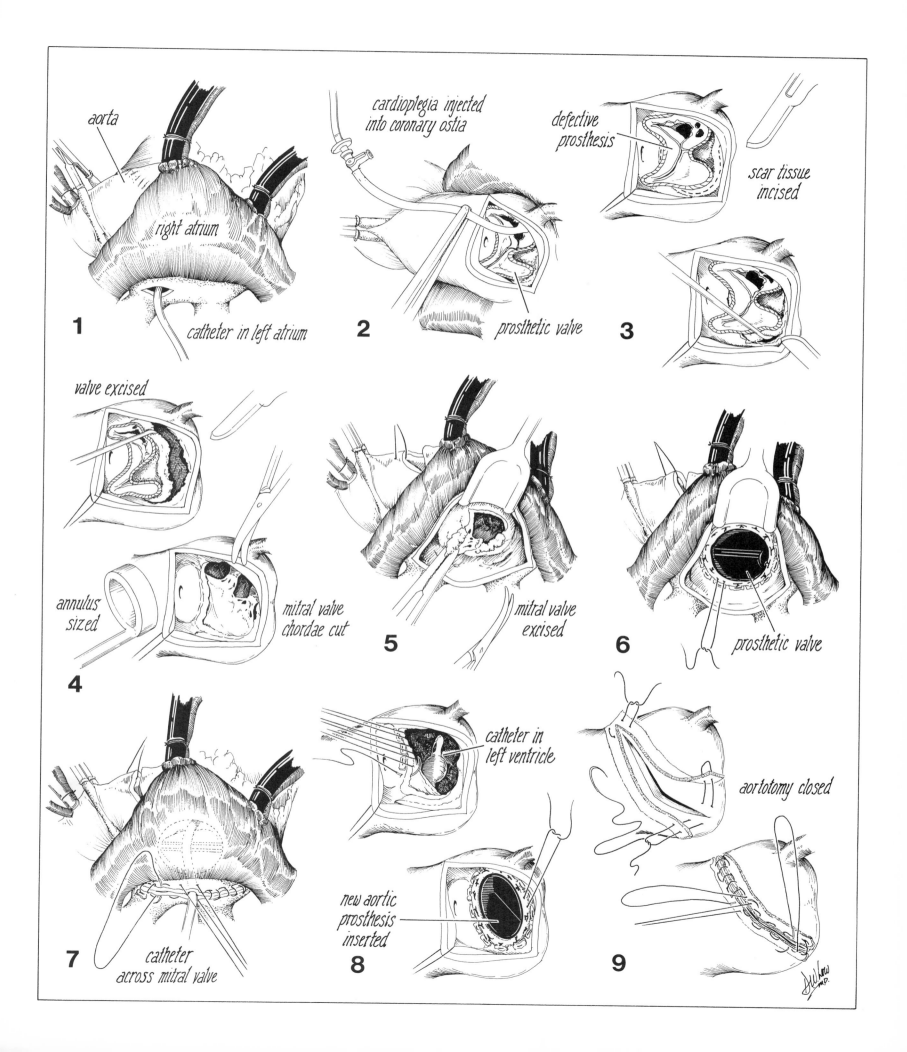

1 aorta / right atrium / catheter in left atrium

2 cardioplegia injected into coronary ostia / prosthetic valve

3 defective prosthesis / scar tissue incised

4 valve excised / annulus sized / mitral valve chordae cut

5 mitral valve excised

6 prosthetic valve

7 catheter across mitral valve

8 catheter in left ventricle / new aortic prosthesis inserted

9 aortotomy closed

Combinations

MITRAL VALVE REPLACEMENT, TRICUSPID ANNULOPLASTY

The heart is usually exposed by means of a median sternotomy, but the operation can also be done from a right thoracotomy. The aorta and both cavae are cannulated. Slings are required around both cavae to produce a dry right atrium. Aortic clamping and cold cardioplegia are used.

(1) The mitral valve is usually exposed through a lateral left atriotomy placed posterior to the interatrial septum. The tricuspid valve is exposed through a separate incision in the right atrium.

(2) Alternatively, the mitral valve may be exposed through a right atriotomy and an incision in the interatrial septum. Retraction sutures in the lip of the incised septum anteriorly are useful for exposure during insertion of the mitral prosthesis, which is performed as described previously.

(3) After the mitral prosthesis is tied down, a Foley catheter is placed through the prosthesis to keep it incompetent and prevent distension of the left ventricle. If a bioprosthesis is used in the mitral position, a second hole is cut in the Foley catheter to permit blood to exit the ventricle through the catheter into the atrium. Without this hole, leaflets of the bioprosthesis may not be rendered incompetent by the presence of the catheter.

(4) The interatrial septum or left atriotomy is closed but not tied until the tricuspid annuloplasty is completed and all air is evacuated from the left heart. The tricuspid annuloplasty may be performed by any of the techniques illustrated previously.

(5) The right atriotomy is closed and air is evacuated from the right atrium by releasing the caval tourniquets and partially occluding the venous line. The right atrial sutures are tied. After all air is removed from the left atrium, ventricle, and aortic root, the aortic cross-clamp is released. The ascending aorta is vented with a No. 19 needle. After cardiac contractions return, the Foley catheter is removed. The left atrial sutures are held until bypass is successfully stopped and the heart has taken over the circulation.

TRIPLE VALVE REPLACEMENT

The ascending aorta is cannulated, and both cavae are cannulated through the right atrium. Caval tourniquets are used. After initiating bypass and hypothermia to 26 to 28° C, the heart is arrested by aortic root or direct coronary ostial injection of cold cardioplegia. An incision in the left atrium and insertion of a suction catheter into the left atrium or ventricle facilitate exposure.

(6) The aortic valve is excised and sized first, and mitral chordae are cut by way of the aortic root.

(7) The mitral valve is exposed, usually by a left atriotomy posterior to the interatrial septum. The valve is excised, sized, and replaced. A Foley catheter is placed through the valve. The left atrium is closed but not tied.

(8) The aortic prosthesis is inserted next. The aortotomy is closed after the prosthesis is inserted. Air is evacuated from the left heart and aortic root through the aortic suture line before it is tied. The aortic crossclamp is not removed at this time. After closure of the aorta, cardioplegic solution is injected into the aortic root through a No. 14 angiocatheter. Rewarming is usually started after the aortotomy is closed.

(9) The tricuspid valve is excised and replaced, using pledgeted interrupted sutures along the septal annulus. Continuous sutures may be used for the remainder of the valve if desired. The right atrium is closed immediately and tied after air is evacuated from the right atrium and ventricle.

(10) The cardioplegic catheter is used to vent the ascending aorta as the aortic cross-clamp is removed. Before the clamp is removed, maneuvers to remove all air from the left heart and aortic root are repeated and gentle suction is applied to the angiocatheter as the aortic clamp is released. The Foley catheter through the mitral prosthesis is removed after reliable cardiac contractions return. The left atrial sutures are tied after bypass is stopped.

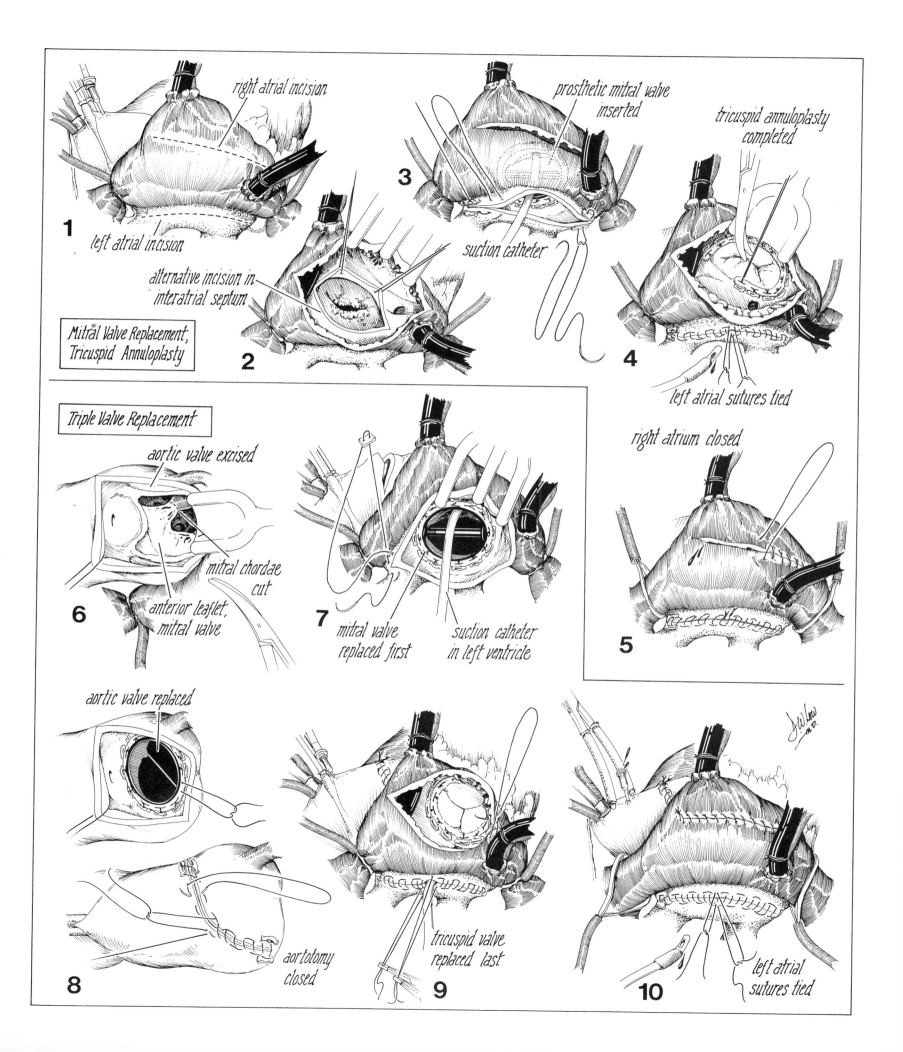

1 right atrial incision

left atrial incision

Mitral Valve Replacement, Tricuspid Annuloplasty

2 alternative incision in interatrial septum

3 prosthetic mitral valve inserted

suction catheter

tricuspid annuloplasty completed

4 left atrial sutures tied

5 right atrium closed

Triple Valve Replacement

6 aortic valve excised

mitral chordae cut

anterior leaflet, mitral valve

7 mitral valve replaced first

suction catheter in left ventricle

8 aortic valve replaced

aortotomy closed

9 tricuspid valve replaced last

10 left atrial sutures tied

Valve Replacement and Coronary Revascularization

1 The heart is exposed through a midline sternotomy and usually two caval catheters are placed. If the aortic valve is insufficient, cardioplegia is achieved by direct injection into both coronary ostia from the aortotomy. The left atrium is opened at the right superior pulmonary vein–left atrial junction to decompress the ventricle. With the heart arrested, vein segments are anastomosed to the obstructed coronary arteries. When this is completed, cardioplegic solution can be injected into the grafts as well as the native coronary vessels to ensure myocardial preservation.

2 The diseased aortic valve is excised and the annulus is sized.

3 The left atrium is opened wide by an incision posterior to the interatrial septum. The mitral valve is excised and is replaced first. After the valve is tied down, a catheter is left through the valve into the left ventricle. The left atrium is closed, but the sutures are not tied until after the heart is contracting well.

4 The aortic prosthesis is inserted next. The aortotomy is closed after this prosthesis is inserted. Air is evacuated from the left heart and aortic root before the aortotomy sutures are tied. The aortic clamp is not released. Further doses of cardioplegic solution are given through a #14 angiocatheter inserted at the site of a planned proximal saphenous vein anastomosis.

5 The right atrium is opened and the right tricuspid valve is repaired as described elsewhere.

6 The right atrium is closed and, after evacuation of all air, the sutures are tied.

7 Maneuvers to remove all air from the left heart are repeated and the aortic cross-clamp is removed. Rewarming is started. A side-biting (Hunter, Satinsky, Beck) clamp is placed on the ascending aorta for construction of the proximal vein graft anastomoses. Before cardiac contractions begin, the left ventricle is kept decompressed by allowing blood to escape through the left atrial suture line. This suture line is kept under blood.

INTERNAL MAMMARY ARTERY GRAFTS

8 If either or both internal mammary arteries are preferred for revascularization, the anastomoses are made only to anterior coronary vessels (for example, distal right coronary, left anterior descending, diagonal arteries). Circumflex coronary arteries are revascularized using the vein *before* valve prostheses are inserted to avoid retraction injuries caused by the rigid valve prostheses.

9 After valves are inserted and the heart is closed (except for venting the left ventricle), the internal mammary artery anastomoses are made to the distal coronary arteries. Proximal vein anastomoses are made last. This sequence precludes the chance of injury to the internal mammary arterial pedicles, which may occur during insertion of valve prostheses.

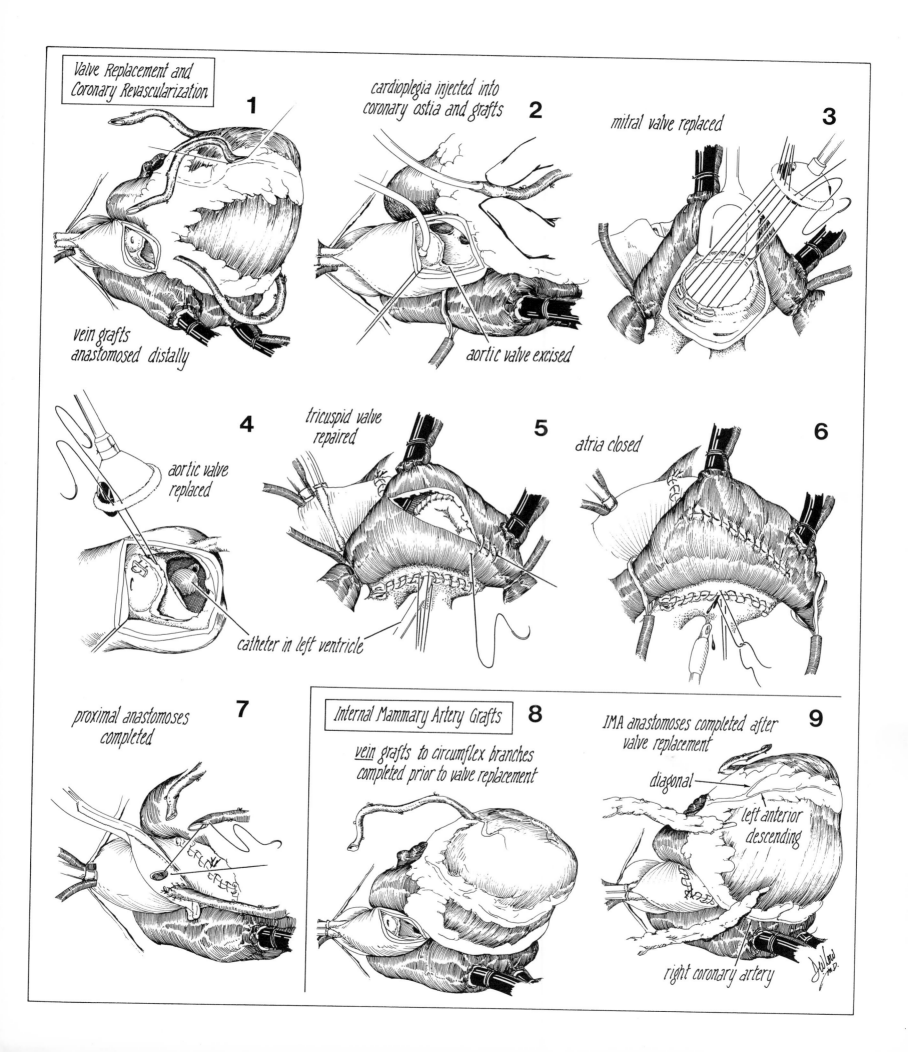

Valve Replacement and Coronary Revascularization

1 vein grafts anastomosed distally

2 cardioplegia injected into coronary ostia and grafts
aortic valve excised

3 mitral valve replaced

4 aortic valve replaced
catheter in left ventricle

5 tricuspid valve repaired

6 atria closed

7 proximal anastomoses completed

8 Internal Mammary Artery Grafts
vein grafts to circumflex branches completed prior to valve replacement

9 IMA anastomoses completed after valve replacement
diagonal
left anterior descending
right coronary artery

Excision Asymmetric Septal Hypertrophy

Asymmetric septal hypertrophy (ASH) is a form of hypertrophic cardiomyopathy characterized by localized hypertrophy of the ventricular septum. Hypertrophied, abnormally shaped, and bizarrely arranged muscle fibers in the ventricular septum obstruct the outflow of the left ventricle during systole. The anterior leaflet of the mitral valve may become thickened and mitral regurgitation may occur. Although relatively few individuals now require operation, refractory patients require surgical relief of the obstructing muscle mass. Myomectomy (Morrow operation) is recommended; replacement of the mitral valve is not recommended. The myomectomy carves a trough through the obstructing muscle mass and, if successful, reduces apical left ventricular pressure and relieves mitral insufficiency.

(1) The pathology is illustrated. The abnormal muscle mass may involve the entire septum and even parts of the ventricular free wall. The anterior leaflet of the mitral valve abuts against the abnormal septum to obstruct egress of blood from the ventricular cavity.

(2) The heart and aortic valve are exposed as for aortic valve replacement. The initial dose of cardioplegic solution can be injected into the aortic root; subsequent doses are given directly into the coronary arteries.

(3) The aortic valve leaflets are carefully retracted to observe the hypertrophied septal muscle mass that may or may not have a fibrous tissue component. The right coronary aortic leaflet is conveniently retracted by placing a 7-0 monofilament suture in the nodule of Arantii and suturing the leaflet against the adjacent aortic wall.

(4) The myomectomy consists of two parallel incisions approximately 2 cm deep and 1.5 to 2 cm apart. One incision is placed slightly counterclockwise and below the ostium of the right coronary artery, which is anterior, and at approximately 12 o'clock on a hypothetic clockface.

(5) The second incision is in the junction of septum and left ventricular free wall and is counterclockwise from the first incision and roughly below the commissure between the right and left coronary aortic valvular cusps. Incisions in this area of the septum divide the left bundle branch but do not cause heart block. The depth of the incisions is guided by echocardiographic estimates of the localized thickening. A No. 15 scalpel blade on a long handle is convenient; great care is taken not to injure the valve cusp at its attachment to the annulus at the sinus of Valsalva or the anterior papillary muscle of the mitral valve.

(6) The parallel incisions are connected just below the aorta annulus. Either a knife or scissors can be used to carve the intervening block of muscle out. Pressure on the anterior ventricular wall and septum facilitates this part of the block removal. Care must be exercised to avoid perforating the septum or inadequately resecting the localized hypertrophic muscle.

(7) When the muscle block is removed, a relatively wide and deep trough should be present between the body of the left ventricle and aortic valve. Bits and pieces of loose muscle strands are carefully debrided to prevent emboli. Nothing is done to the anterior mitral leaflet.

(8) The operation is completed by removal of valve retraction sutures, closure of the aorta, evacuation of air, stopping of bypass, and closure of the chest.

(9) The adequacy of the trough can be assessed by measuring left ventricular pressure (No. 20 spinal needle) passed across right ventricle and septum into the body of the left ventricle of bypass under different conditions of volume loading and isoproterenol infusion.

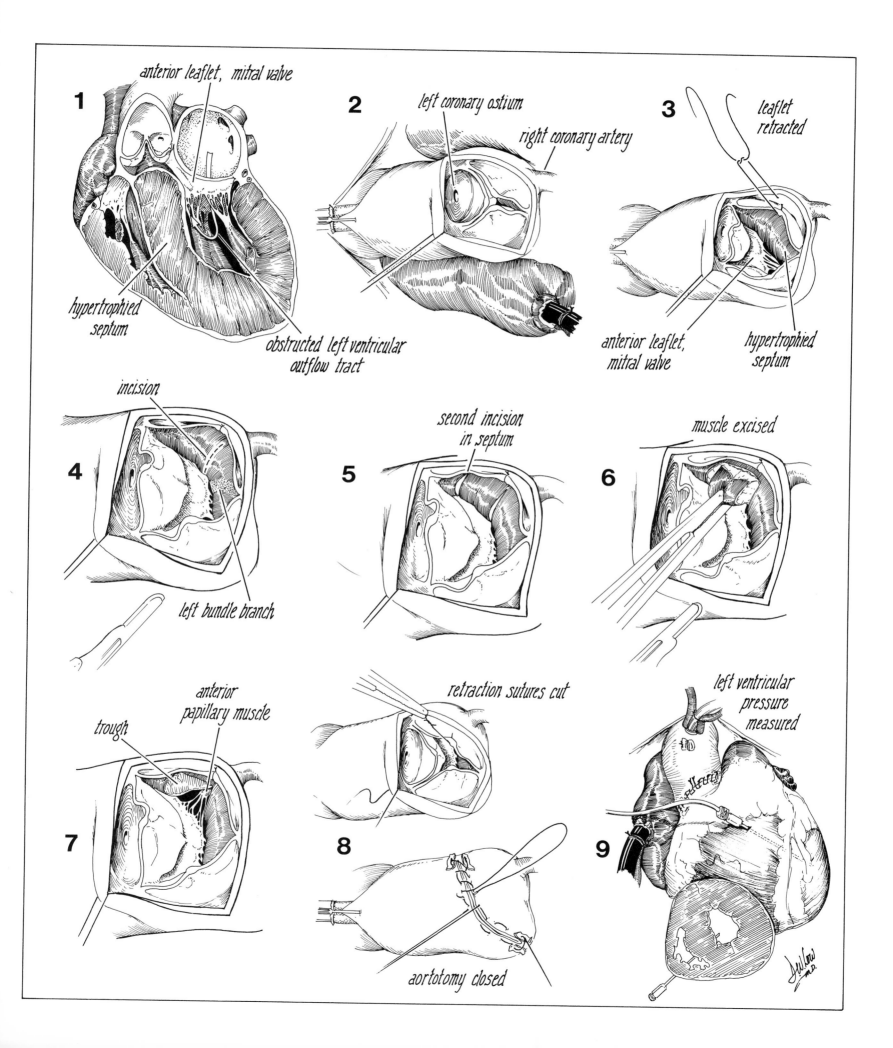

1 anterior leaflet, mitral valve

hypertrophied septum

obstructed left ventricular outflow tract

2 left coronary ostium

right coronary artery

3 leaflet retracted

anterior leaflet, mitral valve

hypertrophied septum

4 incision

left bundle branch

5 second incision in septum

6 muscle excised

7 trough

anterior papillary muscle

8 retraction sutures cut

aortotomy closed

9 left ventricular pressure measured

Myocardial Revascularization with Venous Segments

The greater saphenous vein is universally the preferred venous conduit for aortocoronary bypass grafts. When the vein is not available because of prior stripping or previous use, either the cephalic vein or the lesser saphenous vein may be used. In patients with large varicose veins or very large proximal saphenous veins, sometimes branches of the saphenous vein in the thigh may provide enough vein of suitable length for the construction of a graft. On rare occasions, a segment of varicose saphenous vein has been placed inside a 6 mm diameter polytetrafluoroethylene tube that constricts the vein diameter, prevents rupture, and still provides an endothelial cell-lined conduit. Cryopreserved venous allograft segments are also available.

1 Both legs are prepped with antiseptic solution from below the middle malleolus to above the groin circumferentially. The feet are wrapped in sterile stockinette and then placed on the sterile operating room table.

2 Alternatively, the legs can be placed in a frog-leg position supported by a pillow, with the feet taped together. In this position, just the medial portion of both legs can be prepped and covered with an adhesive sterile drape. The lesser saphenous veins are harvested from the frog-leg position, but the legs are prepped circumferentially and placed on a sterile pillow with the knees spread wide apart.

3 The greater saphenous vein is easily located at the ankle between the medial malleolus and the extensor hallucis longus. In most patients, the saphenous vein in the lower leg is sufficiently large in diameter to be used for aortocoronary saphenous bypass grafts. The incision can be made over the vein from the ankle upward (or slightly to one side to avoid injury to the vein if it is superficial). In most patients, it is convenient to use blunt dissection or a finger to separate the overlying skin and subcutaneous tissue from the plane of the vein. As the skin and subcutaneous tissue are lifted from the vein, the incision is progressively extended cephalad until the desired length of vein is exposed. This produces a long, continuous incision which is well tolerated but more unsightly than multiple short incisions of about 3 to 4 inches in length.

4 When multiple incisions are used, they are placed over the vein but separated by 3 to 4 inch bridges of intact skin. The exposed vein is dissected out from the surrounding structures including the saphenous nerve by a combination of blunt and sharp dissection. All branches are ligated with 5-0 or 3-0 polyester ligatures. It is convenient to clip the opposite end with small hemoclips before dividing the branch. When all branches have been ligated and divided, the vein is divided at the ankle. The distal (ankle) end of the vein is marked with a suture ligature. The marked vein is lifted out of the wound and divided at the opposite end. Suture ligatures are used to tie off the two in situ ends of the saphenous vein.

5 The harvested vein is injected gently with saline solution to slightly dilate the vein and to locate any untied branches or leaks. These are oversewn with 6-0 or 7-0 monofilament figure-of-eight sutures. The harvested vein is placed in saline to await use. The cautery and appropriate hemoclips, ligatures, and suture ligatures are used to achieve complete hemostasis in the leg. Occasionally, a hemovac catheter is placed in a fat thigh to prevent hematoma. Running 3-0 absorbable sutures are used to close the leg wound or wounds. The tissue should be reapproximated carefully to avoid dead space within the wound. The skin is usually closed with a subcuticular stitch of 4-0 absorbable suture. Occasionally, skin clips are used.

6 The cephalic vein is harvested by prepping one or both arms from the shoulder, neck, and upper chest to the forearm. A sterile stockinette is used to cover the unprepped hand and wrist. This vein runs from the lateral area of the antecubital space cephalad in the delto-pectoral groove to approximately the junction between the outer and middle thirds of the clavicle. After the vein is located in the antecubital space, it is followed proximally by dividing the skin and overlying subcutaneous tissue with either a continuous long incision or multiple short incisions. The exposed vein is harvested by ligating all branches and by marking the distal end with a suture. The cephalic vein is generally more thin-walled than the greater saphenous vein and therefore somewhat more difficult to handle.

7 The lesser saphenous vein is rarely used, but is occasionally the only vein available. This vein is posterior and runs with the sural nerve in the lower third of the leg. An incision slightly lateral to the Achilles tendon and placed about two or three inches above the lateral malleolus is used to locate the vein. Once located, a continuous incision is used to expose the vein up to the popliteal space, where it runs with the posterior cutaneous nerve of the thigh. The lesser saphenous vein usually has many branches that must be ligated and divided. The lower portion of this vein may be too small in some patients, but usually enough vein is available for one or two grafts.

8 The heart is exposed through a midline sternotomy incision, and the divided pericardial edges are tacked to the edges of the incision. The patient is cannulated, placed on cardiopulmonary bypass, and generally cooled to a nasopharyngeal temperature of 26 to 34° C. The degree of cooling is directly proportional to the estimated time of aortic crossclamping. After starting bypass, cold saline with saline slush is poured into the pericardial cavity and the heart manipulated until a ventricular fibrillation occurs. At that moment, the aorta is clamped and cold cardioplegia is infused through a No. 14 plastic catheter inserted at one of the planned graft sites on the proximal aorta.

9 The heart should not become distended during the period when cardioplegic solution is infused. If dilatation occurs, the junction of the right superior pulmonary vein and left atrium is incised, and a No. 18 Ferguson catheter is inserted past the mitral valve to decompress the left ventricle. Alternatively, the catheter may be inserted into the main pulmonary artery to decompress the left heart. The latter method reduces the risk of air embolism.

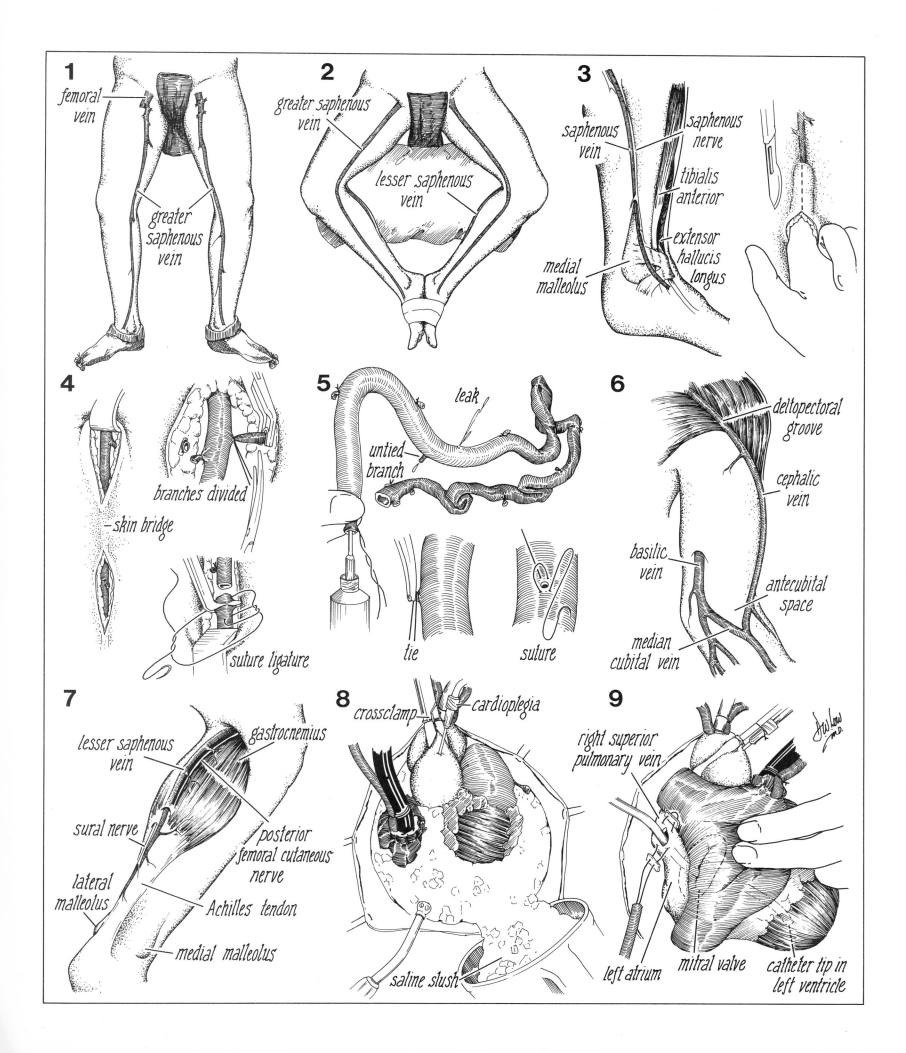

The heart is kept cold by periodic reinfusion of cold cardioplegic solution into the aortic root and reapplication of cold saline slush around the heart. A myocardial temperature probe is used to monitor septal temperature continuously. This probe is inserted after arrest rightward of the left anterior descending coronary artery at the junction of the right ventricle and septum. It enters the ventricular septum and generally stays in place without sutures. Cardioplegic solution is renewed every 20 minutes or when septal temperature rises above 18° C. Usually 200 to 300 ml of cardioplegic solution is used for each renewal.

With the heart arrested, the coronary arteries are inspected. For this part of the operation, both surgeon and assistant need 2.5 to 3.5 power magnification loupes. The target vessels for bypass are positively identified, and any sizeable vessels that are not seen on the angiogram but may perfuse viable myocardium are also identified. The surgeon determines the proposed sites of anastomoses and the arrangement of the various bypass grafts. In general, we prefer three separate grafts for five or more distal anastomoses, two or three separate grafts for two to four distal anastomoses, and a single sequential graft for two distal anastomoses that are near each other.

(10) The order of distal graft construction is not important. The target distal vessel is incised using a Beaver or a No. 11 knife blade. The arteriotomy is extended to a distance of 5 to 6 mm with Potts scissors. If back-bleeding from the coronary vessel occurs, it may be occluded by a small bulldog clamp placed across the proximal vessel. Small retraction sutures in the adjacent myocardial fat may facilitate exposure of the coronary arteriotomy.

(11) The anastomosis is done with either 6-0 or 7-0 monofilament suture. A continuous anastomosis is almost always used except in unusual circumstances. The segment of saphenous vein is cut straight across rather than beveled. The anastomotic diameter may be enlarged by a small incision in the heel of the transected vein.

Sometimes the anastomosis begins at the heel. The needle is passed from outside the vein to inside, and then from inside to outside the proximal portion of the coronary artery. A keeper is placed on this suture and, using the opposite end, a similar stitch is placed through the vein from outside in and through the artery from inside out. When pulled up, this stitch approximates the apex of the venotomy to the proximal apex of the coronary arteriotomy.

(12) The anastomosis is completed by continuous over-and-over sutures. The sutures pass from intima to adventitia through the artery to avoid raising any atheromatous material. Fine bites are placed near the distal (downstream) apex of the arteriotomy to avoid constriction of the vessel. After passing the apex, this suture is held while the opposite suture is used to complete the anastomosis. The two ends are tied with six knots. The anastomosis is tested for leaks by injecting saline or blood. Leaks are repaired with fine simple or mattress sutures.

(13) Preferably, the anastomosis starts at the toe. This method has the advantage of minimizing any constriction of the distal native coronary artery. A mattress suture that starts at the toe of the vein is run towards the heel for four sutures. This suture is held and the opposite suture is passed outside in through the vein and inside out through the artery at the apex, and then run down the opposite side for four sutures.

(14) The vein is drawn over the toe of the anastomosis to expose an open triangle of vein and an open triangle of artery. With this exposure, the suture is continued around the proximal apex of the arteriotomy to the first suture. The two sutures are pulled up and tied.

SIDE-TO-SIDE ANASTOMOSIS

(15) Side-to-side anastomoses are used in the construction of sequential bypass grafts. A longitudinal arteriotomy is usually made, definitely if the diameter of the vein is small (<3.5 mm). A 4.0 to 5.0 mm arteriotomy is made. If the diameter of the vein is larger, a 6 mm arteriotomy is used. The incision in the vein is made after first laying the distended vein graft over the arteriotomy. Care is taken to ensure that the distal anastomosis and the vein are not kinked or twisted. The venotomy may be made parallel to or perpendicular to the direction of the arteriotomy. A parallel venotomy is preferred because the vein is not pulled down into the anastomosis to produce indentation of the anterior wall.

(16) The incised vein is twisted 180 degrees so that the arteriotomy and venotomy face each other like pages in a book. With 7-0 monofilament suture, the anastomosis is begun by passing the suture outside in through the vein and then inside out through the artery at the proximal apex of the arteriotomy incision. The suture is started at either the upstream or downstream apex of the arteriotomy as determined by how the vein is twisted. The needle passes outside in through that part of the venotomy incision opposite the arterial suture without concern or reference to the apices of the venotomy incision. The suture is continued in this fashion for three or four stitches on the vessel walls nearest the distal end-to-side anastomosis. This suture is held and the other end is passed through the vein outside in, and then through the opposite wall of the artery near the starting arterial apex. This suture is then continued around the vein and arterial edges past the opposite apex of the arteriotomy, to be tied to the first suture. It is important that the venotomy and arteriotomy not be so long as to flatten or indent the vein graft at the side-to-side anastomosis. Therefore, the incision generally used in both vein and artery is shorter for side-to-side anastomosis than for end-to-side anastomoses. In setting up the side-to-side anastomosis, the surgeon should position the "back of the book" away from himself and sew toward himself, gradually bringing the two vessels into opposition. Before tying the suture, he places a bulldog clamp on the segment of vein between the side-to-side and distal anastomoses and injects the graft with saline to remove air prior to tying down the suture. The anastomosis is checked for leaks before moving to the next anastomosis.

(17) The proximal anastomosis in the ascending aorta is made during the period of rewarming after releasing the aortic crossclamp. If the left atrium has been opened to decompress the heart, it is imperative that steps be taken to remove all possible air from within the heart before releasing the aortic crossclamp (see Air Maneuvers, this section). After the aortic crossclamp is removed, a side-biting clamp is placed on the anterior surface of the ascending aorta for the construction of the proximal anastomoses. The heart is defibrillated, electrically if necessary, as soon as possible to avoid the detrimental effects of prolonged ventricular defibrillation.

(18) With the side-biting clamp in place, one to three 3 mm incisions are made in the ascending aorta with a No. 11 blade. A 4.8 mm aortic punch (occasionally a 4.0 mm punch is needed) is used to make precise holes in the anterior wall of the ascending aorta. With the heart slightly distended by partial occlusion of the venous line, the length of the vein graft is carefully measured and trimmed for the proximal anastomosis. The vein graft is injected with blood or saline for this measurement and care is taken to ensure that the vein is not twisted or kinked. The proximal end of the vein is incised 2 to 6 mm at the heel to "fishmouth" the opening. The anastomosis is made with 6-0 monofilament suture.

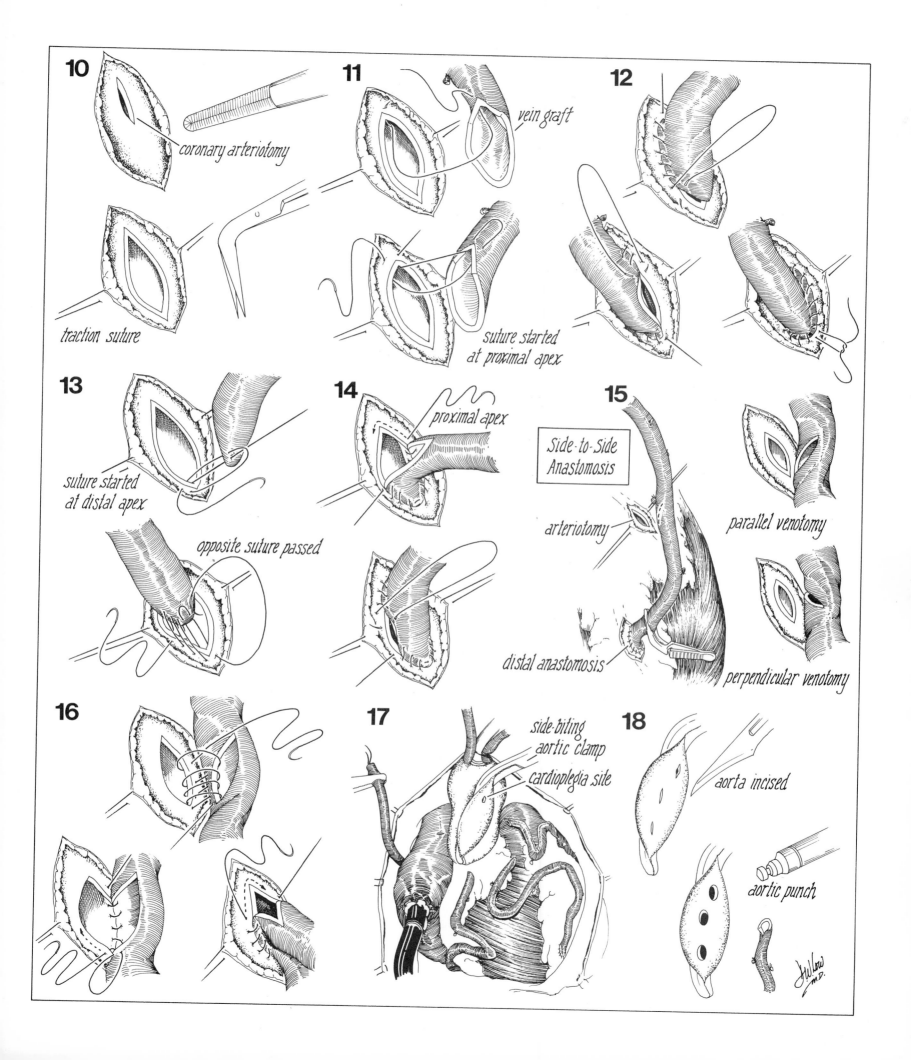

(19) Just as with the distal coronary anastomoses, various techniques can be used for the construction of the proximal anastomoses. We usually start the anastomosis by passing the suture outside in through the vein at the apex or heel of the venotomy. The suture is then passed inside out through the aorta and again outside in through the vein on the other side of the apex. When the suture is again passed inside out through the aorta, the vein is pulled down to the aorta. The assistant grasps the vein about 1.5 cm from the tip with forceps in one hand and the standing suture in the other. The surgeon aligns the edge of the vein closest to him, and proceeds with a continuous anastomosis, passing the needle from the outside of the vein through to the inside of the aorta until about two-thirds of the circumference is completed.

(20) The process is repeated using the opposite needle. The two ends are tied with six knots. A medium hemoclip is attached to the completed tie and secured with additional knots. The clip, which is visible on x-ray, marks the site of the proximal anastomosis. All the proximal anastomoses are completed before the side-biting clamp is removed. Before removal of the side-biting clamp, a bulldog clamp is placed on each vein graft to trap any air that might be present in the aorta or proximal grafts. The air is removed after the side-biting clamp is removed by inserting a 25 gauge needle into the vein graft and massaging the air out through the small needle hole. The bulldog clamps are removed after each graft is rendered air-free. Before stopping cardiopulmonary bypass, the distal anastomoses and veins are inspected for leaks.

(21) The order of construction of the distal anastomoses is not critical. Exposure of the left anterior descending and diagonal branches is facilitated by placing one or two wet lap pads behind the heart to elevate the heart and rotate it slightly towards the operator who stands on the patient's right side.

Troublesome leaks at the proximal anastomosis are conveniently controlled with one or more mattress sutures of 6-0 monofilament using a 1 x 3 mm wide pledget of vein. When tied, the vein pledget controls the leak without compromising the ostium of the anastomosis.

(22) To view the circumflex vessels and the obtuse margin and posterior surface of the heart, the apex of the heart must be lifted after the patient has been rotated toward the right. It is helpful to bring the venous line cephalad to prevent potential kinking of the line and obstruction of venous return when the heart is held up. An assistant standing toward the surgeon's left may be used to hold the heart up while the circumflex anastomoses are constructed. When the heart is held in this way, the circumflex anastomoses can easily be made with the surgeon standing on either the patient's left or right.

(23) For exposure of the posterior descending coronary artery and distal right coronary artery, the apex of the heart need not be dislocated. Usually a lap pad behind the heart is helpful in elevating it. Heavy polyester stay sutures passed through a plastic button can be used to retract the acute margin of the heart cephalad to provide good exposure of the posterior descending and distal right coronary vessels. Alternatively, the heart can be held.

(24) A wide number of variations can be used in the construction of saphenous vein bypass grafts. Single and sequential grafts have been described. Because of the large diameter of the vein, the proximal ends of only one vein graft need be anastomosed to the ascending aorta. The proximal ends of other grafts can then be sewn end-to-side to the primary vein graft to form "Y" anastomoses. This may be necessary if the ascending aorta is heavily calcified or contains soft atheromatous material, or is otherwise unavailable for multiple proximal anastomoses. In unusual circumstances, the proximal portion of the innominate artery can be used for the proximal anastomosis if the ascending aorta is not suitable.

(25) Coronary artery bypass vein grafts can also be made by construction of the proximal anastomoses first. This technique shortens the period of bypass because the proximal anastomoses can usually be constructed before starting bypass. Moreover, this technique facilitates the distribution of cold cardioplegic solution, because each obstructed coronary artery is perfused after construction of each anastomosis.

After placement of the bypass cannulas, a side-biting clamp is placed on the ascending aorta, and one to three holes are made in the ascending aorta. The harvested vein is cut into segments, and each segment is anastomosed to the ascending aorta as described for the proximal anastomosis. After completion of the proximal anastomoses, the side-biting clamp is removed, leaks are repaired, and cardiopulmonary bypass is started. The patient is cooled to an appropriate temperature, the heart is fibrillated, the aorta is crossclamped, and the heart is arrested with cold cardioplegic solution and external cold saline. When proximal anastomoses are done first, the cardioplegic solution should be delivered through a "Y" catheter with one limb attached to the cardioplegic solution system and the other to gravity drainage.

With the heart arrested, the sites for arteriotomy in the distal vessels are identified and the revascularization pattern is determined. The surgeon proceeds from the proximal anastomosis at the aorta to the final distal anastomosis of the graft. Thus in the construction of a sequential vein graft, the side-to-side anastomoses are completed before the distal end-to-side anastomosis is made. With the heart moderately distended by partial venous occlusion, the site of the venotomy is determined for the first anastomosis. Care is taken to determine that the vein graft is not obstructed or kinked.

(26) After the anastomosis is completed but before it is tied, the bulldog clamp on the vein graft is removed and cardioplegic solution is started to flush all air out of the graft. The anastomosis is tied. Either a full dose of cardioplegic solution with external cold saline is administered, or the bulldog clamp is replaced just distal to the completed anastomosis and a second anastomosis is made.

(27) In this fashion, all of the anastomoses are completed, working from the proximal anastomosis to the distal end-to-side anastomosis.

The disadvantage of doing the proximal anastomoses first is that rewarming is started before the last two distal anastomoses are completed. Furthermore, the surgeon has less leeway in adjusting to changes in sites of distal anastomoses if the proposed site is found unsuitable. There is more difficulty in determining the length of vein segments between anastomotic sites. These disadvantages, however, are easily overcome by surgeons who routinely construct proximal anastomoses first, and who are able to orchestrate the operation smoothly.

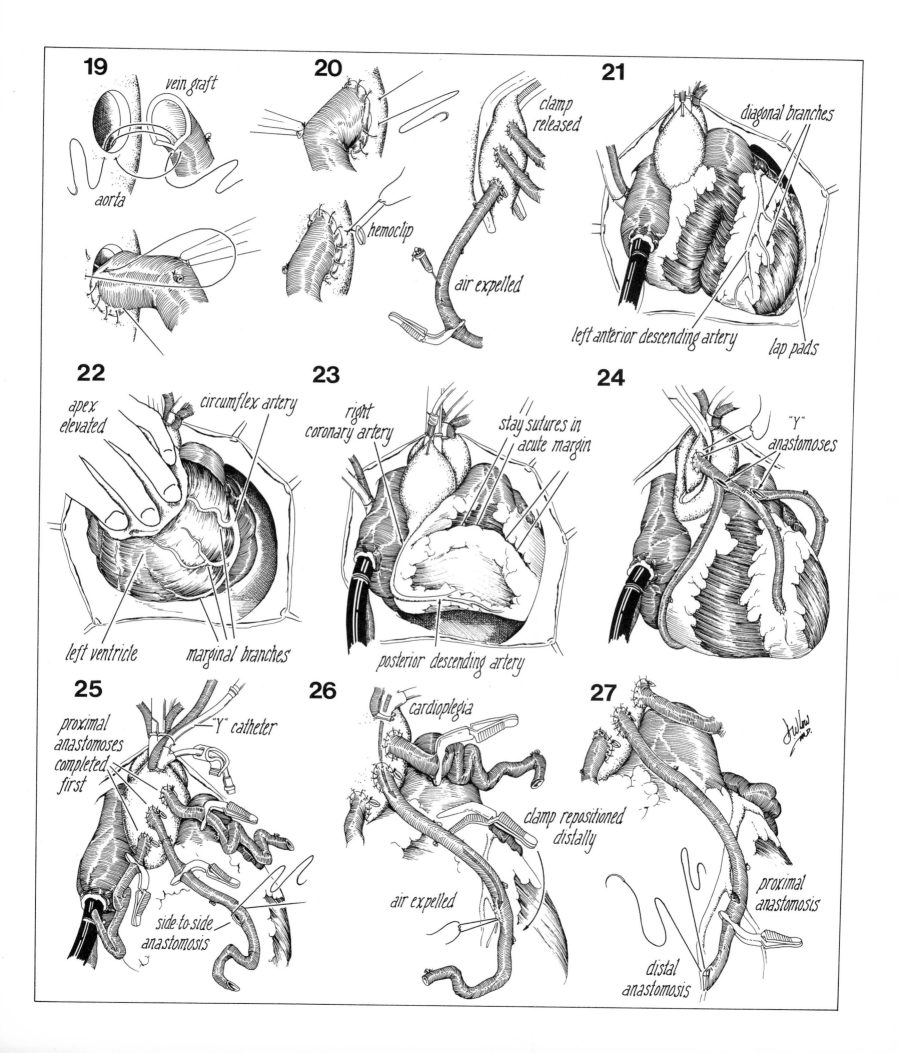

19

vein graft

aorta

20

hemoclip

clamp released

air expelled

21

diagonal branches

left anterior descending artery

lap pads

22

apex elevated

circumflex artery

left ventricle

marginal branches

23

right coronary artery

stay sutures in acute margin

posterior descending artery

24

"Y" anastomoses

25

proximal anastomoses completed first

"Y" catheter

side-to-side anastomosis

26

cardioplegia

clamp repositioned distally

air expelled

27

proximal anastomosis

distal anastomosis

Myocardial Revascularization with Internal Mammary Arteries

The left, right, and both internal mammary arteries may be anastomosed to obstructed coronary arteries.

1 The pedicled right internal mammary artery reaches the right coronary artery at the acute cardiac margin, the proximal half of the left anterior descending, or a high diagonal branch. The left internal mammary artery reaches most of the left anterior descending coronary artery, the diagonal vessels, and the proximal segments of circumflex marginal vessels. The length of the pedicled internal mammary artery is roughly proportional to the length of the sternum from notch to xiphoid.

2 If the right internal mammary artery is passed behind the aorta through the transverse sinus, it reaches a high circumflex marginal vessel.

3 A long midline sternotomy incision is made to open the chest wide. The chest wall on the side of the internal mammary artery to be taken (left for this description) is retracted upward using Favaloro retractors. The table is raised and rotated away from the operator so that the anterior chest is approximately at the level of the surgeon's shoulders. Binocular loupes facilitate the dissection. The left parietal pleura is bluntly stripped away from the underside of the chest wall. Sometimes it is punctured, and if so, the puncture site is extended the full length of the internal mammary artery. Two parallel incisions are made in the endothoracic fascia on each side of the internal mammary artery and vein. Dissection begins at approximately the midpoint of the artery on the undersurface of a rib. The artery, vein, and surrounding fat are gently separated from the rib with forceps and the unactivated cautery blade. The cautery blade is used both without current as a dissecting instrument and with coagulation (noncutting) current.

4 After separating both artery and vein from the rib, the dissection proceeds in both directions. Intercostal branches are carefully dissected out, clipped (if relatively large), or cauterized and divided. No loops or ties are passed around the pedicle. The dissection continues from the first rib to the caudal end of the sternum. Often the artery bifurcates near the end of the sternum. The larger branch is dissected free; if both are small, the dissection ends at the bifurcation. The pedicle is not divided until heparin has been given.

Bleeding from the distal end of the divided mammary vessels is controlled by hemostatic clips. Blood flow from the mammary artery is inspected and may be measured. The cut end of the vessel is "fishmouthed." A No. 22 angiocatheter is carefully introduced into the lumen of the artery and dilute papaverine solution is injected to dilate the artery. Probes are never introduced into the vessel. If doubtful, blood flow is observed and measured a few minutes after instillation of papaverine. The pericardium is incised or slit to bring the untwisted pedicle onto the epicardial surface of the heart. The Favaloro retractor is removed.

If indicated, the opposite internal mammary artery and vein are dissected free of the chest wall in a similar manner.

To avoid injury to mammary pedicles, concomitant saphenous vein bypass grafts are constructed before mammary–coronary anastomoses. All distal coronary arterial anastomoses are made during cardiopulmonary bypass while the heart is arrested with cold cardioplegic solution.

5 Epicardium and fat over the selected segment of coronary artery are incised, and a longitudinal incision is made with a Beaver blade or coronary arterial knife. The incision is extended with angled Potts scissors for a total length of 4 to 5 mm. The mammary pedicle is laid over the site of the proposed anastomosis and divided at the appropriate length after the heart has first been filled to approximate its normal working volume. Excess fat, fascia, and muscle are trimmed for approximately 1 cm from the end of the divided mammary artery. A 3 to 4 mm incision is made to enlarge the circumference of the anastomosis.

INTERRUPTED ANASTOMOSIS

6 The interrupted suture technique is less likely to result in constriction at the anastomosis, but takes longer than the continuous suture method, which is more commonly used. Either siliconized silk or monofilament 7-0 sutures are used. Silk sutures require only three throws in the knot, and are preferred for interrupted anastomoses. Silk sutures also lie easily on the drapes surrounding the wound and are less apt to become twisted or tangled.

Two double (needle)-ended traction sutures are placed inside-to-outside through the coronary artery wall on opposite sides of the incision at the approximate midpoint. Two sutures are then placed inside-to-outside on either side of the proximal apex of the coronary arterial incision. A third suture is passed inside out through the apex of the coronary arterial incision inside; then the opposite end is passed inside out through the heel of the internal mammary artery orifice.

7 The pedicle is brought down to the coronary artery and this apical suture is tied and cut. The opposite end of the previously placed suture on the near side is passed inside out through the internal mammary artery and tied.

8 The far side suture is similarly passed through the internal mammary artery, but is not tied.

9 Three more sutures are now passed inside out through the apex of the distal coronary arterial incision. The opposite ends are passed inside out through the toe of the internal mammary artery, and these three sutures are tied and cut. The near side of the anastomosis is completed by placing 1 or 2 more interrupted sutures (including the traction suture) inside out between the two vessels.

10 The far side of the anastomosis is completed with 1 or 2 interrupted sutures. Before placement of the far-side sutures, a 1 or 1.5 mm probe may be passed into the coronary artery across the toe and heel of the anastomosis. Sometimes it is convenient to pass one or two of the far-side sutures outside in through the two vessels, after first passing the traction suture inside out through the mammary artery to ensure an everting anastomosis. The pedicle bulldog clamp is released briefly to check for leaks and then replaced to maintain cardioplegic arrest. The pedicle of the internal mammary artery is sutured with fine sutures to the adjacent epicardium to reduce tension on the anastomosis and prevent twisting of the pedicle.

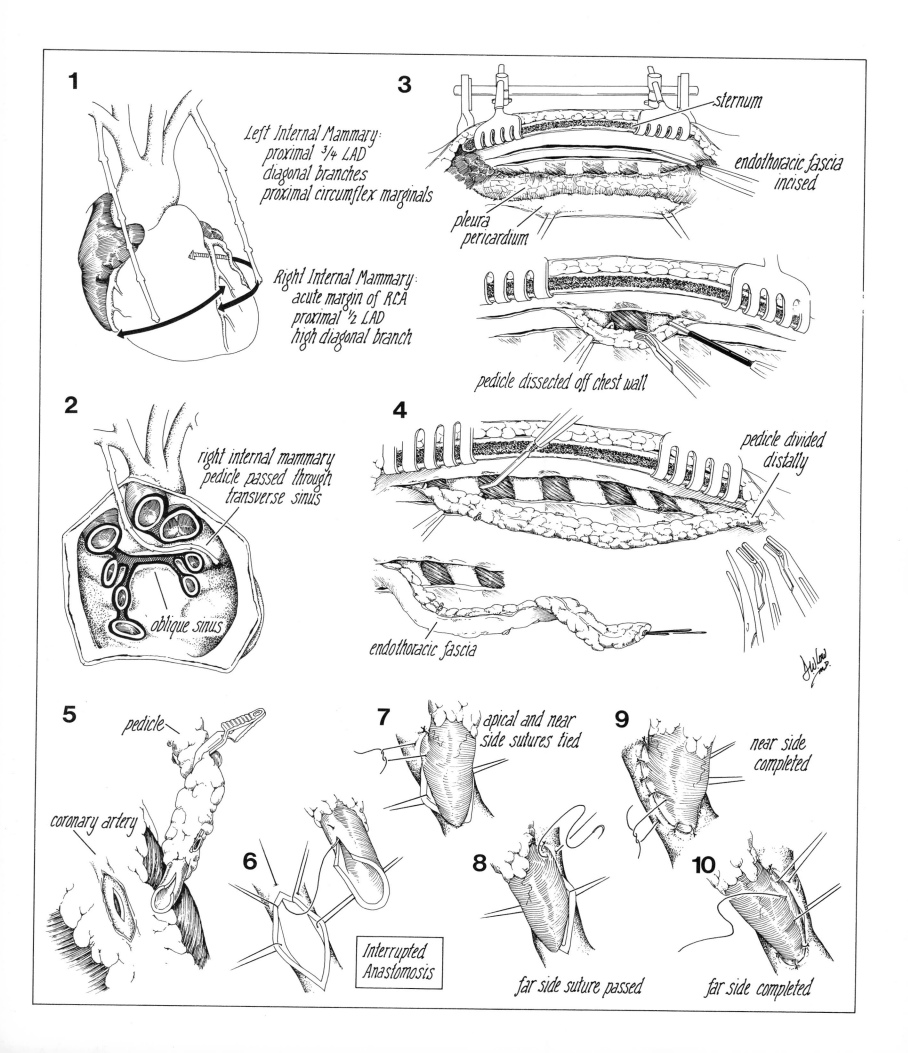

1

Left Internal Mammary:
proximal ¾ LAD
diagonal branches
proximal circumflex marginals

Right Internal Mammary:
acute margin of RCA
proximal ½ LAD
high diagonal branch

2

right internal mammary
pedicle passed through
transverse sinus

oblique sinus

3

sternum

endothoracic fascia
incised

pleura
pericardium

pedicle dissected off chest wall

4

pedicle divided
distally

endothoracic fascia

5

pedicle

coronary artery

6

Interrupted
Anastomosis

7

apical and near
side sutures tied

8

far side suture passed

9

near side
completed

10

far side completed

CONTINUOUS ANASTOMOSIS

(11) The end-to-side anastomosis of the internal mammary artery is more commonly made with a continuous 7-0 monofilament suture. Both ends of the suture are passed outside in through the heel of the mammary artery and then through the proximal (upstream) apex of the coronary arteriotomy.

(12) The near side suture is continued to the apex as a continuous over-and-over suture passing the needle through the mammary artery outside in and through the coronary artery inside out.

(13) With the opposite needle, the suture line of the far side is completed. Sutures around the apex are closely spaced, so as not to narrow the coronary artery. Moreover, this part of the anastomosis is usually made with the sutures slightly loose so that the entire path of the needle can be closely observed.

(14) When the suture reaches the opposite end, it is pulled up and tied. The mammary pedicle is tacked to the ventricular epicardium with one or two 6-0 simple sutures.

SIDE-TO-SIDE ANASTOMOSIS

(15) When the internal mammary artery is 2 mm or more in diameter (after dilatation with papaverine) and has a flow greater than 80 ml/min, it can be used as a sequential graft. Usually this anastomosis is made to a high diagonal branch, and the distal end-to-side anastomosis is made to the left anterior descending coronary artery; however, the opposite sequence (side-to-side to LAD) is also acceptable. The side-to-side anastomosis is made first after selecting the sites for both anastomoses and opening both coronary arteries. The incision in the diagonal branch is 2.5 to 3.0 mm long.

The internal mammary artery is separated from the other tissues of the pedicle at the site of the side-to-side anastomosis. Excluding the artery, the other tissues of the pedicle are transected to leave approximately 1 cm of the artery denuded of surrounding tissue. A longitudinal incision is made in the internal mammary artery. The incision is slightly longer than the incision in the coronary artery, and is made with a Beaver or No. 11 knife blade to prevent the anastomosis from pulling the mammary artery into the coronary artery and possibly reducing flow to the distal end-to-side anastomosis.

(16) For the continuous suture technique, the two arteriotomies are positioned like "pages in a book." The 7-0 monofilament suture begins at the midpoint of the coronary arteriotomy, and the needle passes into the adjacent wall of the mammary arteriotomy.

(17) The proximal segment of the far suture line is completed by bringing the suture around the apices of the coronary arteriotomy. With the opposite needle, the row nearest to the surgeon is completed.

(18) The suture is continued around the coronary apices and along the near arterial wall to the opposite end of the suture. The loops are pulled up and tied. When the pedicle bulldog clamp is released, good blood flow should emerge from the distal mammary artery.

(19) The interrupted suture technique is more likely to yield a technically perfect, unconstricted anastomosis, particularly if the coronary vessel is less than 2 mm in diameter. Two traction sutures are placed on opposite walls of the coronary artery at the midpoint of the incision. Three sutures are then passed inside out through the coronary artery around the apex of the incision, and the opposite ends are passed inside out through the mammary arterial incision. The untied sutures are laid on drapes around the wound.

(20) Three sutures are now passed inside out around the apex of the distal coronary arterial incision; the opposite ends are passed through the mammary artery inside out. The inside needles of the two traction sutures are passed inside out through the mammary artery inside so that a total of eight sutures have been placed around the two arterial openings.

(21) The heel suture is tied first as an assistant approximates the two vessels with traction on the pedicle. The remaining sutures are tied in order and cut. The bulldog clamp on the pedicle is released as the distal end of the pedicle is gently compressed by fingers to test for leaks. The proximal portion of the pedicle upstream to the anastomosis is sutured to the epicardium with one or two fine sutures.

The distal anastomosis is completed as previously described.

Free IMA Graft

(22) Pedicled internal mammary arterial (IMA) grafts are preferred to free grafts. Free grafts, however, are excellent conduits. The mammary pedicle is clamped and divided near the first rib. The proximal pedicle is ligated. Approximately 1 cm of the internal mammary artery is dissected free of the surrounding pedicle tissues. The posterior side of the artery is incised 3 to 4 mm to "fishmouth" the vessel.

(23) Adventitia is removed from the ascending aorta around the site of the proposed anastomosis. A side-biting (Cooley or Hunter) clamp is placed on the aorta. The aortotomy is made free-hand with a No. 11 knife blade or a small 4 mm arterial punch. The anastomosis is made with continuous 7-0 monofilament or interrupted siliconized silk sutures.

(24) The free mammary arterial pedicle may be anastomosed to a short segment of vein. The vein is anastomosed first to the aortotomy, which is made with either a 4.8 mm or 4.0 mm arterial punch. Excess vein is amputated. The end-to-end vein-to-artery anastomosis is made as illustrated with two mattress sutures placed 180 degrees apart. The suture ends are continued toward each other as continuous over-and-over sutures.

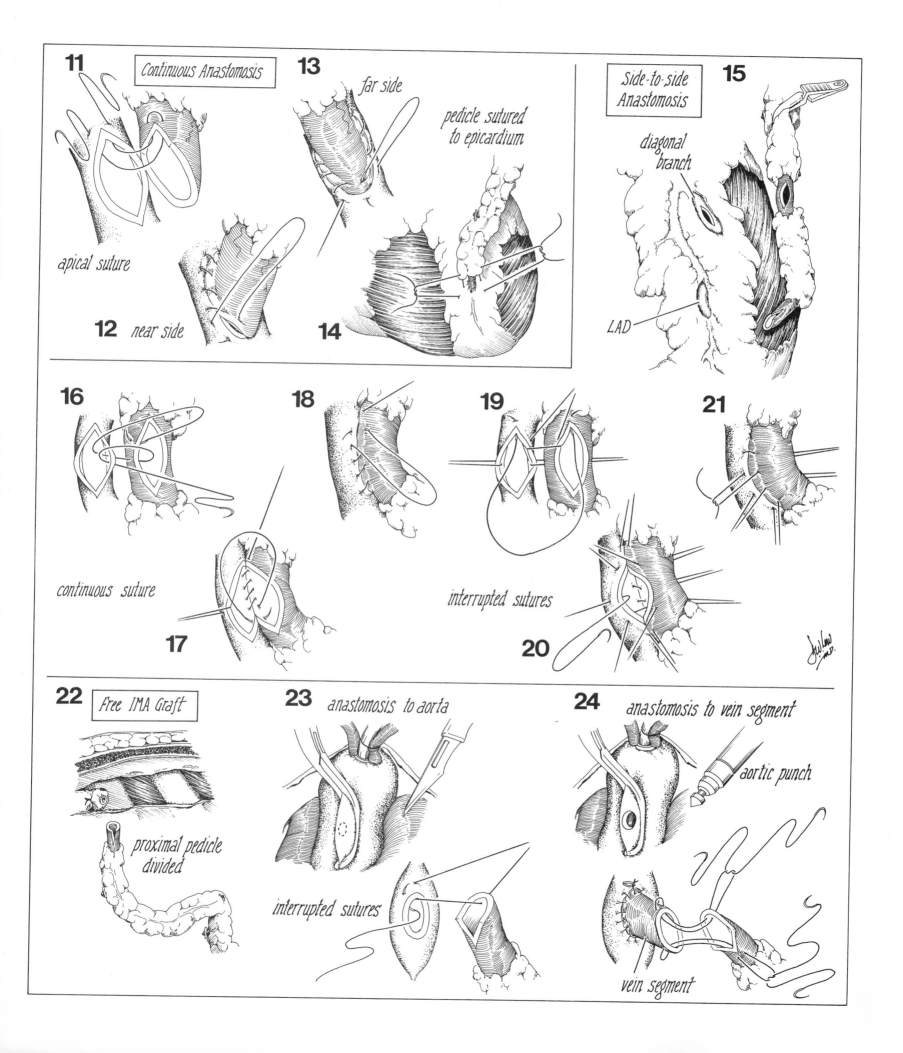

11 | Continuous Anastomosis

13 far side

pedicle sutured to epicardium

apical suture

12 near side

14

15 | Side-to-side Anastomosis

diagonal branch

LAD

16

18

19

21

continuous suture

17

interrupted sutures

20

22 | Free IMA Graft

proximal pedicle divided

23 anastomosis to aorta

interrupted sutures

24 anastomosis to vein segment

aortic punch

vein segment

Resection of Left Ventricular Aneurysm, Endocardial Mapping and Resection, Replacement of the Mitral Valve through the Ventricle

Myocardial infarction may result in left ventricular aneurysm, recurrent ventricular tachycardia, and/or ischemic mitral insufficiency. Most often, excision of left ventricular aneurysm is combined with myocardial revascularization. In patients with recurrent ventricular tachycardia, endocardial resection is added. Occasionally, patients have mitral insufficiency and require replacement of the valve. The combined operation of endocardial mapping and resection, replacement of the mitral valve, and resection of left ventricular aneurysm is illustrated.

1 The location of the tachycardic focus or foci is determined in the operating room by endocardial mapping. Surface ECG leads for the mapping recorder are placed on the patient before operation. After the heart is exposed and the patient is cannulated for bypass, plunge electrodes are placed in the lateral wall of the left ventricle and anterior wall of the right ventricle. A single or two-stage right atrial catheter is used unless the patient also has a postinfarction ventricular septal defect.

2 Cardiopulmonary bypass is started and maintained at 37 degrees during the mapping period, which is limited to 50 minutes. A No. 18 Fr Ferguson catheter is inserted into the left ventricle to maintain a blood-free field. An incision is made in the thin, fibrous portion of the ventricular aneurysm to expose the endocardial surface of the ventricle. Any clot or thrombus is removed. If only an infarct is present, the incision is made in the infarct area with the heart beating. Air embolism must be avoided, but the aorta is not clamped.

3 The general area of the tachycardic focus is determined in the electrophysiologic laboratory preoperatively by catheterization. With the ventricle held wide open by traction sutures, ventricular tachycardia is induced by rapid electrical stimulation of a plunge electrode. When sustained ventricular tachycardia is induced, the surgeon maps the endocardial surface of the ventricular septum and ventricular cavity using a hand-held electrode. By prearrangement, the ventriculotomy is viewed as a clock face. During induced tachycardia, the hand-held probe is placed at each hour position near the edge of the ventriculotomy while recordings are obtained from all electrodes. Usually three or four concentric circles, separated by 1 or 2 cm, are mapped. Location of each papillary muscle is noted during mapping of the deeper circles.

4 The septum, which is partially mapped during cavity mapping, is also mapped separately. This may be done with special multi-electrode pads placed against the septum. From the recordings, the site of the earliest activation of the tachycardia is determined. If the patient has more than one focus, as recognized by a different pattern of tachycardia, all are resected. The site of the first focus is resected by endocardial resection (see 5 below). The second tachycardia is then induced and mapping repeated until the second earliest site of activation is located. The process is repeated until all sites of inducible tachycardia are located and ablated by resection or cryoprobe.

5 Endocardial resection removes the sheet of fibrous tissue that lines the inside of the aneurysm and adjacent contracting myocardium. A plane is developed between the fibrous endocardial sheet and the overlying ventricular muscle. This endocardial scar is separated by knife or scissors for at least 2 cm around the tachycardic focus.

6 If the endocardial scar is discrete, the entire sheet is removed circumferentially from the base of the aneurysm to the base of the papillary muscles. Injury to the papillary muscles is avoided.

7 Early activation foci on or near papillary muscles or high in the ventricular septum are ablated by cryoablation. The precise location of the focus to be ablated is determined by mapping. The probe is cooled and, when frost appears, placed on the focus and held there for 120 seconds. The probe must be warmed before detachment from the endocardium. The process may be repeated.

After the endocardial resection is completed and plunge electrodes are removed, the patient is cooled to 26° to 30° C. The aorta is clamped and the heart is arrested. All obstructed coronary vessels suitable for bypass are identified and bypassed with venous segments or internal mammary arteries.

8 If the mitral valve must be replaced, this can be done through the ventriculotomy. Traditionally, the valve is excised. More recently, some chordal attachments and leaflet tissue are retained to improve ventricular function. If the valve is excised, a 2 to 3 mm rim of valve tissue is left attached to the annulus. Pledgeted 0 polyester sutures are passed from ventricle to atrium through this rim (or the retained valve leaflet), through the annulus into the atrium. The suture then passes through the sewing ring and is tied on the ventricular side. Although obvious, the prosthesis must not be inserted upside down. Sutures are tied after interrupted mattress sutures are placed. With a ventricular view, any obstructing valve tissue is easily removed.

9 When all distal anastomoses are completed and the mitral valve dealt with, rewarming is started and the ventriculotomy is closed. The thin fibrous walls of the aneurysm are excised to a rim approximately 1 cm wide. Three 1 cm wide strips of Teflon felt are cut. Beginning at the apex, the ventricle is closed between two felt strips using a horizontal mattress suture of heavy monofilament. Allis clamps placed at the two apices of the ventriculotomy facilitate this running suture. When the cephalad apex is reached, the third felt strip is placed over the suture line and the same suture is run back to the ventricular apex as an over-and-over suture with bites about 5 mm apart.

Before the ventriculotomy suture line is tied down and the aortic clamp is released, lungs are expanded and all air is removed from the ventricle, left atrium, and aortic root. The suture line is tied because the ventricle is still decompressed. The heart is electrically defibrillated and temporary ventricular pacemaker wires are placed. The proximal anastomoses of the coronary venous grafts are made. A No. 19 needle is placed in the ascending aorta to aspirate air.

Many patients require catecholamine, amrinone, vasodilator, and/or intra-aortic balloon support to discontinue cardiopulmonary bypass. During this critical period, distention of the ventricle and unnecessary manipulation and stimulation must be avoided. Antiarrythmic drugs may be required for the first few hours or days. When the circulation is stable off bypass, cannulas are removed, protamine is given, and very careful hemostasis is achieved before the standard closure over drainage tubes.

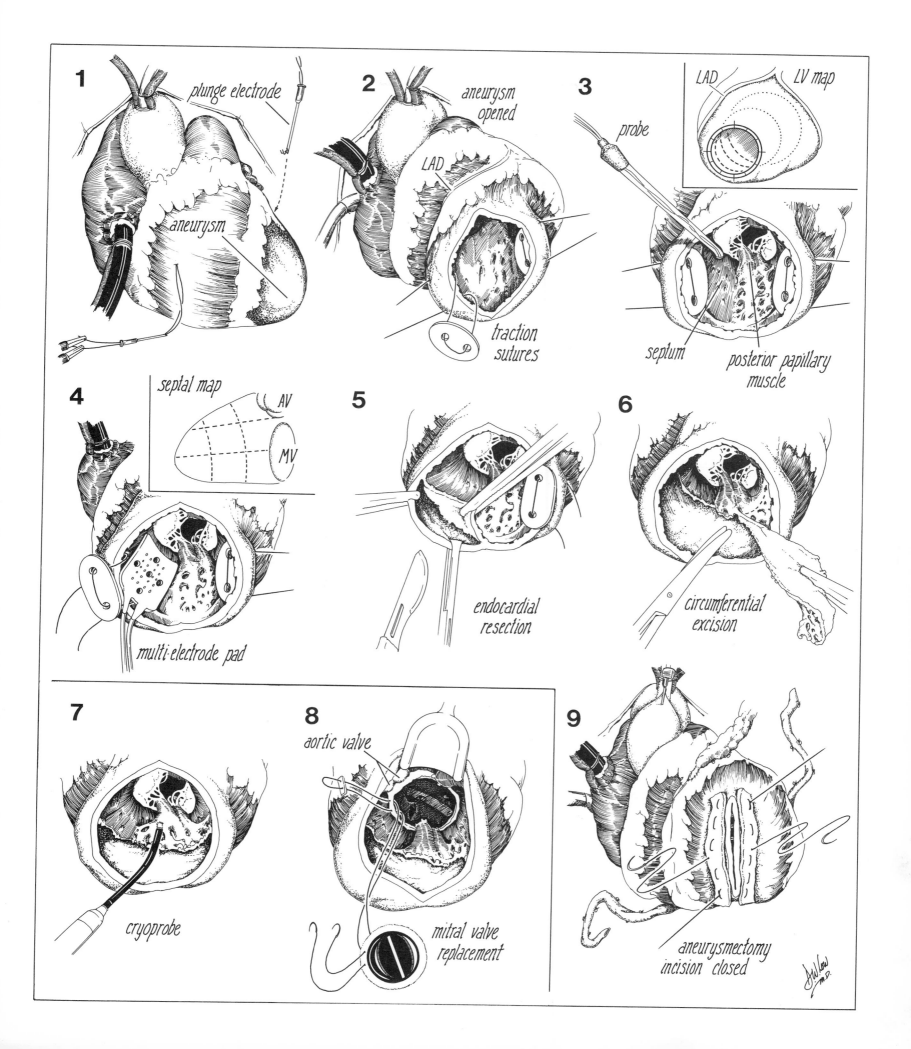

1
plunge electrode
aneurysm

2
aneurysm opened
LAD
traction sutures

3
probe
LAD   LV map
septum
posterior papillary muscle

4
septal map
AV
MV
multi-electrode pad

5
endocardial resection

6
circumferential excision

7
cryoprobe

8
aortic valve
mitral valve replacement

9
aneurysmectomy incision closed

Posterior Postinfarction Ventricular Septal Defect

The additional hemodynamic burden of a left-to-right shunt may produce both acute pulmonary edema and cardiogenic shock. Early surgery, before failure of other organ systems develops, is recommended for all patients except those with hemodynamically trivial shunts. About two-thirds of the ventricular septal defects are in the anterior septum; the remainder are posterior.

The patient may develop circulatory insufficiency and require endotracheal intubation and pharmacologic and mechanical (intra-aortic balloon pump) circulatory support before reaching the operating room. Usually cardiac catheterization and coronary angiograms are obtained before operation, but can be omitted in life-threatening situations.

The chest, groins, and both legs are prepped and draped into the operative field. After a midline sternotomy, heparin is given before opening the pericardium (particularly if blood is visible through the pericardium). The ascending aorta is cannulated near the base of the innominate artery. Both cavae are cannulated separately through the right atrium. If coronary artery bypass grafts are also planned, the saphenous vein is harvested by a separate team during sternotomy and cannulation.

Moderate hypothermia (28° to 30° C) is used.

1 Cardiopulmonary bypass is established, but the heart is not manipulated, to reduce the risk of dislodging a ventricular thrombus. Cold saline is poured into the pericardial well. The aorta is clamped when the heart fibrillates. Fibrinous adhesions are taken down and the heart is arrested by infusion of cold cardioplegic solution into the aortic root.

2 The apex of the heart is elevated to expose the occluded posterior descending coronary artery and hemorrhagic and discolored infarcted myocardium. An incision is made close to and parallel to the posterior descending coronary artery into the *left* ventricular cavity. The artery marks the ventricular septum. The posterior papillary muscle of the mitral valve is attached to the posterior ventricular wall more laterally.

3 The incision is enlarged within the infarcted muscle to expose the left ventricular cavity, posterior papillary muscle, mitral valve, ventricular septum, and ventricular septal defect. The edges of the infarct are incised to within 1 cm of adjacent viable muscle. Any adherent clot or potential embolus is removed. The ragged edges of the ventricular septal defect are not debrided. The amount of infarcted septum surrounding the ventricular septal defect is estimated, however, and a Teflon felt or woven Dacron patch is cut to include this infarcted tissue beneath the patch.

4 The patch is inserted with Teflon felt pledgeted mattress sutures of 3-0 polypropylene. The sutures are placed in the viable muscle at the edge of the infarct (not the edges of the defect) and passed through the patch. The mattress sutures are placed in a semicircle around the septal portion of the infarct from free wall to ventricular free wall. These sutures are tied firmly, but not tightly, to avoid cutting the muscle. A continuous over-and-over suture may be placed around the edge of the patch to reinforce this suture line.

Alternatively, two patches of Teflon felt may be used on either side of the ventricular septum. A parallel incision is made to the *right* of the posterior descending coronary artery to expose the right ventricular surface of the septum. Teflon felt patches are cut for each side of the septum. Interrupted mattress sutures passed through both patches and the intervening septum essentially replace the infarcted septum with Teflon felt. Alternatively, a running horizontal mattress suture, run up and back, may be used to anchor the two patches to the septal edge adjacent to the infarct and to each other.

5 The unsutured edge of the patch (or patches) extends out of the ventriculotomy (or ventriculotomies) and will be incorporated in the closure.

6 The ventriculotomy is closed with No. 1 polypropylene over strips of Teflon felt. A line of horizontal mattress sutures is first placed through the viable muscle edges of the infarct. Sutures must avoid the posterior papillary muscle and closure of the ventricular cavity must not distort the mitral valve and cause valvular dysfunction. A continuous horizontal mattress suture can also be used.

7 When this line of sutures is tied down, the ventricle is closed between two broad strips of Teflon felt. Before the ventricle is closed, air is removed by gently inflating the lungs and compressing the ventricular walls.

8 The ventriculotomy repair is completed by a continuous No. 1 over-and-over polypropylene suture passed between the two felt strips and intervening muscle, and over a third felt strip covering the suture line. When this suture is tied firmly down, complete hemostasis should be achieved.

9 If coronary artery bypass grafts are added, the distal anastomoses are performed before the ventriculotomy is completely closed. This practice permits decompression of the ventricle until rewarming, defibrillation (if necessary), and the resumption of cardiac contractions. After release of the aortic clamp, the ventricle should be kept decompressed manually until effective cardiac contractions resume. Occasionally, a small incision in the right superior pulmonary vein-left atrial junction is made to decompress the left heart until effective contractions return.

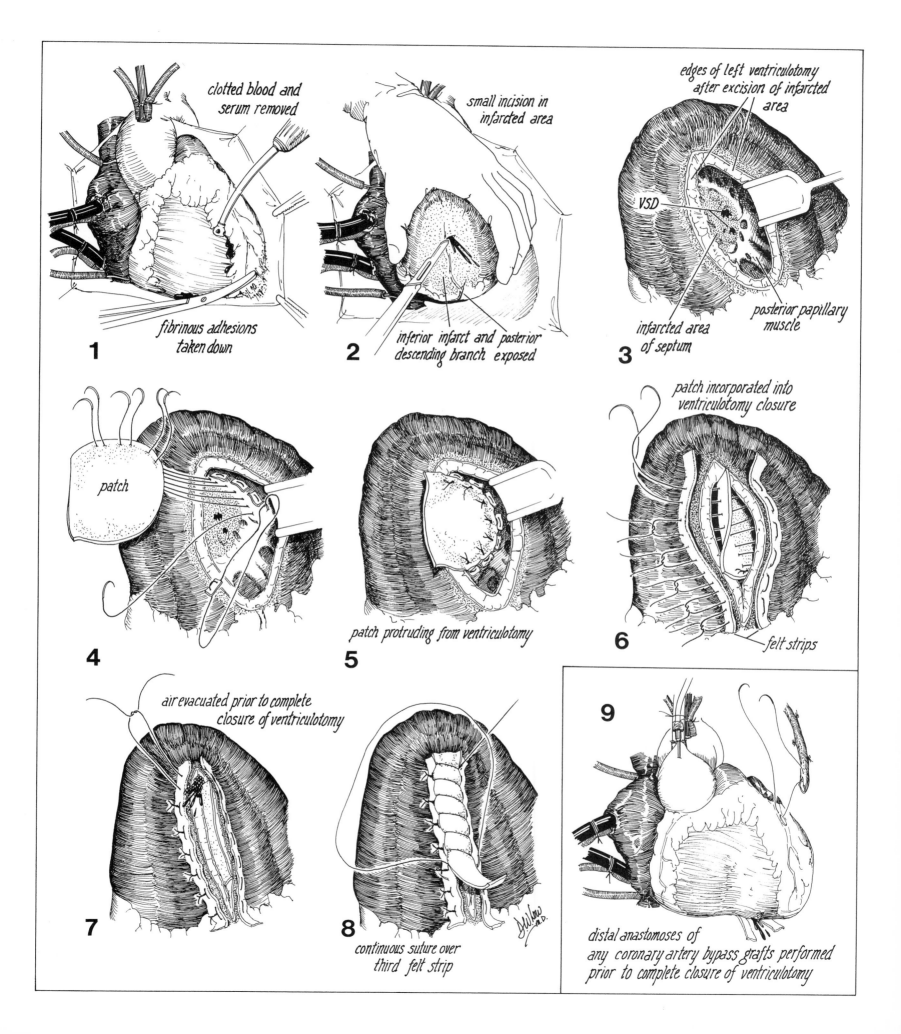

1 clotted blood and serum removed / fibrinous adhesions taken down

2 small incision in infarcted area / inferior infarct and posterior descending branch exposed

3 edges of left ventriculotomy after excision of infarcted area / VSD / infarcted area of septum / posterior papillary muscle

4 patch

5 patch protruding from ventriculotomy

6 patch incorporated into ventriculotomy closure / felt strips

7 air evacuated prior to complete closure of ventriculotomy

8 continuous suture over third felt strip

9 distal anastomoses of any coronary artery bypass grafts performed prior to complete closure of ventriculotomy

Anterior Postinfarction Ventricular Septal Defect

The more common anterior postinfarction VSD is managed similarly. The superior and inferior cavae are both cannulated; caval tapes are rarely necessary. The aorta is cannulated.

1 If the patient is hemodynamically stable before bypass, proximal ends of planned coronary artery bypass grafts may be anastomosed to the ascending aorta using a side-biting aortic clamp. After bypass starts, the aorta is clamped and the heart is arrested.

2 The infarcted myocardium is incised just lateral to the occluded left anterior descending coronary artery. The incision is made parallel to the artery within the infarct and may extend around the apex of the ventricle in some patients. Extension of the incision into viable muscle is avoided.

3 The incision is extended after the left ventricle is entered to expose the ventricular septum, the anterior VSD, and the anterior papillary muscle of the mitral valve. Infarcted ventricular septum is *not* removed, although thrombus and loose necrotic debris are excised.

4 The infarcted ventricular free wall is excised to within 1 cm of the healthy muscle. Necrotic muscle and healthy muscle are generally easily differentiated several days after an acute infarction. Excision of the infarcted left ventricular free wall may remove the distal left anterior descending coronary artery and part of the right ventricle. Too-aggressive excision of the infarct may compromise left ventricular cavity size; therefore, we prefer not to excise the infarcted anterior septum, which can heal by fibrosis beneath a large woven Dacron or Teflon felt patch.

5 The patch is cut to cover the entire infarcted septum and sewn to the healthy posterior septum with either pledgeted interrupted mattress sutures or two continuous 3-0

monofilament sutures with deep bites into healthy muscle. Alternatively, the two-patch technique described for a posterior defect may be used if a parallel incision is made in the right ventricle.

6 Patch sutures are continued until the ventricular free wall is reached at the proximal and distal ends of the free wall defect.

7 Before closure, the ventricular cavity is carefully inspected for loose debris. The free ventricular wall defect is closed with a continuous horizontal mattress suture of No. 1 monofilament buttressed with wide Teflon felt strips. This is followed by a continuous suture over a third felt strip as described and illustrated for a posterior VSD.

8 Rarely, the amount of excised free wall infarcted muscle may produce a dangerously small left ventricle or cause mitral insufficiency by interference with the anterior mitral papillary muscle if the trimmed edges are approximated as described above. An elliptical patch of thick Teflon felt (two thicknesses) is cut to size, but the size of the patch should be made as small as possible to reduce systolic bulging and an elastic anchorage for healthy myocardial fibers.

9 When a free wall patch is used, the Dacron patch used to cover the left ventricular face of the ventricular septum is sewn along with the edge of the right ventricular free wall to the patch. The patch is sewn in place using two continuous, over-and-over running 2-0 monofilament sutures buttressed with felt strips on the endocardial and epicardial surfaces of the edges of the defect. All air is removed from *both* ventricles before suture lines are tied. When a free wall patch is used, a small incision at the junction of the right superior pulmonary vein–left atrial junction is wise to keep the left ventricle decompressed while the heart recovers contractile strength.

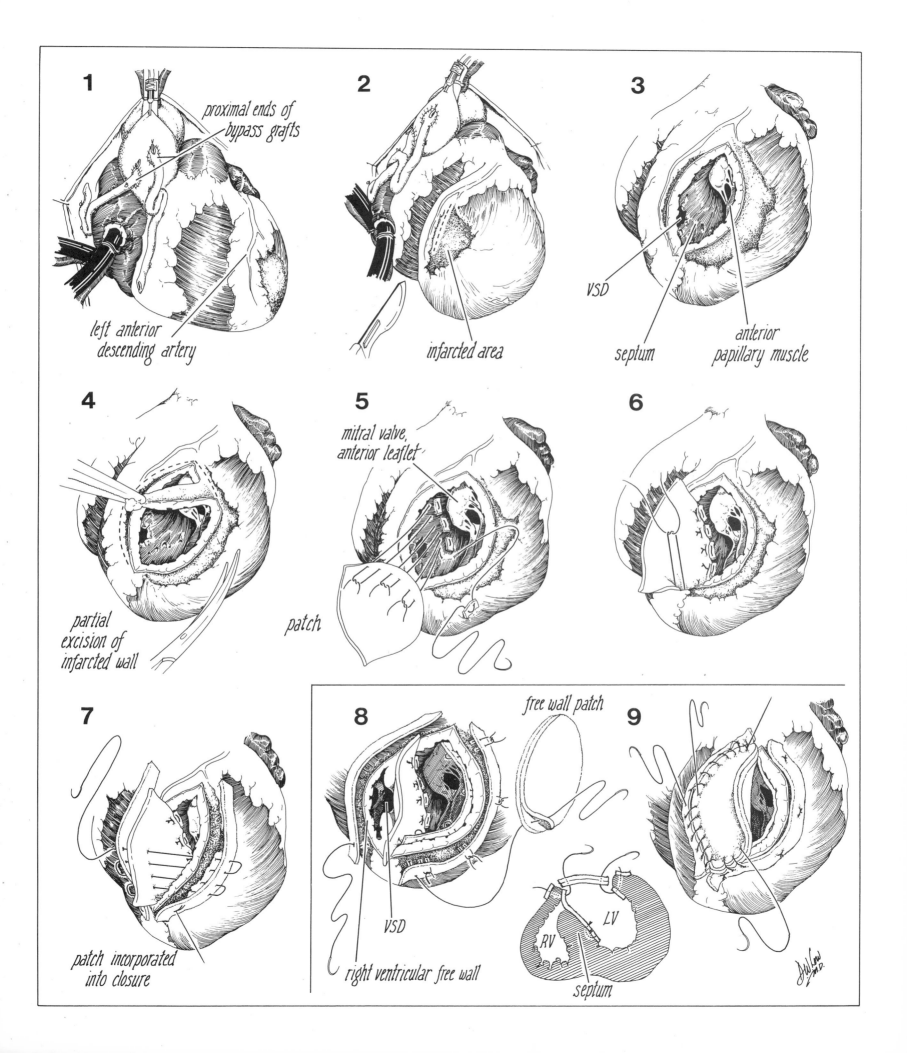

1 proximal ends of bypass grafts

left anterior descending artery

2 infarcted area

3 VSD

septum

anterior papillary muscle

4 partial excision of infarcted wall

5 mitral valve, anterior leaflet

patch

6

7 patch incorporated into closure

8 free wall patch

VSD

right ventricular free wall

LV

RV

septum

9

Wolff-Parkinson-White (WPW) Syndrome

Patients with the WPW syndrome have one or more anomalous strands of conducting muscular tissue between the atrium and ventricle. These strands, termed bypass tracts or Kent bundles, may be anywhere along the atrioventricular rings except in the central fibrous portion where the fibrous annuli of the aortic and mitral valves are in continuity. Atrial impulses travel antegrade down these bypass tracts to adjacent ventricular myocardium and bypass the atrioventricular (AV) node, which normally slows impulse conduction. Rapid propagation of the impulse over the bypass tracts causes premature depolarization or pre-excitation of the ventricle. The differential conduction properties of the bypass tracts and AV node predispose the patient to re-entrant supraventricular tachycardias (SVT).

In patients with WPW, the bypass tract serves as the retrograde limb of the reentrant circuit in 95% of SVT. The AV node-His bundle serves as the antegrade limb. Approximately 20% of patients have bypass tracts that conduct only retrograde. Surgical treatment of the WPW syndrome requires division or ablation of all conducting bypass tracts. Approximately 20 to 25% of patients have two or more tracts.

1 The atrioventricular rings may be divided into four distinct segments, which are designated anterior and posterior *septal* and right and left *free wall*. The cross-sectional view of the heart at the atrioventricular rings illustrates the location of these segments and their relationships to other structures. Location of the anomalous bypass tracts requires good preoperative and intraoperative electrophysiologic mapping.

2 The heart is exposed through a midline sternotomy and the patient is cannulated for bypass. Right-angled venous cannulas are inserted in either the lateral caval walls or lateral atrial-caval junctions. Slings are passed around each cava. Manipulation of the heart is avoided to eliminate temporary loss of conduction in the bypass tracts. Mapping reference electrodes are placed in both atria and in the right ventricle.

3 A multielectrode strip pad may be used instead of a single hand-held bipolar or quadripolar probe. The strip pad facilitates mapping the posterior surface of the heart. The ventricular side of the atrioventricular rings is mapped during sinus rhythm to determine the earliest site of ventricular depolarization and the ventricular location of the bypass tract. Mapping is repeated during left and right atrial pacing to enhance preexcitation of the ventricle. The atria are mapped around the AV groove during induced SVT, or during ventricular pacing if SVT cannot be induced. Cardiopulmonary bypass at 37° C may be started if mapping causes hemodynamic instability. Otherwise, bypass is used only during the dissection portion of the operation.

4 A cross-section of the atrioventricular groove is illustrated. The endocardial approach permits division of bypass tracts in all four locations and is the only approach to the anteroseptal space. We prefer the epicardial approach for posteroseptal and right free wall tracts but it can also be used for left free wall tracts.

Cardioplegic arrest is used for endocardial dissections. Anterior septal, right free wall, and posterior septal tracts are approached through the right atrium. Left free wall tracts are approached through the left atrium. The plane of the endocardial dissection is between the top of the ventricular wall below and the fat pad that contains the coronary vessels above. Binocular loupes (× 2.5) are helpful. The endocardium is incised 2 mm above the valve annulus with a No. 15 scalpel and the plane between the top of the ventricular wall and fat pad is entered.

Using careful dissection, a cautery for small vessels and a thin nerve hook, the dissection is deepened until the epicardium is reached. The entire sector of the AV groove is dissected before the patient is rewarmed. Mapping is repeated after rewarming.

Epicardial dissections are done during warm (37° C) cardiopulmonary bypass. The plane for epicardial dissection is between the atrial wall above and the fat pad below. The dissection technique is similar.

5 The posterior septal space is shaped like a pyramid toppled on its side. The central fibrous body of the heart represents the apex of the pyramid, where injury to the AV node and His bundle may cause permanent atrioventricular block. During dissection, AV conduction is monitored with the heart beating during warm bypass.

The heart is elevated by traction sutures. The epicardial incision is made upstream to the origin of the posterior descending coronary artery in the posterior portion of the right free wall. The incision extends posteriorly beyond but superior to the entrance of the middle cardiac vein, which may be divided to improve exposure. The dissection continues along the atrial wall until the annulus of the tricuspid valve, the ostium of the coronary sinus into the right atrium, and the annulus of the mitral valve. The dissection proceeds superior to the coronary sinus within the crux. Vessels to the atrium are ligated, clipped, or cauterized; all muscle fibers that are not part of the atrial wall are divided.

6 Epicardial dissection of the left ventricular free wall is illustrated. This requires elevation of the heart; therefore we prefer the endocardial approach (panel 8). The dissection occurs along the superior border of the circumflex coronary artery and coronary sinus to the base of the left atrial appendage and reaches the annulus of the mitral valve.

7 The anterior septal region can be reached only by the endocardial approach. The right atrium is opened to expose the interatrial septum and tricuspid valve. The locations of the AV node, tricuspid valve, and proximal right coronary artery are illustrated. The endocardial incision is made around the anterior commissure of the tricuspid valve and deepened to the top of the ventricle. Dissection continues in this plane beneath the right coronary artery adjacent to the noncoronary and right coronary cusps of the aorta until the atrial epicardium is reached.

8 The endocardial approach to the left ventricular free wall is illustrated. The left atrium is opened widely by an incision posterior to the interatrial septum. An incision is made 2 mm from the annulus of the posterior (mural) leaflet and extends in both directions from the left fibrous trigone to the posterior commissure. The dissection continues to the epicardium between the fat pad and circumflex vessels and top of the ventricular septum.

9 The use of the cryoprobe is illustrated during epicardial dissection of the right ventricular free wall. Usually the cryoprobe is not needed, but if a bypass tract persists after an apparent complete dissection, the probe is applied for 120 seconds to the area of the anomalous tract as determined by postdissection mapping.

Both endocardial and epicardial dissections are closed with a fine monofilament continuous suture after the dissection is completed. After bypass stops, mapping during sinus rhythm, right and left atrial pacing, and ventricular pacing is repeated. Attempts are also made to induce SVT.

70

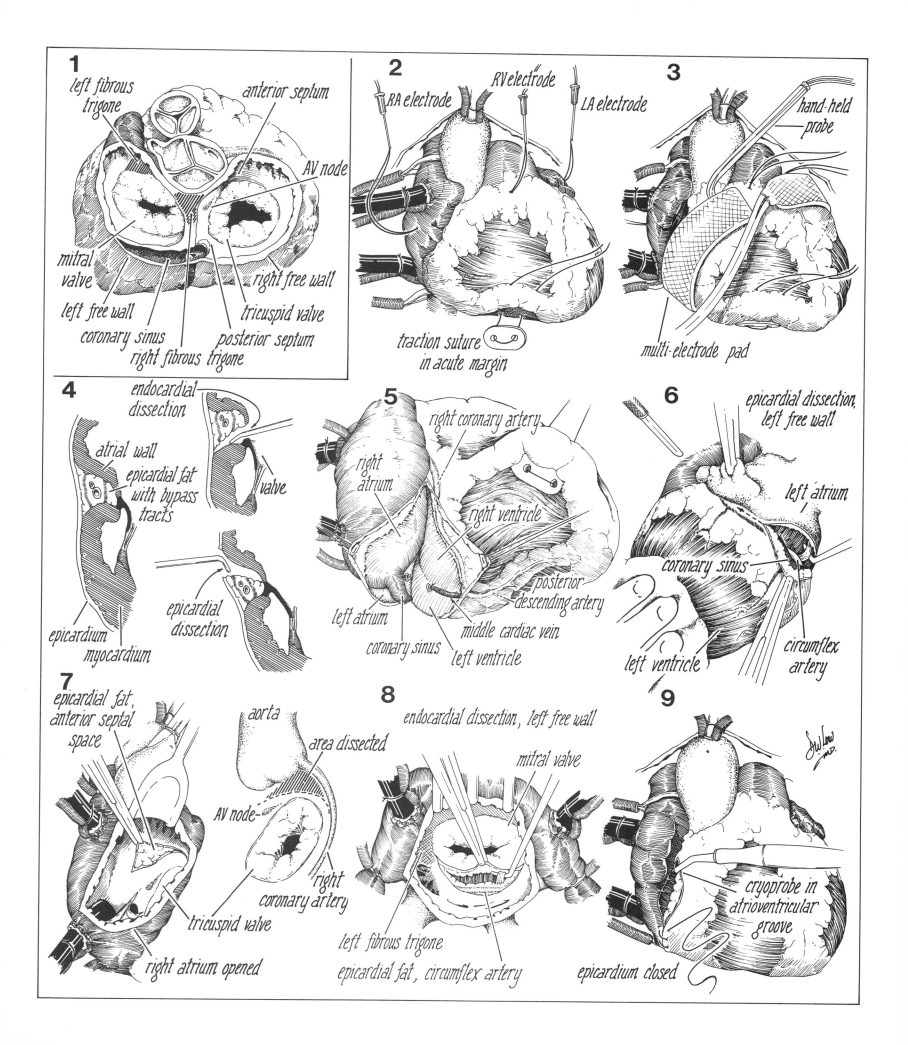

1
left fibrous trigone
anterior septum
AV node
mitral valve
left free wall
coronary sinus
right fibrous trigone
posterior septum
right free wall
tricuspid valve

2
RA electrode
RV electrode
LA electrode
traction suture in acute margin

3
hand-held probe
multi-electrode pad

4
endocardial dissection
atrial wall
epicardial fat with bypass tracts
valve
epicardial dissection
epicardium
myocardium

5
right coronary artery
right atrium
right ventricle
left atrium
coronary sinus
posterior descending artery
middle cardiac vein
left ventricle

6
epicardial dissection, left free wall
left atrium
coronary sinus
left ventricle
circumflex artery

7
epicardial fat, anterior septal space
aorta
area dissected
AV node
right coronary artery
tricuspid valve
right atrium opened

8
endocardial dissection, left free wall
mitral valve
left fibrous trigone
epicardial fat, circumflex artery

9
cryoprobe in atrioventricular groove
epicardium closed

Heart Transplantation

Ideally, the donor heart should arrive in the operating room just as cardiopulmonary bypass begins in the recipient. This goal minimizes the ischemic time of the donor heart. Periodic communications from the procurement team are needed to coordinate the recipient's operation with harvest of the heart and preparations for bypass.

The donor heart is usually obtained by a surgical team sent out from the recipient hospital. Donors are living, brain-dead individuals whose next-of-kin have consented to the harvest of the heart and usually other organs as well. Harvest operations are often performed at night with full operating teams in the donor hospital. Although the heart is harvested first, the dissection of other organs is completed before any organs are removed.

Under sterile conditions, a midline incision is made from sternal notch to pubis. The heart is inspected for injury, unsuspected disease, or lack of vigor. A final decision is made to accept or reject the heart and the message is transmitted to the recipient team. The heart is covered during the dissection of liver, pancreas, and kidneys.

When the heart team returns, the pericardium is tacked up and the ascending aorta and superior cava are dissected free. Ligatures are passed around the cava, and monitoring catheters in the heart or lungs are withdrawn. Heparin (3 mg/kg) is given intravenously. A No. 14 angiocatheter is inserted and tied into the ascending aorta. Cold cardioplegic solution is prepared; two suction lines are made available.

When the other harvest teams are ready, the superior cava is divided between ligatures. The inferior vena cava is transected at the diaphragm and at least one of the right pulmonary veins is opened. A previously placed linear cutting stapler is closed across the ascending aorta just upstream to the innominate artery. Infusion of cardioplegic solution is started as blood is aspirated from the pericardial cavity. The quiet heart is retracted cephalad to facilitate transection of the pulmonary veins at the pericardium. With a finger in the transverse sinus, the main pulmonary artery is transected at its bifurcation. The heart is transferred to a basin of cold saline slush and additional cardioplegic solution is infused for a total of 1 to 1.5 L. The cold, quiet heart is packaged with 150 ml of cold saline into two sterile bags and placed under ice in a portable styrofoam ice chest for transport. A sample of the donor's blood and a few lymph nodes are taken with the heart for retrospective tissue typing.

The recipient surgical team opens the chest through a midline sternotomy. After heparin, the ascending aorta is cannulated near the base of the innominate artery and both cavae are cannulated by means of purse-string sutures placed on the lateral wall of the right atrium away from the atrioventricular groove. Umbilical tapes are placed around both cavae near the atrial junctions.

(1) Cardiopulmonary bypass begins and the recipient is cooled to 28 to 30° C. The caval tourniquets are snugged down and a small incision is made in the right atrium near the atrioventricular groove. The ascending aorta is clamped.

(2) With the heart partially decompressed, the ascending aorta and main pulmonary artery are transected just above their respective valves. This exposes the superior wall of the left atrium. The left atrium is entered and, with scissors, the incision in the atrium is continued rightward along the atrioventricular groove across the interatrial septum into the right atrium down to the coronary sinus. Usually, the recipient right atrial appendage is removed. The incision in the left atrium is continued along the atrioventricular groove near the base of the left atrial appendage and the mural annulus of the mitral valve.

(3) The recipient heart is removed by dividing the posterior atrioventricular junction, following the coronary sinus. The left atrial appendage is usually removed, but is retained in the illustration for orientation.

(4) The donor team unpackages the heart into a basin of cold saline. The right atrium is incised from the inferior vena cava to the base of the right atrial appendage. The orifices of the pulmonary veins are connected and the resulting piece of atrium and tags of vein are trimmed away. The interatrial septum is inspected for a patent foramen ovale which is sutured closed. Lastly, six biopsies are taken from the right ventricle with the biotome.

(5) The suture line begins at the base of the left atrial appendage. A continuous 3-0 monofilament (48 inch) suture is used. The needle is passed through the tissue 6 to 7 mm from the edges of the cut atria and run as a continuous over-and-over suture to the caudad end of the interatrial septa.

(6) The opposite needle is used to anastomose the superior wall of the left atria and the left atrial wall of the interatrial septa. The two sutures are tied and held after the left atrium is filled with cold saline to displace air.

(7) The right atrial anastomosis begins at the cephalad end of the interatrial septa. The suture line continues down the two septa and around the inferior border of the right atria. With the opposite needle, the superior and anterior borders of the right atria are joined. About 2 to 3 cm is left unsutured to permit decompression of the heart later.

(8) Cold cardioplegia is renewed and rewarming is usually started. The pulmonary arteries are trimmed to match. With a 30-inch 3-0 monofilament suture, the anastomosis is started as a continuous over-and-over stitch on the lateral wall of the pulmonary artery. The suture line continues posteriorly and then anteriorly to complete the anastomosis.

(9) The two aortas are trimmed appropriately and anastomosed with a continuous 3-0 monofilament suture. Before the aortic clamp is released, air maneuvers are completed. The heart is kept decompressed by way of the open right atrium or pulmonary artery and by manual compression until coordinated contractions are reestablished. An isoproterenol infusion is started. Suture lines are inspected for leaks, which are sutured closed. When the patient is rewarmed, and when the heart is beating forcefully, bypass is stopped. Temporary atrial and ventricular pacing wires are left.

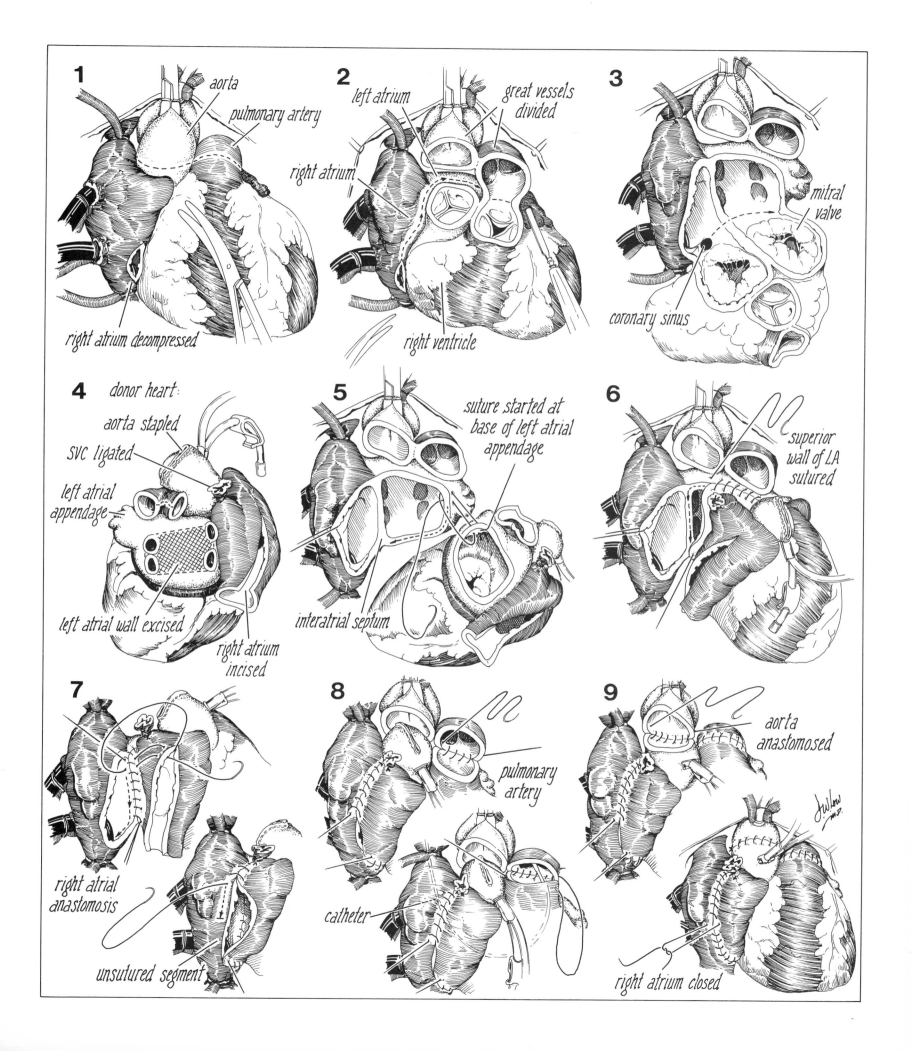

1 aorta — pulmonary artery — right atrium decompressed

2 left atrium — great vessels divided — right atrium — right ventricle

3 mitral valve — coronary sinus

4 donor heart: aorta stapled — SVC ligated — left atrial appendage — left atrial wall excised — right atrium incised

5 suture started at base of left atrial appendage — interatrial septum

6 superior wall of LA sutured

7 right atrial anastomosis — unsutured segment

8 pulmonary artery — catheter

9 aorta anastomosed — right atrium closed

Section 3

Aorta

The various segments of the thoracic aorta may be replaced with prosthetic grafts, but during these operations, the duration of ischemia to the tissues and organs supplied by the various aortic branch vessels must be limited to safe intervals. For aneurysms of the ascending thoracic aorta, full cardiopulmonary bypass is required. Arch aneurysms can be replaced during a period of circulatory arrest at low temperature (20° C) or by using some end-to-side anastomoses so that the ischemic time to the cerebral vessels is limited to only a few minutes. For descending thoracic and thoracoabdominal aneurysms, intraluminal grafts, rapid insertion techniques, Gott shunts, and partial venoarterial bypass are methods used to prevent organ ischemia. All of these techniques will be described and illustrated, but the reader must realize that selection and application of each method or combination of methods must be individualized. The fact that prosthetic grafts are available and can be used to route blood to downstream organs by way of unusual anatomic pathways offers the surgeon imaginative opportunities to solve individual problems created by diseases of the thoracic aorta.

For descriptive purposes, the aorta may be divided into five segments: ascending aorta, arch, descending thoracic, thoracoabdominal and abdominal. The ascending aorta is between the aortic valve and origin of the innominate artery. The aortic arch extends to and includes the origin of the left subclavian artery. The descending thoracic aorta is the segment between the origin of the left subclavian artery and T8 through 10 above the diaphragm. The thoracoabdominal aorta includes the origins of the blood supply to the spinal cord, celiac, superior mesenteric, and renal arteries and describes the segment between T8 through 10 and L2. The abdominal aorta begins below the renal arteries and extends to the aortic bifurcation.

Aneurysms may involve any or all of these segments in virtually any combination because the aorta is one continuous tube and not five anatomically demarcated segments. Because of the importance of their branches, any aneurysm involving the aortic arch or thoracoabdominal aorta is usually labeled as such regardless of its extent into adjacent segments.

Ascending Aortic Aneurysm

Aneurysms of the ascending aorta often involve the aortic annulus and coronary ostia. When the aortic valve is intact and coronary ostia are not involved, however, the proximal suture line can be placed just downstream to the coronary ostia and valve commissures.

(1) The aneurysm is exposed through a midline sternotomy. Prior exposure of the femoral artery and vein in the groin is prudent for large aneurysms that may abut the underside of the sternum. Pericardium generally covers only part of the aneurysm. After the chest is entered, heparin is given and the right atrium and a femoral artery are cannulated.

For false or infected aneurysms, administration of heparin and cannulation of the right internal jugular vein (catheter tip advanced to right atrium), femoral vein, and femoral artery are recommended. Bypass is established and the patient is cooled with the heart beating before the sternum (and aneurysm) is opened.

(2) After bypass is started, the patient is cooled to 28 to 30° C and a catheter is inserted into the right superior pulmonary vein-left atrial junction to vent the left ventricle. During cooling, the pericardial reflection is dissected off the aortic aneurysm and the origin and first centimeter or so of the innominate artery is exposed. As cooling continues, a Crafoord clamp is placed across the aorta just upstream to the origin of the innominate artery. When the heart fibrillates, the heart is arrested with cold cardioplegic solution injected into the aneurysm.

(3) The aneurysm is opened in a longitudinal direction. The valve, coronary ostia, and aortic diameter at the prospective suture lines are inspected.

The prosthetic graft is chosen and prepared before bypass starts. The aortic diameter just beyond the annulus is estimated from the angiogram, and the diameter at the origin of the innominate artery is estimated directly. The woven Dacron graft is preclotted by either forcing nonheparinized blood through the interstices of the graft until coagulation occurs or rinsing the graft in 5% albumin and then placing the soaked graft in the autoclave for 3 minutes. Gross fibrinous material, which could embolize, is removed from the inside of the graft by carefully rinsing in saline.

(4) The proximal anastomosis is made first using a double-ended 3-0 monofilament suture. The first suture is placed outside in through the Dacron graft and then through the medial aortic wall just above the commissure.

(5) The aortic bite proceeds caudad (inside) to cephalad (outside) and is reasonably deep and secure. Stitches continue to develop a continuous posterior suture line to the lateral wall of the aorta.

(6) With the other needle, the anterior suture line is completed, passing the needle deeply through the anterior aortic wall from cephalad (outside) to caudad (inside) and through the graft inside to outside. If the aortic wall is thin, strips of Teflon felt are used to strengthen the suture line. After all loops are tightened, the two ends are tied to complete the anastomosis.

Usually rewarming is started at the beginning of the distal anastomosis. If technical difficulties require renewal of cardioplegic solution, it is injected directly into the coronary ostia using Spencer-Malette catheters.

(7) The distal end of the graft is cut. Because the posterior-medial aortic wall is shorter than the anterior-lateral wall, the graft must be beveled. The distal anastomosis is similarly made with a continuous 3-0 monofilament suture with or without strips of Teflon felt beginning outside (caudad) in (cephalad) on the posteromedial wall of the aorta near the aortic clamp. A Swan-Ganz catheter in the pulmonary artery should be withdrawn into the right atrium to avoid catching the catheter in a stitch.

(8) Before the distal anastomosis is tied down, all air is removed from the left heart and aortic root. Perfusion flow is temporarily reduced with the patient tipped head down as the aortic clamp is removed. The distal suture is tied as blood under low pressure leaks from the suture line. A No. 19 needle is placed in the aorta distal to the anastomosis.

(9) Any leaks in either suture line are closed with individual sutures with or without Teflon pledgets. Bypass is stopped after rewarming is complete, suture lines are secure, and the heart is beating well. The walls of the aneurysm are trimmed and then sutured together over the graft with a continuous stitch. Part of the aneurysmal wall is sent for microscopy.

Routine decannulation and closure of the chest follow.

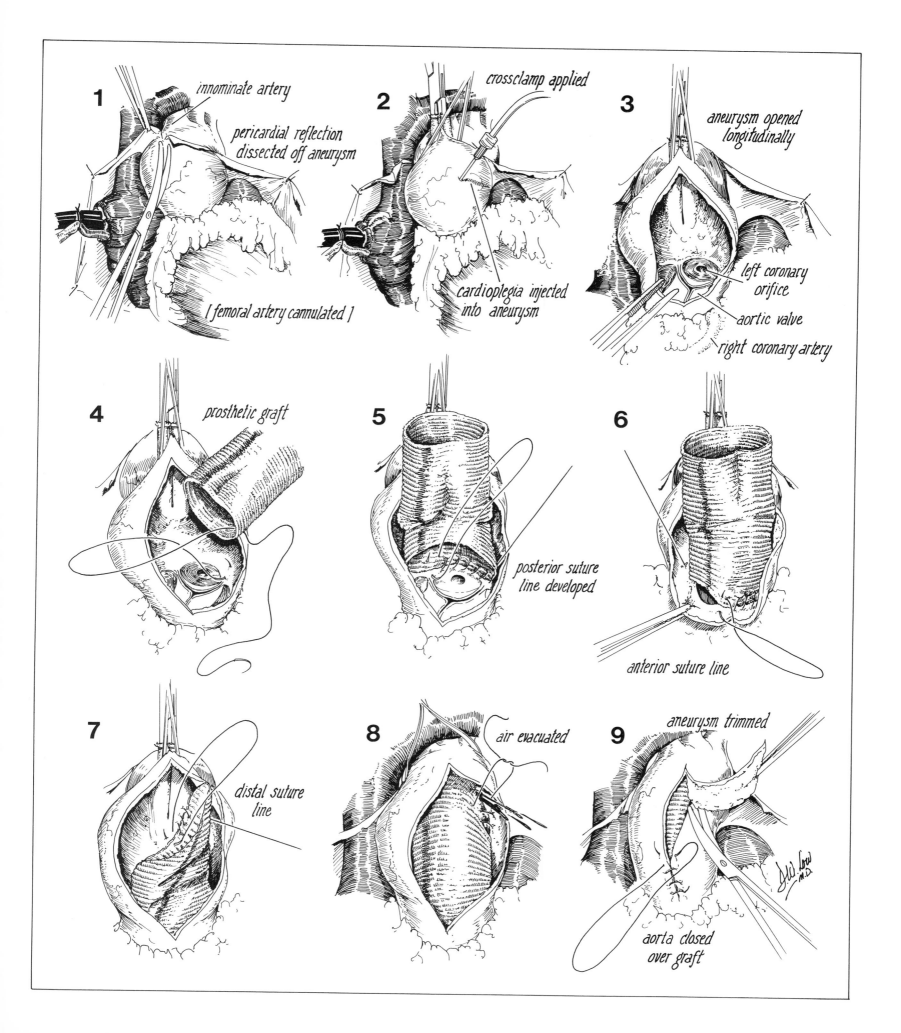

1 innominate artery

pericardial reflection dissected off aneurysm

[femoral artery cannulated]

2 crossclamp applied

cardioplegia injected into aneurysm

3 aneurysm opened longitudinally

left coronary orifice

aortic valve

right coronary artery

4 prosthetic graft

5 posterior suture line developed

6 anterior suture line

7 distal suture line

8 air evacuated

9 aneurysm trimmed

aorta closed over graft

Replacement of Ascending Aorta and Aortic Valve

In this operation, the proximal end of the aortic prosthesis and the aortic prosthetic sewing ring are sutured to the aortic annulus upstream to the coronary ostia. The coronary ostia are sutured to holes made in the prosthetic graft, and the distal end of the graft is anastomosed to the ascending aorta upstream to the innominate artery.

A common femoral artery is exposed through an oblique incision in the groin and prepared for subsequent cannulation. A midline sternotomy is made and the pericardium opened vertically. Pericardial edges are tacked to the wound. A simple purse-string suture is placed in the right atrium, and a second purse-string suture is placed at the junction of the left atrium and right superior pulmonary vein.

1 While the chest is opened, the prosthetic valve is sutured to one end of a preclotted woven Dacron aortic prosthesis. The valve size is slightly smaller than the diameter of the graft (for example, No. 29 valve, No. 30 woven Dacron prosthesis), and either a bioprosthesis or a mechanical valve may be used. Graft and valve size are determined from preoperative angiograms; most patients who require this operation have large aortic annuli. The valve is inserted into the graft. Three fine (4-0 monofilament) sutures are placed equidistant around the circumference of the valve sewing ring and the end of the graft and tied. The sewing ring and graft are sutured together with running sutures to securely anchor the valve within the graft.

2 After heparin, the common femoral artery is cannulated. The right atrium is cannulated, cardiopulmonary bypass is started, and the patient is cooled to 28° C. A left atrial vent catheter is inserted. The aorta is dissected free of the main and right pulmonary arteries, encircled with an umbilical tape, and clamped just upstream to the origin of the innominate artery.

3 The ascending aorta, which is usually aneurysmal, is opened through a vertical incision which is curved slightly toward the noncoronary sinus Valsalva at the aortic root. Cold crystalloid cardioplegic solution is injected through Spencer-Malette catheters into the right and left coronary ostia to achieve cardiac arrest. Simultaneously, the heart is bathed in external cold saline. Cold cardioplegia is renewed every 20 to 25 minutes during the period of cardiac ischemia.

4 The aortic valve is excised. The composite prosthesis is sutured to the aortic annulus with pledgeted 2-0 polyester mattress sutures. Sutures are passed from above downward through the aortic annulus beginning at the commissure between the left and right sinuses of Valsalva. The needles are passed from below upward through both the valvular sewing ring and Dacron graft. The posterior annulus is done first, followed by the right lateral (noncoronary) annulus. The anterior (right coronary) annulus is sutured last. The valve and graft unit is slid into the aortic root and the sutures are tied and cut.

5 The spot on the Dacron prosthesis opposite the left coronary ostium is marked. Gentle downward traction on the heart may be needed to properly align the folded aneurysmal aorta and the prosthetic graft. A 7 to 8 mm hole is burned into the Dacron graft opposite the left coronary ostium with a battery-powered cautery (Storz Instrument Co., St. Louis, MO). The anastomosis is made with a running 4-0 monofilament suture. The first stitch is passed substantially into the aortic wall to exit near, but not within, the coronary ostium on the left side of the coronary ostium.

6 The suture then passes inside out through the graft and is continued as an over-and-over stitch around the posterior edge of the coronary ostium. The opposite end of the same stitch is continued around the anterior superior edge of the coronary ostium to the first stitch. The suture line is tightened using a nerve hook to pull up loose loops and is tied.

7 The ostium of the right coronary artery is sutured to a hole in the Dacron prosthesis in a similar manner using one continuous suture. Rewarming is begun after completing this anastomosis.

8 With the Dacron graft gently pulled straight, excess length is trimmed. Because the length of the posterior wall of the ascending aorta is shorter than the anterior wall, the distal cut is beveled. If the wall of the ascending aorta is thin or friable, a strip of Teflon felt is used to buttress the distal anastomosis. The Swan-Ganz catheter in the pulmonary artery is withdrawn into the right atrium.

A 3-0 monofilament suture is used. The first stitch is passed from proximal to distal aorta (from within the opened vessel) at the medial wall. The suture then passes from inside out, through the graft and felt strip, and is continued as an over-and-over suture along the posterior wall approximately 180 degrees around the circumference. After pulling up loops to tighten the suture line, the opposite needle is used to complete the anterior portion of the anastomosis. Before tying the suture, the heart is filled with blood and all air is evacuated. Perfusion flow is reduced with the patient tipped head down as the aortic clamp is released. The distal suture is tied. A No. 19 needle is inserted into the aorta to remove any residual air.

Any suture line leaks are closed at this time with additional mattress or figure-of-eight sutures. The heart is electrically defibrillated if necessary, but remains decompressed by means of the left atrial vent catheter.

9 Redundant aneurysmal aorta is trimmed and submitted for histologic examination. The host aorta is closed over the Dacron graft with running 3-0 monofilament suture buttressed with Teflon felt strips.

When good cardiac contractions return and rewarming is complete, bypass is discontinued. The femoral arterial cannulation site is repaired with a 5-0 monofilament continuous suture.

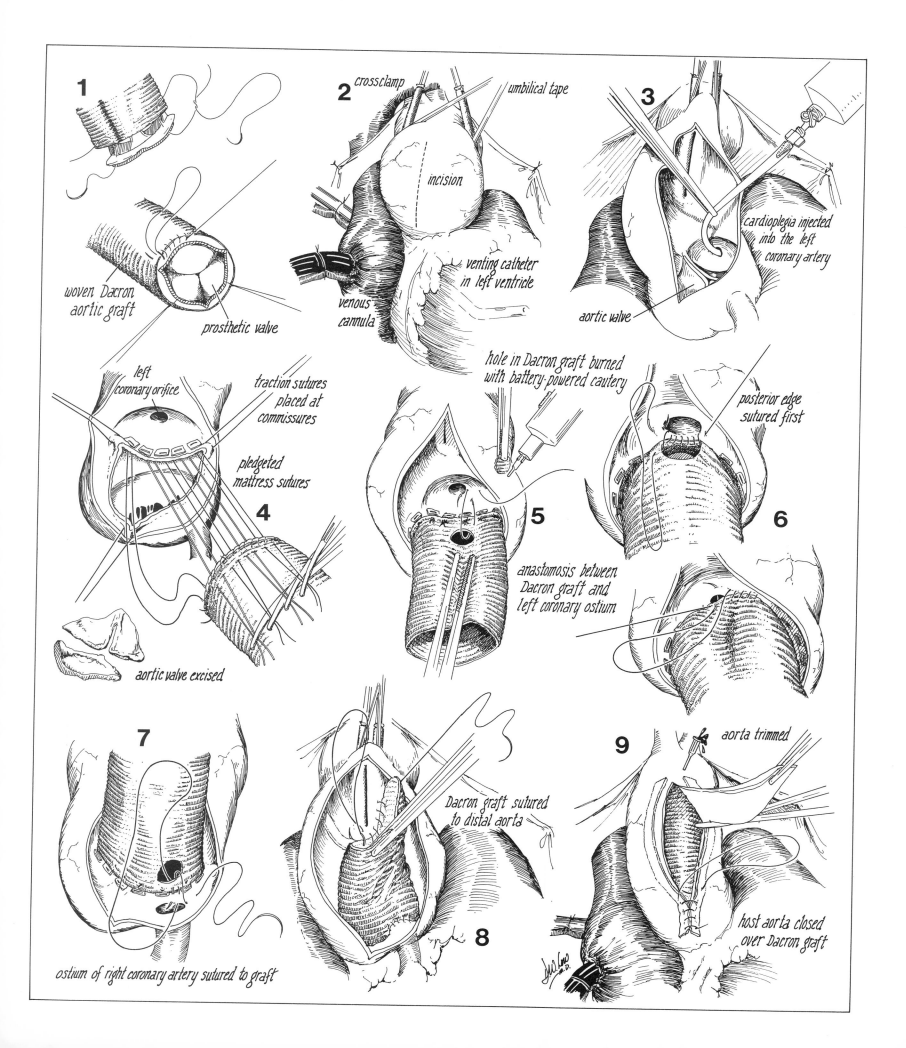

1

woven Dacron
aortic graft

prosthetic valve

2 crossclamp

umbilical tape

incision

venting catheter
in left ventricle

venous
cannula

3

cardioplegia injected
into the left
coronary artery

aortic valve

4

left
coronary orifice

traction sutures
placed at
commissures

pledgeted
mattress sutures

aortic valve excised

5

hole in Dacron graft burned
with battery-powered cautery

anastomosis between
Dacron graft and
left coronary ostium

6

posterior edge
sutured first

7

ostium of right coronary artery sutured to graft

8

Dacron graft sutured
to distal aorta

9

aorta trimmed

host aorta closed
over Dacron graft

Replacement of Aortic Arch

The warm-safe duration of brain ischemia is only 3 to 5 minutes; therefore, resection of the aortic arch requires special techniques. Methods using extracorporeal perfusion of separately cannulated, carotid vessels are no longer used. Best results have been obtained with the combination of deep hypothermia and cardiopulmonary bypass. Alternatively, the aortic arch can be replaced using multiple end-to-side anastomoses.

1 For arch aneurysms that do not extend beyond the ligamentum arteriosum (aortic isthmus), a midline sternotomy provides adequate exposure. This incision may be extended along the anterior border of either the left or right sternocleidomastoid muscle with detachment of the sternal insertion of the muscle to provide additional exposure of the innominate or left carotid and proximal left subclavian artery.

2 If the aneurysm extends beyond the ligamentum arteriosum, a transverse incision is recommended. The patient should be rotated 45 degrees anteriorly with sandbags beneath the left shoulder and hip. This incision is placed in the right fourth intercostal space, and in either the left third or fourth intercostal space, as necessary to provide adequate exposure. Both mammary vessels are ligated and divided, and the sternum is transected horizontally or obliquely to allow the edges of the incision to be retracted widely. If the descending thoracic aortic anastomosis must be made low, a second left thoracotomy incision with resection of the sixth rib is made. The skin and chest wall muscles are reflected off the sixth rib to avoid a second skin incision in the left chest.

After heparin, the femoral artery (usually the left) is cannulated and a large single venous cannula is placed in the right atrium. Cardiopulmonary bypass is started and the patient is cooled to a nasopharyngeal temperature of 18 to 20° C. This usually requires 30 minutes and may be hastened slightly by a high flow rate and vasodilators. A venting catheter is passed through the junction of the left atrium and right superior pulmonary vein into the left ventricle to prevent ventricular distension.

3 While the patient is being cooled, the left pleural cavity is entered and a tape is passed around the proximal descending thoracic aorta distal to the aneurysm. The left phrenic nerve is dissected free and gently retracted laterally; the vagus nerve is retracted medially. The proximal segments of the left subclavian, left carotid, and innominate artery are dissected out and encircled with tapes. Both the left phrenic nerve and innominate vein are protected.

4 As the target temperature is approached, the ascending aorta upstream to the aneurysm is clamped and the heart is vented and decompressed and is completely arrested with cold cardioplegic solution injected into the aortic root. Bulldog clamps are separately applied to the innominate, left carotid and left subclavian vessels as bypass continues briefly. When the descending thoracic aorta is clamped, bypass stops; both the venous and arterial lines are clamped to maintain blood within the patient during the period of arrest.

5 The anterior wall of the arch aneurysm is now opened with a longitudinal incision and blood and any thrombus is removed. The distal anastomosis is made first, placing the preclotted, presized woven Dacron graft within the opened aorta at the junction of the normal aorta and aneurysm. A continuous 2-0 or 3-0 monofilament double-ended suture is used. The posterior suture line is done first.

6 Because the anastomosis is down and away, sutures are placed through the aortic wall from upstream to downstream and then inside to outside through the graft. Often these sutures, placed with a backhand motion, are more easily passed than forehand sutures.

The suture line is continued anteriorly with a forehand stroke, by invaginating the anterior wall of the graft into the distal aorta so that the needle is easily retrieved. After completing the anastomosis, loops are pulled up and the two ends are tied. The completed anastomosis is not tested for leaks at this time.

7 An elliptical hole is cut into the superior margin of the graft with the battery-operated cautery opposite the orifices of the innominate, left carotid and left subclavian arteries. These vessels are sewn to the graft as a unit. The posterior suture line begins at the point opposite the left subclavian artery, passing the needle through the aortic wall toward the orifice of the vessel. The 3-0 monofilament suture passes inside out through the graft. After the posterior row is finished, the anterior row is made passing the needle outside-in through the graft and inside-out through the aortic wall.

8 After pulling up of any slack loops, perfusion is restarted before the anastomotic suture is tied. When the graft is filled with blood and any trapped air is dislodged manually from the orifices of the cerebral vessels, the proximal graft is clamped and the suture is tied. Clamps on the brachiocephalic vessels are removed to restore perfusion. Rewarming now begins. Suture lines are carefully inspected for leaks, which are closed with pledgeted or unpledgeted sutures.

The deep hypothermic intraluminal anastomotic technique requires rapid anastomoses. The safe duration of cerebral ischemia for adults at nasopharyngeal temperatures of 20 to 22° C is not precisely known, but the risk of brain damage increases after 40 minutes of ischemia and there is probably some risk after only 30 minutes of circulatory arrest.

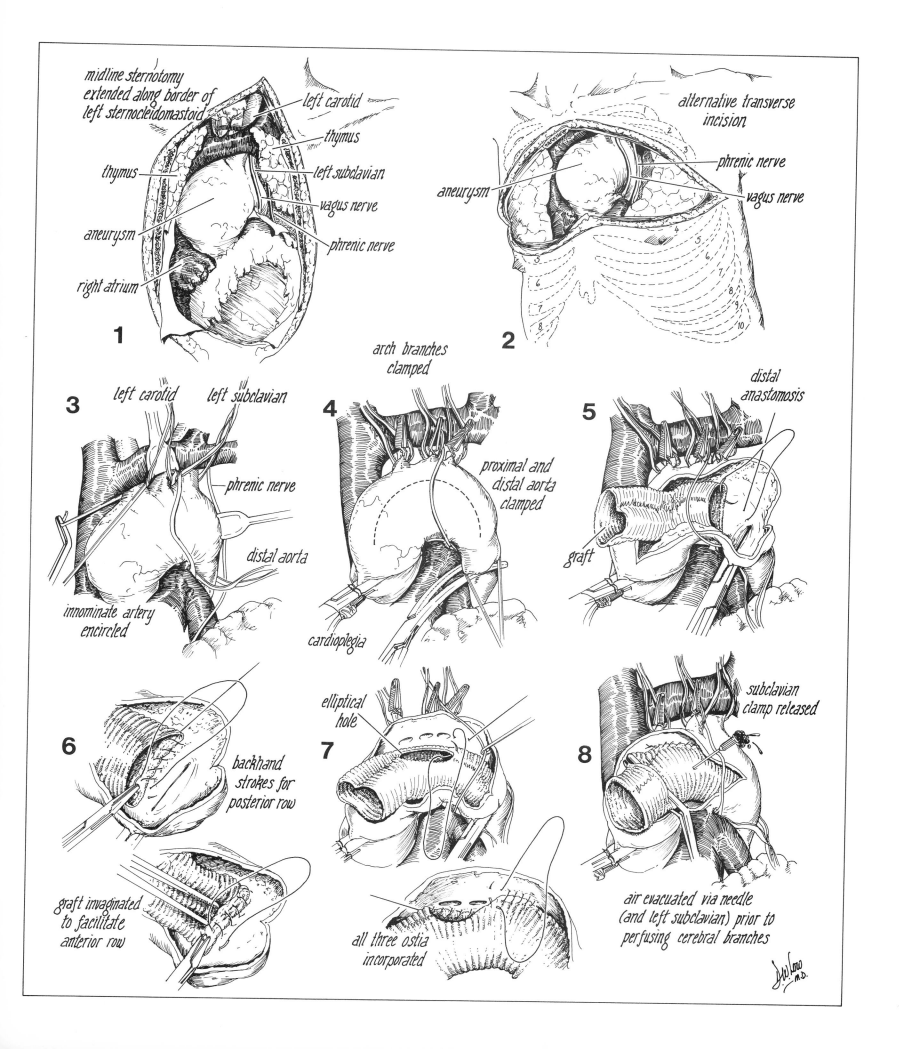

1

midline sternotomy extended along border of left sternocleidomastoid

left carotid

thymus

thymus

left subclavian

vagus nerve

aneurysm

phrenic nerve

right atrium

2

alternative transverse incision

aneurysm

phrenic nerve

vagus nerve

3

left carotid

left subclavian

phrenic nerve

distal aorta

innominate artery encircled

4

arch branches clamped

proximal and distal aorta clamped

cardioplegia

5

distal anastomosis

graft

6

backhand strokes for posterior row

graft invaginated to facilitate anterior row

7

elliptical hole

all three ostia incorporated

8

subclavian clamp released

air evacuated via needle (and left subclavian) prior to perfusing cerebral branches

9 Cold cardioplegia is renewed and the external surface of the heart is bathed with cold saline before the proximal anastomosis is started. The graft is trimmed appropriately. The posterior row is started opposite the surgeon passing the 2-0 or 3-0 monofilament double-ended suture outside in through the graft and from caudad to cephalad through the aortic wall.

10 After the anterior row is completed, the heart is allowed to fill with blood and any air in the left ventricle, atrium, or aortic root is dislodged. It is convenient to slow perfusion flow to decrease blood pressure as the clamp on the graft is released. The anastomotic suture is tied after all air is evacuated; full perfusion flow is resumed.

As rewarming continues, the heart may require defibrillation. Leaks must be closed. The walls of the aneurysm are trimmed and sutured together over the prosthesis.

ALTERNATIVE END-TO-SIDE ANASTOMOSIS

Alternatively, end-to-side anastomoses can be used to replace the aortic arch. This method can be used without cardiopulmonary bypass and produces turned-in vascular stumps, which theoretically and esthetically are less desirable than end-to-end anastomoses. Nevertheless, the method may be useful for special instances.

11 The ascending aorta, arch, and proximal portions of the brachiocephalic vessels and proximal descending thoracic aorta are exposed as previously described by midline sternotomy or bilateral anterior thoracotomy. A preclotted, presized woven Dacron prosthesis is sutured end-to-side to the descending thoracic aorta below the aneurysm or segment of aorta to be replaced. A side-biting Satinsky or similar vascular clamp is used to partially occlude the aorta during construction of the anastomosis. A continuous 2-0 or 3-0 monofilament suture is used. After the anastomosis is tested for leaks, the prosthesis is clamped at the suture line.

12 The proximal ends of the three brachiocephalic vessels are dissected out. Short preclotted 8 to 12 mm diameter segments are now sewn to the superior margin of the arch prosthesis near the proximal brachiocephalic vessels. Continuous 3-0 or 4-0 monofilament sutures are used to construct these prosthesis-to-prosthesis anastomoses, although some surgeons prefer polyester. Holes are made with a battery-powered cautery.

13 The graft to the left subclavian artery is usually made end-to-end because the vessel is usually small and ischemic time is not critical. When this distal anastomosis is completed, air is removed from the arch prosthesis and left subclavian segment and flow is restored to the left arm from the descending thoracic aorta through the distal arch prosthesis.

14 If possible, a side-biting clamp is placed on the left carotid artery so that flow can continue while the anastomosis is made. If the size of the vessel precludes this, the vessel is transected and a rapid end-to-end anastomosis is made. This can usually be done in 5 minutes or less and should not cause brain damage even at 37° C if the other blood supply to the brain is intact. Air is removed and flow is established from the distal prosthetic arch as soon as the anastomosis is completed.

15 The distal anastomosis to the innominate artery may be made end-to-side to the proximal right subclavian artery, end-to-side to the innominate artery, which is partially occluded by a side-biting clamp, or by rapid end-to-end anastomosis to the innominate.

16 A side-biting Satinsky clamp is placed on the ascending aorta below the aneurysm or diseased arch. The arch prosthesis is tailored to fit and then sewn end-to-side to the ascending aorta with a continuous 2-0 or 3-0 monofilament suture. When the clamps are released, the prosthetic and natural aortic arches provide parallel flow to the lower body.

17 The natural arch is transected just beyond the proximal end-to-side anastomosis and oversewn. The thoracic aorta just upstream to the distal end-to-side anastomosis is similarly transected and oversewn. If any end-to-side anastomoses were used for brachiocephalic vessels, the bypassed segments of these vessels are also transected and oversewn. Teflon felt strips may be used to reinforce the oversewn suture lines.

18 The anterior wall of the natural aorta is incised longitudinally. Any bleeding orifices of small anomalous vessels are oversewn. Usually the natural aorta is not completely excised, but part of it is removed for histology and also to permit the prosthetic arch to occupy a more normal position within the chest.

Both methods of replacing the aortic arch risk cerebral ischemia and place unusual time constraints on the surgeon. Although the technique of deep perfusion hypothermia and circulatory arrest requires a long perfusion time to cool and rewarm, operative conditions, the ability to perform intraluminal anastomoses, the absence of vascular turned-in stumps, reduced amount of dissection, generally good results, and low morbidity of bypass favor this method.

Following completion of all arch anastomoses, hemostasis, and stoppage of bypass, the lateral chest incisions are closed. A single drainage catheter is left to drain each opened pleural cavity and the mediastinum. Intercostal muscles are approximated with interrupted 1-0 or 0 absorbable sutures. The cut sternum is reapproximated with wire single and mattress sutures. Remaining chest wall muscles are reapproximated with running absorbable sutures.

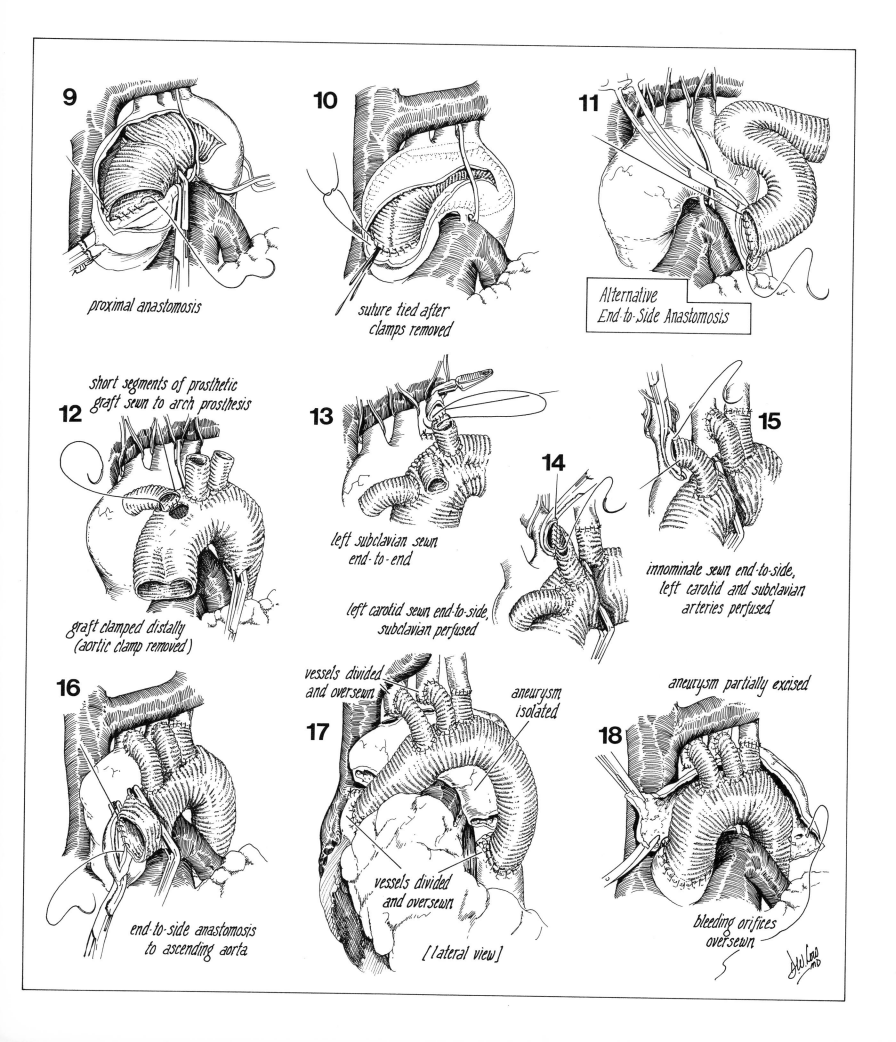

9 proximal anastomosis

10 suture tied after clamps removed

11 Alternative End-to-Side Anastomosis

12 short segments of prosthetic graft sewn to arch prosthesis

graft clamped distally (aortic clamp removed)

13 left subclavian sewn end-to-end

left carotid sewn end-to-side, subclavian perfused

14

15 innominate sewn end-to-side, left carotid and subclavian arteries perfused

16 end-to-side anastomosis to ascending aorta

17 vessels divided and oversewn

aneurysm isolated

vessels divided and oversewn

[lateral view]

18 aneurysm partially excised

bleeding orifices oversewn

Replacement of Descending Thoracic Aorta, Aortic Rupture

The operative techniques described for replacement of the descending thoracic aorta are those used for various congenital and acquired lesions that involve the aortic isthmus, which is the segment of aorta just beyond the origin of the left subclavian artery to which the ligamentum arteriosum attaches. Some of the lesions for which surgery is prescribed include traumatic rupture of the aorta, post-traumatic aneurysm, aneurysm of the ductus arteriosus, adult coarctation, recurrent coarctation, and atherosclerotic aneurysms involving this and often other segments of the aorta.

Occlusion of the proximal descending thoracic aorta causes hypertension in the proximal aorta and hypotension in the lower body. Prolonged lower body hypotension may cause paraplegia; ligation of a critical vessel to the anterior spinal cord above T10 is a rare cause of this complication. Paraplegia has developed after only 18 minutes of distal aortic hypotension; therefore, several different methods have been developed to reduce the incidence of this complication during resection of the descending thoracic aorta. The use of an intraluminal aortic prosthesis, Gott shunt, left heart bypass, partial bypass and rapid anastomosis without shunt or bypass are illustrated.

Both femoral and radial arterial pressures are monitored continuously during operation and vasodilators are available to control proximal hypertension. Evoked potentials of the spinal cord are not monitored.

The patient is positioned for either a straight lateral thoracotomy or an anterolateral thoracotomy if a Gott shunt is used. A posterolateral incision with resection of the fourth rib gives excellent exposure of the proximal portion of the descending thoracic aorta. If a long segment of aorta must be replaced, a second rib, usually the seventh or eighth, is removed through the single skin incision. Tapes are passed around the left subclavian artery, the aortic arch between the left subclavian and left carotid arteries, and the descending thoracic aorta below the aneurysm or diseased segment. The diameter of the aortic prosthesis is chosen and, if necessary, the graft is preclotted.

1 The intraluminal aortic prosthesis permits replacement of an aortic segment with no anastomotic suture lines. The commercially available prosthesis consists of a woven Dacron tube of varying length and diameter, fitted with a semi-rigid ring at either end. The napkin ring ends are designed to fit inside the host aorta, which is then tied tightly around the slightly concave center portion of the ring with Teflon umbilical tapes. The diameter and length of the intraluminal aortic prosthesis are chosen after the descending thoracic aorta is exposed, but before it is opened. Because the adult aorta lacks elasticity and cannot be stretched, the prosthesis chosen must be small enough that the napkin-ring ends can be easily inserted into the host aorta above and below the diseased segment. The advantage of the intraluminal prosthesis is rapid insertion, which precludes the need for measures to avoid lower body hypotension. Teflon umbilical tapes at the planned locations of the intraluminal napkin-rings are passed around the aorta. Tapes for the aortic clamps are also placed. Intercostal vessels to the diseased aortic segment are ligated. The prosthesis is preclotted.

2 Vascular clamps are placed on the distal aortic arch, left subclavian, and descending thoracic aorta below the diseased segment. The aorta is opened longitudinally and bleeding intercostal vessels are oversewn.

3 The preselected intraluminal prosthesis is inserted into the proximal aorta below the clamp and above the top of the aortotomy. The Teflon umbilical tape, which has been previously placed, is tied around the aorta against the saddle of the semi-rigid ring.

4 The distal ring is inserted into the distal aorta below the lesion and similarly tied in place. The distal aortic clamp is released and any trapped air within the graft escapes through the pores of the graft or a needle placed in the graft. The proximal clamp is released slowly to avoid sudden hypotension.

5 With proper exposure and judicious selection of ring diameter and graft length, these prostheses can be inserted during 5 to 10 minutes of aortic clamping. A second tape is often passed around each ring and tied for insurance. The host aorta, after trimming, is closed over the intraluminal prosthesis with a running suture. These prostheses can be used to replace other segments of the aorta; however, they are not wholly satisfactory for dissecting aneurysms involving the ascending aorta.

INSERTION SITES FOR THE GOTT SHUNT

6 The Gott shunt is a polyvinyl tube tapered at either end. The inside surface is coated with a surface-bound heparin complex. One end of the shunt is inserted into the apex of the left ventricle or into the ascending aorta, which requires extension of the thoracotomy incision anteriorly to expose. The other end is inserted into the descending thoracic aorta below the diseased segment or in the left femoral artery exposed in the groin. Gott shunts are available in two sizes. With the shunt open, the aorta may be safely clamped for resection of the aneurysm.

LEFT HEART BYPASS

7 Left heart bypass requires systemic heparin. One cannula is inserted into the left atrial appendage or in the apex of the left ventricle, and the in-flow cannula is inserted into the descending thoracic aorta or the left femoral artery. No oxygenator is included in the system.

PARTIAL CARDIOPULMONARY BYPASS

8 Partial cardiopulmonary bypass also requires systemic heparin, but includes an oxygenator in the circuit. Usually, the venous and arterial cannulas are inserted into the left femoral or external iliac vessels, which are exposed through a retroperitoneal dissection from an oblique incision just above the inguinal ligament

The opened Gott shunt or operating left or partial bypass systems provide perfusion of the lower body during the period of aortic crossclamping. Use of these systems requires additional dissection and operating time and systemic heparin for the bypass systems. These systems, however, permit the aortic anastomoses to be made without time constraints.

A descending thoracic aortic prosthesis may be inserted without shunts or bypass. The surgical technique is the same as when a shunt is used; however, the anastomoses must be made rapidly to minimize the duration of aortic crossclamping. A cell saver or autotransfusion system is used to return shed blood. The selected woven Dacron prosthesis is preclotted. Proximal hypertension during aortic clamping must be controlled pharmacologically.

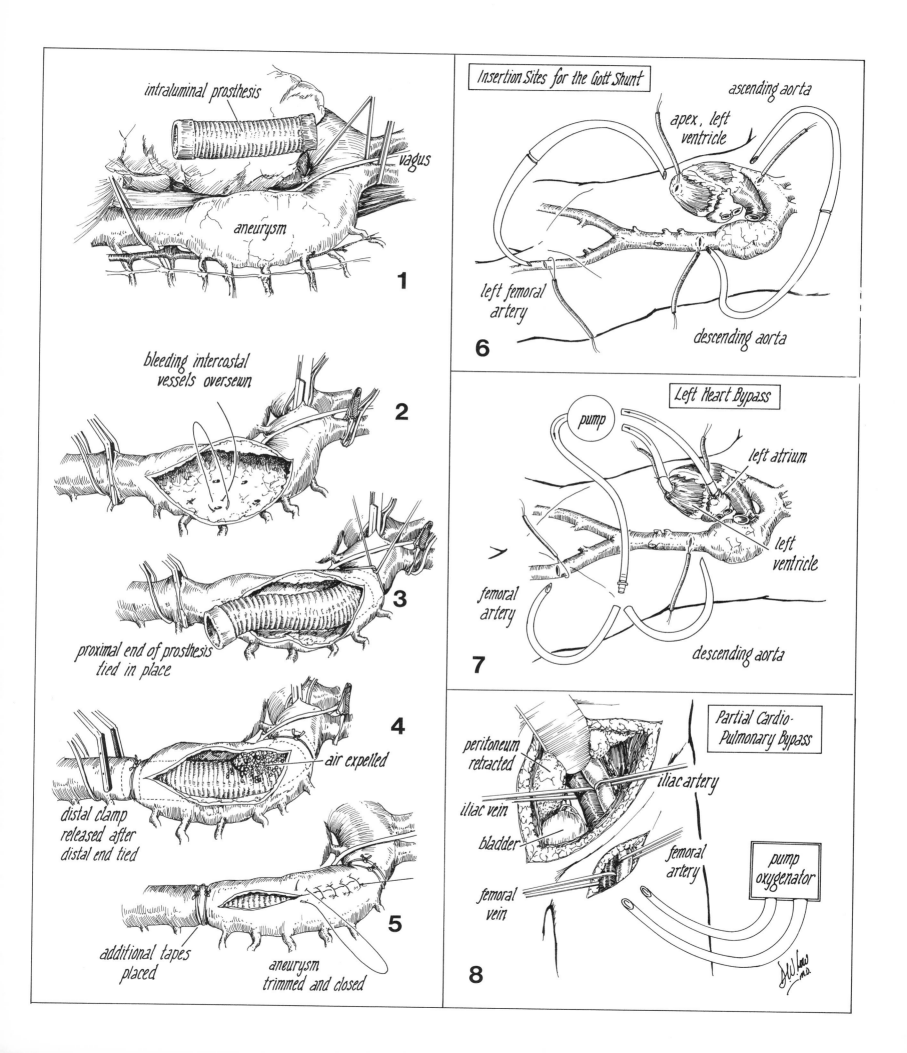

1
intraluminal prosthesis
vagus
aneurysm

2
bleeding intercostal
vessels oversewn

3
proximal end of prosthesis
tied in place

4
air expelled
distal clamp
released after
distal end tied

5
additional tapes
placed
aneurysm
trimmed and closed

6
Insertion Sites for the Gott Shunt
apex, left
ventricle
ascending aorta
left femoral
artery
descending aorta

7
Left Heart Bypass
pump
left atrium
left
ventricle
femoral
artery
descending aorta

8
Partial Cardio-
Pulmonary Bypass
peritoneum
retracted
iliac artery
iliac vein
bladder
femoral
artery
femoral
vein
pump
oxygenator

9 The distal aortic arch is clamped with a Fogarty or Crafoord clamp. The aorta is transected above the diseased segment for an end-to-end anastomosis to the preclotted woven Dacron graft. A large bulldog clamp is placed across the distal diseased aorta to reduce bleeding from intercostal arteries.

10 A continuous 2-0 or 3-0 double-ended monofilament suture is used. The needle is passed outside in through the prosthesis and inside out through the proximal transected aorta on the medial wall of the aorta. When the needle again passes through the prosthesis outside in and the suture is tightened, the posterior row is easily completed as a continuous over-and-over suture.

11 The anterior part of the anastomosis is made similarly, using the opposite needle and passing the suture outside in through the aorta and inside out through the prosthesis. Loops are tightened and the two ends are tied. The anastomosis is tested for leaks by releasing the aortic clamp and clamping the prosthesis. The aortic clamp is replaced to avoid clot formation in the proximal portion of the prosthesis while the distal anastomosis is made.

12 The distal anastomosis is made similarly. The suture starts outside in through the medial wall of the distal aorta and passes inside out through the prosthesis. After the second stitch through the aortic wall, the surgeon can easily pass the needle through the prosthesis and aortic wall in one stroke. This anastomosis is tested by releasing the distal aortic clamp; if no leaks are present, the proximal clamp is released slowly.

13 The bypassed segment of diseased aorta may be excised after each intercostal artery is ligated. Usually the segment is opened longitudinally, and the orifices of bleeding intercostal arteries are oversewn.

14 The native aorta is sutured around the prosthesis, as is done when the aorta is not transected and an intraluminal prosthesis or intraluminal anastomosis is used.

15 The woven Dacron prosthesis may also be inserted by intraluminal anastomoses. The diseased segment is isolated by aortic clamps and opened longitudinally. Bleeding intercostal vessels that have not been ligated before the aortotomy are oversewn.

16 The preclotted graft is sutured to the posteromedial aortic wall with a continuous over-and-over 3-0 monofilament suture. The anastomosis begins on the medial wall as illustrated. The anterior wall is completed using the opposite needle. The distal anastomosis is made in a similar manner. The needle passes through the distal aortic wall cephalad to caudad and then through the prosthesis inside to outside. The graft is covered with the aneurysmal wall (see 14) after the clamps are removed and leaks are controlled.

The chest is closed with one chest tube for drainage. Usually the mediastinal pleura is not closed over the aorta. If two ribs have been resected, both incisions are closed with interrupted 0 or No. 1 absorbable sutures. Reflected chest wall muscles are reattached with interrupted sutures. Remaining transected chest wall muscles are closed with continuous absorbable sutures.

AORTIC RUPTURE

Most traumatic tears of the aorta in patients who survive the initial injury occur at or near the aortic isthmus near the insertion of the ligamentum arteriosum. Many of these patients have other injuries, including head injuries; therefore systemic heparin may be contraindicated

The patient is positioned on his right side for a straight posterolateral thoracotomy incision. A right radial arterial, a femoral arterial, and a central venous catheter and the electrocardiogram are necessary for intraoperative monitoring. An autotransfusion or cell-saver system is desirable. The chest is entered after excision of the fourth rib.

17 The left lung is gently retracted forward. If a Robertshaw divided endotracheal tube has been passed, the left lung is collapsed. The aorta below the tear is exposed and encircled with a cloth tape. The apex of the left lung is retracted downward to permit identification of the left subclavian artery. This vessel is followed to the aorta. The mediastinal pleura between the left carotid and left subclavian arteries is opened, and a clamp and tape are gently passed around the distal aortic arch upstream to the left subclavian artery and torn aorta. A bulldog clamp is placed on the left subclavian artery.

18 The aorta above and below the isthmus is clamped and the mediastinal pleura over the isthmus is incised. Often, extravasated blood surrounds the isthmus. The aorta is inspected, and although the adventitial bulge can be easily found, the exact site of the transverse intimal tear cannot. Therefore, a short prosthesis with two anastomotic suture lines is usually required for repair.

19 The aorta is transected and then recut across normal aorta at or slightly above the intimal tear. The distal aorta just below the tear is transected similarly. The short preclotted prosthesis is rapidly sutured to the two cut ends with running 3-0 monofilament suture. With good exposure, the two anastomoses can be completed rapidly since the untorn aorta is normal and the graft is short.

In most instances, left heart or partial cardiopulmonary bypass is not used for repair of traumatic rupture of the aorta. Systemic heparin and the longer operation are often contraindicated by other associated injuries. An intraluminal prosthesis can be used, but necessarily the semi-rigid rings narrow the lumen of the aorta below the diameter of the normal aorta. Most often, the repair is made by rapid anastomosis; occasionally a Gott shunt is used.

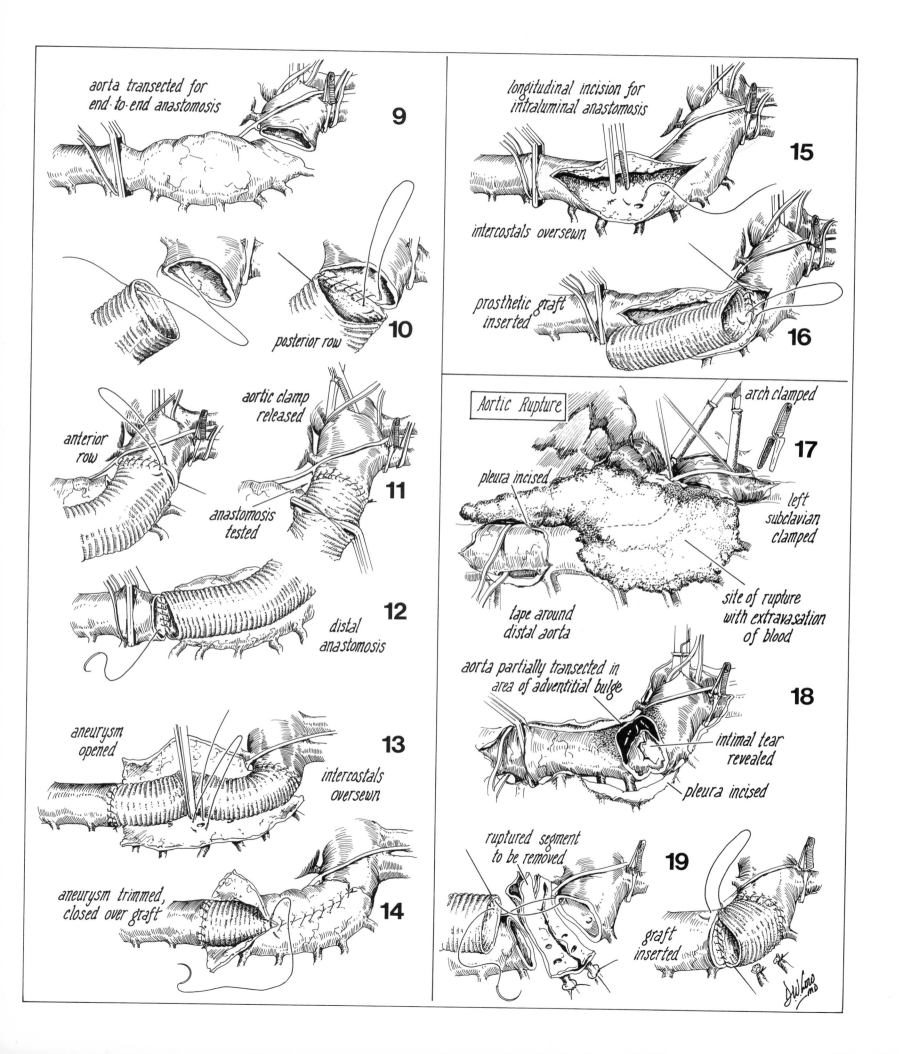

Saccular Aneurysm, Adult Coarctation

Saccular aneurysms by definition involve one wall rather than the entire circumference of the aorta, and therefore do not necessarily require resection. Some saccular aneurysms may be excised with direct closure of the aortic wall; others require insertion of a woven Dacron patch. Insertion of an intraluminal prosthesis or replacement of a segment of the aorta are other alternatives to the management of a saccular aneurysm.

The use of cardiopulmonary bypass or variations of bypass is optional. Bypass may be helpful in the treatment of saccular aneurysms of the ascending aorta or arch, particularly if patch closure is required. Saccular aneurysms of the descending thoracic aorta are usually managed within the safe time limits of aortic crossclamping.

SACCULAR ANEURYSM

1 Because saccular aneurysms may contain thrombus, embolization must be prevented. Clamps may be placed above and below the aneurysm before it is opened, or it may be opened as a previously positioned side-biting clamp is closed over the neck of the aneurysm.

2 If the anatomy of the aneurysm permits, the majority of the aneurysm is excised and the edges are closed flush with aortic wall with a continuous 3-0 monofilament suture. Usually a running mattress suture buttressed with Teflon felt strips followed by an over-and-over continuous suture is used. This relatively simple and safe operation is particularly applicable for elderly patients. Often the site of the aneurysm is wrapped circumferentially with a segment of woven Dacron to help strengthen the aortic wall.

3 When the neck of the saccular aneurysm is large, the segment of aorta containing the aneurysm is isolated between clamps. The aneurysm is opened wide and trimmed back to the normal aortic wall. The patch of preclotted woven Dacron is cut to size, leaving 3 to 4 mm around the edge for sewing. The patch is inserted with a single 3-0 monofilament suture. Teflon felt strips may be used to strengthen the aortic wall if necessary. After the anastomosis is completed, the distal clamp is removed first to express air trapped in the aortic segment and to identify leaks. The proximal clamp is released slowly.

ADULT COARCTATION

The amount of collateral circulation between the upper and lower body in adults with coarctation of the aorta varies, but is often considerable. If the narrowing is not severe, however, as may be the case in patients with recoarctation, collaterals may not be sufficient to ensure perfusion of the lower body during aortic clamping. Collaterals arise from branches of the subclavian arteries.

Adult coarctation differs from juvenile or infant coarctation primarily in the inelasticity of the aorta. In adults, the development of aneurysmal dilatation of the aorta below the coarctation, atherosclerotic changes in the aortic wall, and the occurrence of thin-walled aneuryms at the origin of one or more intercostal arteries below the coarctation make the need for a prosthesis more likely.

A posterolateral thoracotomy incision is made and the fourth rib is excised. If collateral vessels are poorly developed, a Gott shunt is placed in the left ventricular apex and in the descending thoracic aorta to provide blood to the lower body while the aorta is clamped. Dissection of the isthmus may be difficult because of fibrous tissue, and rupture of the thin-walled aorta or an intercostal aneurysm may occur. Tapes should be passed around the aorta above and below the pathologic segment before this segment is dissected out. If a Gott shunt is used, this should be placed and opened before the coarcted segment is dissected. A cell saver or autotransfusion system is recommended.

4 The mediastinal pleura over the aortic isthmus, proximal descending thoracic aorta, and proximal left subclavian artery is incised and the highest thoracic vein is ligated and divided. If one or more left intercostal arteries are aneurysmal, these aneurysmal walls are often thin, and bleeding can be torrential from either end if rupture occurs.

5 The normal aorta below the coarctation and post-stenotic dilated segment is dissected out and encircled with a cloth tape. The proximal left subclavian artery is also dissected out. A clamp is passed around the aorta between the left subclavian and left carotid arteries, and the aorta here is encircled with a tape.

6 The coarcted segment is dissected free; the ligamentum arteriosum and recurrent laryngeal nerve are identified. Intercostal vessels are dissected out and the peripheral ends of those that will be excised with the coarctation are ligated. Clamps are placed above and below the coarcted segment 2 to 3 cm away from the proposed line of resection. Occlusion of the left subclavian artery reduces collateral flow and may mandate use of a Gott shunt.

7 The ligamentum arteriosum is divided first and the pulmonary arterial end is oversewn with 3-0 monofilament suture. The aorta is transected obliquely just above the coarctation so that the cross-sectional area is similar to that of the distal arch and descending thoracic aorta. The coarctation and part of the dilated post-stenotic aorta are transected.

8 A segment of preclotted woven Dacron is inserted between the two ends with continuous 3-0 monofilament suture. The proximal end is done first. The end-to-end anastomosis begins at the medial wall of the distal end of prosthesis. The suture passes outside in and then inside out of the adjacent proximal aorta. This sets up an easy over-and-over continuous suture line for the posterior anastomosis. The anterior suture line is completed with the other end of the double-ended suture. The distal anastomosis is made in a similar manner. Strips of Teflon felt may be incorporated in the anastomosis if the distal aortic wall is thin.

ALTERNATIVES TO RESECTION

9 Alternatively, a preclotted woven Dacron or polyfluoro-tetraethylene patch may be used to widen the coarcted segment. After clamps are applied, the coarcted aorta is incised longitudinally. The patch is cut to fit and sewn to the edges of the aortic wall with running 3-0 monofilament suture. Any membranous portion of the coarcted aorta is excised before the graft is placed.

10 If the proximal aorta between the left subclavian and isthmic narrowing is long enough and of sufficient diameter, an intraluminal tube graft can be inserted. Usually these prostheses cannot be easily inserted without compromising the orifice of the left subclavian artery or the diameter of the aortic isthmus.

11 Although not elegant, placement of a bypass graft around a densely fibrosed, aneurysmal recoarctation may be a safer option than resection and graft reconstruction. A side-biting clamp is applied to the left subclavian-aortic junction and a preclotted woven Dacron graft is sutured to the edges of a longitudinal incision in the lateral-superior aortic wall. The distal end of the Dacron graft is sutured to the edges of a longitudinal incision in the lateral aortic wall below the coarctation. If large intercostal aneurysms are present or if aneurysmal dilation of the postcoarctation segment has occurred, the coarcted aneurysmal segment of the aorta should be isolated from the circulation to reduce the risk of late rupture and hemorrhage.

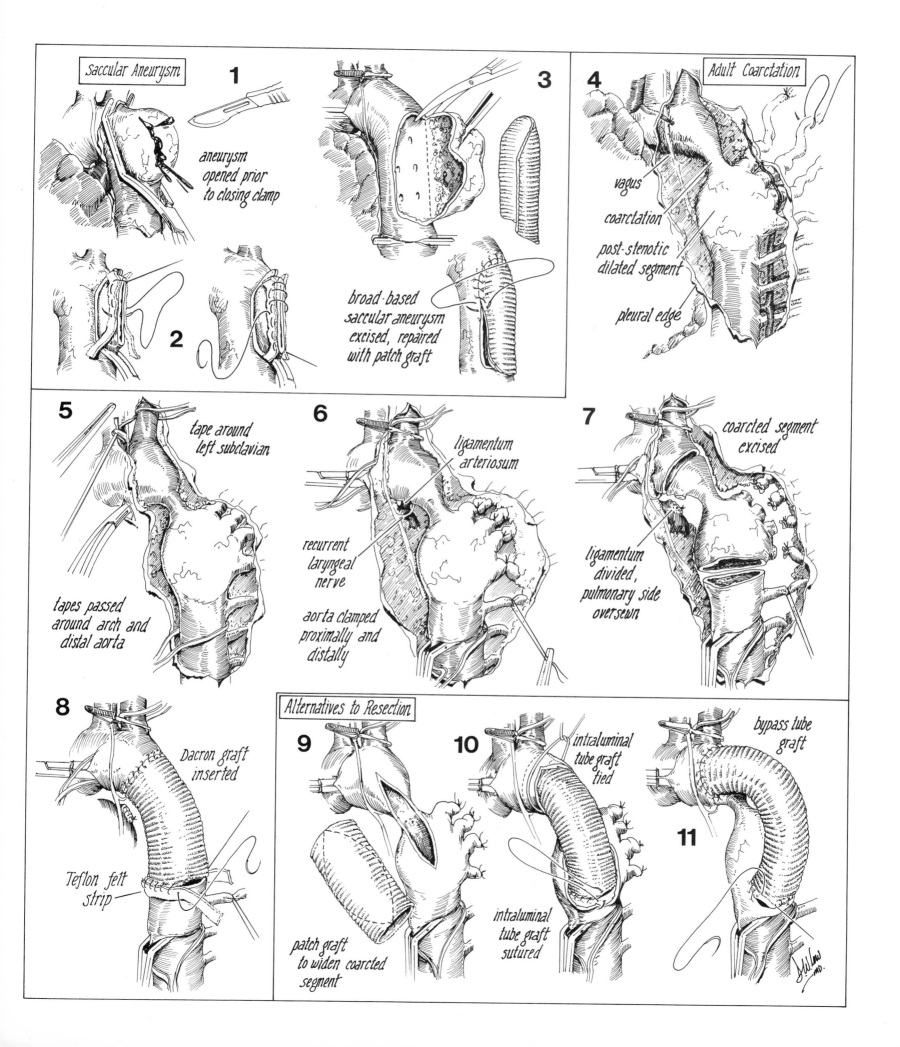

Saccular Aneurysm

1 aneurysm opened prior to closing clamp

2

3 broad-based saccular aneurysm excised, repaired with patch graft

Adult Coarctation

4 vagus
coarctation
post-stenotic dilated segment
pleural edge

5 tape around left subclavian
tapes passed around arch and distal aorta

6 ligamentum arteriosum
recurrent laryngeal nerve
aorta clamped proximally and distally

7 coarcted segment excised
ligamentum divided, pulmonary side oversewn

8 Dacron graft inserted
Teflon felt strip

Alternatives to Resection

9 patch graft to widen coarcted segment

10 intraluminal tube graft tied
intraluminal tube graft sutured

11 bypass tube graft

Thoracoabdominal Aortic Aneurysm

Thoracoabdominal aneurysms may extend from the left subclavian artery to the bifurcation of the abdominal aorta or involve smaller segments of the aorta above and below the diaphragm. The celiac, superior mesenteric, both renal arteries, and the blood supply to the lumbar segment of the spinal cord (arteria radicularis magna; artery of Adamciewicz) arise from the thoracoabdominal aorta.

The thoracoabdominal aorta is exposed from the left side through a thoracoabdominal incision, which is varied depending upon the length and location of aorta to be replaced. The patient is intubated with a Robertshaw divided endotracheal tube and positioned partially on the right side midway between straight lateral and supine (about 45 degrees). Sandbags are placed beneath the left hip and shoulder and the left arm is placed anteriorly across the face and neck. The electrocardiogram and the right radial arterial and central venous pressures (by means of a Swan-Ganz catheter placed in the pulmonary artery) are monitored. A cell saver is used.

1 A full thoracotomy incision, resecting one of the sixth through ninth ribs as determined by the proximal extent of the aneurysm, is made. Low thoracic incisions (eighth or ninth rib) may be extended obliquely across the costal margin and continued obliquely across the upper abdomen to provide exposure of the upper abdominal aorta. For the longer aneurysms, the higher thoracotomy incision is carried across the costal margin and continued as a left paramedian or midline incision to a point just above the pubis. If the aneurysm extends to the aortic isthmus proximally, exposure can be improved by removing the fourth and seventh ribs, leaving the fifth and sixth in place. Both ribs can be removed through the same skin incision and the chest wall muscles over the fourth rib are lifted off the chest wall and retracted rather than cut. Placement of the chest retractor in the upper incision exposes the proximal descending thoracic aorta; placement in the lower incision exposes the most distal thoracic aorta.

2 The peritoneal cavity is NOT entered. The plane between the peritoneum and abdominal wall is carefully developed laterally, and by a combination of blunt and sharp dissection, the abdominal contents, left colon, and left kidney and adrenal gland are reflected off the lateral and posterior abdominal walls toward the right. The diaphragm is incised either radially to the aorta hiatus or circumferentially from the costal margin to the aorta hiatus. A 1 cm cuff or diaphragm is left attached to the chest and abdominal wall if the circumferential incision is used. Extraperitoneal reflection of the viscera off the left psoas muscle exposes the left lateral wall of the thoracoabdominal aorta, which may be surrounded by some retroperitoneal fat. It is possible to expose the entire descending thoracoabdominal aorta from the left subclavian to the aortic bifurcation through this incision.

At this point, one of three methods can be used to protect the kidneys, intestines, and spinal cord from ischemic injury while the thoracoabdominal aorta is replaced. Crawford has developed a highly successful intraluminal technique that requires rapid anastomoses, but that provides excellent exposure for each anastomosis. Alternatively, left heart bypass from the apex of the left ventricle to a femoral artery may be used. Left heart or partial cardiopulmonary bypass, which requires an oxygenator, requires systemic heparin. A Gott surface-bound heparinized shunt may be used instead of left heart or partial bypass to protect distal organs from ischemia while proximal anastomoses are made. The third method uses end-to-side anastomoses of the graft to the aorta above and below the aneurysm. Once this parallel graft is in place, separate woven Dacron grafts can be placed to individual aortic branch vessels one at a time. After all anastomoses are completed, the natural aorta is transected near each end-to-side anastomosis and turned in.

3 The intraluminal method will be described first. Tapes are passed around the aorta above and below the aneurysm. The woven Dacron graft has previously been selected according to the diameters of the aorta at the planned proximal and distal anastomoses and preclotted. Clamps are placed across the proximal and distal aorta and across each exposed major branch. The aneurysm is opened longitudinally just below the planned proximal anastomosis. Any bleeding intercostal vessels are oversewn.

4 The prosthetic graft is sewn to the proximal aorta using a continuous 3-0 monofilament suture. After this anastomosis is completed, the graft is clamped and the aortic clamp is removed. Any leaks are sutured closed.

5 Opposite the celiac artery, a hole is made in the prosthesis with the battery-operated cautery.

6 The ostium of the celiac artery is sutured to the Dacron graft around the hole with running 3-0 monofilament suture.

7 The ostium of the superior mesenteric vessel is similarly sutured to a second hole in the graft. If a large intercostal vessel is encountered between T10 and L2, it too is sutured to a hole in the prosthesis in hope of preserving the blood supply to the spinal cord.

8 After completing the superior mesenteric anastomosis, the clamp on the prosthesis is moved down to restore blood flow to the abdominal viscera.

9 The renal arteries are next anastomosed to the graft. Often it is not feasible to dissect out the right renal artery. To control back-bleeding, a small Fogarty catheter (No. 3 or 4) is inserted into the ostium and removed after the anastomosis is nearly completed.

10 The left renal artery anastomosis is made last. Although the excellent exposure permits rapid suturing, the method requires completion of the proximal aortic anastomosis and 4 or 5 branch anastomoses within 40 to 60 minutes, which is the safe duration of warm ischemia for kidneys.

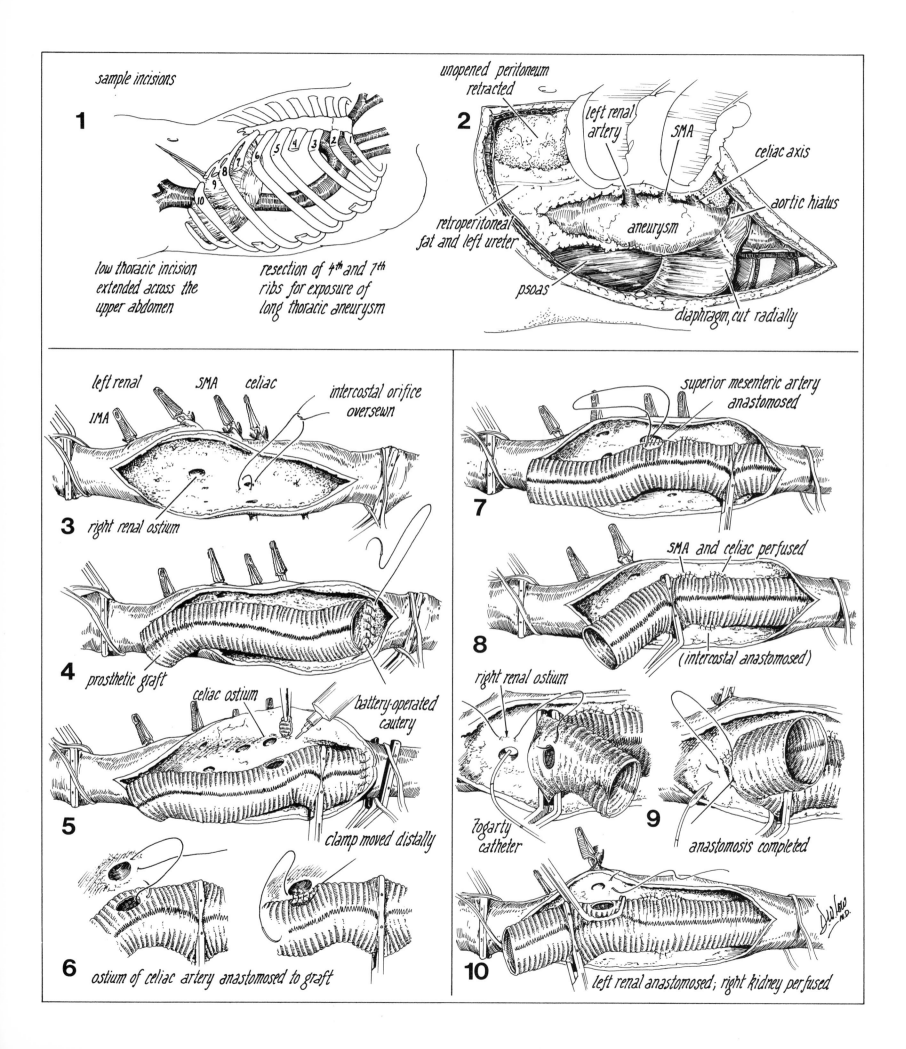

1 sample incisions

low thoracic incision extended across the upper abdomen

resection of 4th and 7th ribs for exposure of long thoracic aneurysm

2 unopened peritoneum retracted

left renal artery

SMA

celiac axis

aortic hiatus

aneurysm

retroperitoneal fat and left ureter

psoas

diaphragm, cut radially

3 left renal

IMA

SMA

celiac

intercostal orifice oversewn

right renal ostium

4 prosthetic graft

5 celiac ostium

battery-operated cautery

clamp moved distally

6 ostium of celiac artery anastomosed to graft

7 superior mesenteric artery anastomosed

8 SMA and celiac perfused

(intercostal anastomosed)

9 right renal ostium

Fogarty catheter

anastomosis completed

10 left renal anastomosed; right kidney perfused

(11) Anastomosis of the inferior mesenteric vessel to the graft is optional. The distal anastomosis is made last, and after removal of all clamps, it restores blood flow to the pelvic organs and legs. It is wise to release the last aortic clamp slowly to avoid precipitous hypotension and excessive washout of potassium and acid metabolites.

During resection of thoracoabdominal aneurysms, the anesthesiologist must control blood pressure in the upper body with appropriate vasodilators. The use of autotransfusion to recover lost red cells is advisable. The time constraints that this method imposes on the surgeon require careful management of blood volume, and replacement and careful management of cardiac performance.

When left heart bypass or a Gott shunt is used, perfusion of the viscera and kidneys continues from below while each anastomosis is performed. The intraluminal technique can still be used. Left heart bypass and the Gott shunt require cannulation of the left ventricle because it is not feasible to cannulate the left atrium or ascending aorta from a sixth rib thoracotomy incision.

(12) To cannulate the left ventricle of the beating heart, the pericardium is opened over the apex. A purse-string suture of 0 or 2-0 polyester is placed in the bare area of the apex just to the left of the distal left anterior descending coronary artery. Often the loops of this suture are buttressed with Teflon felt pledgets. A stab wound is made and the cannula is inserted a distance of 2 cm parallel to the longitudinal axis of the heart. The purse-string is drawn up, held with a tourniquet choke, and secured. After all air is removed from the system, the arterial cannula is inserted into the left femoral artery, which is exposed by an incision over the vessel. When partial cardiopulmonary bypass is used, both common femoral vessels are cannulated. Although the Gott shunt does not require systemic heparin, usually 0.5 to 1.0 mg/kg is given to ensure that the shunt does not clot during use. Blood losses are increased when systemic heparin is used; therefore, a method to recover and reinfuse shed red cells is recommended.

(13) Use of end-to-side anastomoses does not impose the time constraints of the intraluminal technique and does not add the problems of left heart or partial bypass, but does require additional suture lines. The graft is first anastomosed to the proximal aorta above the aneurysm. A side-biting clamp on the anterior or lateral aorta near the left subclavian artery is placed, and a continuous 3-0 monofilament suture is used. The distal end of the graft is sutured end-to-side to the distal abdominal aorta or the proximal left common iliac artery. Flow is established through the graft.

(14) The proximal end of the aorta below the graft anastomosis and above the aneurysm is clamped. Temporary bulldog clamps are placed on the celiac, superior mesenteric, and left renal arteries, and the distal aorta is clamped while the aneurysm is opened longitudinally to a point opposite the ostium of the celiac artery. Potential embolic material is removed from the aneurysm, and bleeding intercostal vessels are sutured closed.

(15) The aorta is clamped just distal to the celiac artery, and the temporary clamps on the distal aorta and the left renal and superior mesenteric vessels are removed to restore perfusion of these vessels. The celiac artery is anastomosed to the graft using the intraluminal technique. Blood flow is restored to the celiac artery and then the mesenteric and both renal arteries are connected to the graft in turn.

After completion of the visceral anastomoses, the surgeon may elect to convert the proximal and distal end-to-side anastomoses to end-to-end anastomoses, or to transect the ends of the aneurysm and turn in the segment of aorta between the line of transection and the end-to-side anastomosis.

CONVERSION OF END-TO-END ANASTOMOSIS

(16) If conversion to an end-to-end anastomosis is chosen, the aorta is clamped proximal to the proximal end-to-side anastomosis. The graft is transected, leaving a small cuff for later closure.

(17) The end of the graft is then sewn end-to-end to the lumen of the proximal aorta with a continuous 3-0 monofilament suture. If the proximal segment of descending thoracic aorta is long enough, the aorta may be transected just above the end-to-side anastomosis and sutured end-to-end at this level. If the anastomosis is below the cuff, it is closed with a continuous suture. The process is repeated at the distal end-to-side anastomosis. The graft can then be placed within the native aorta which, after trimming, is closed over the graft.

END-TO-SIDE ANASTOMOSIS MAINTAINED

(18) If the surgeon elects not to convert the proximal and distal aortic anastomoses to end-to-end, the native aorta is transected just beyond the proximal end-to-side anastomosis.

(19) The transected end of the proximal aorta is sutured closed with a running mattress suture of 3-0 monofilament followed by an over-and-over stitch. If the aortic wall is friable, Teflon felt strips are used to reinforce this suture line. The procedure is repeated at the distal aorta. The technique leaves two blind stumps of aorta; this is esthetically displeasing and creates pockets of stagnant flow and turbulence. Nevertheless, few complications have been associated with these stumps on the few occasions when they have been left.

After completion of the thoracoabdominal graft, the wound is closed. The diaphragm is closed with interrupted mattress sutures of 0 polyester. The costal margin is reapproximated with one or more mattress sutures to hold the cut ends of cartilage together. A single chest tube is placed for drainage. The abdominal and chest incisions can be closed with continuous sutures in routine fashion.

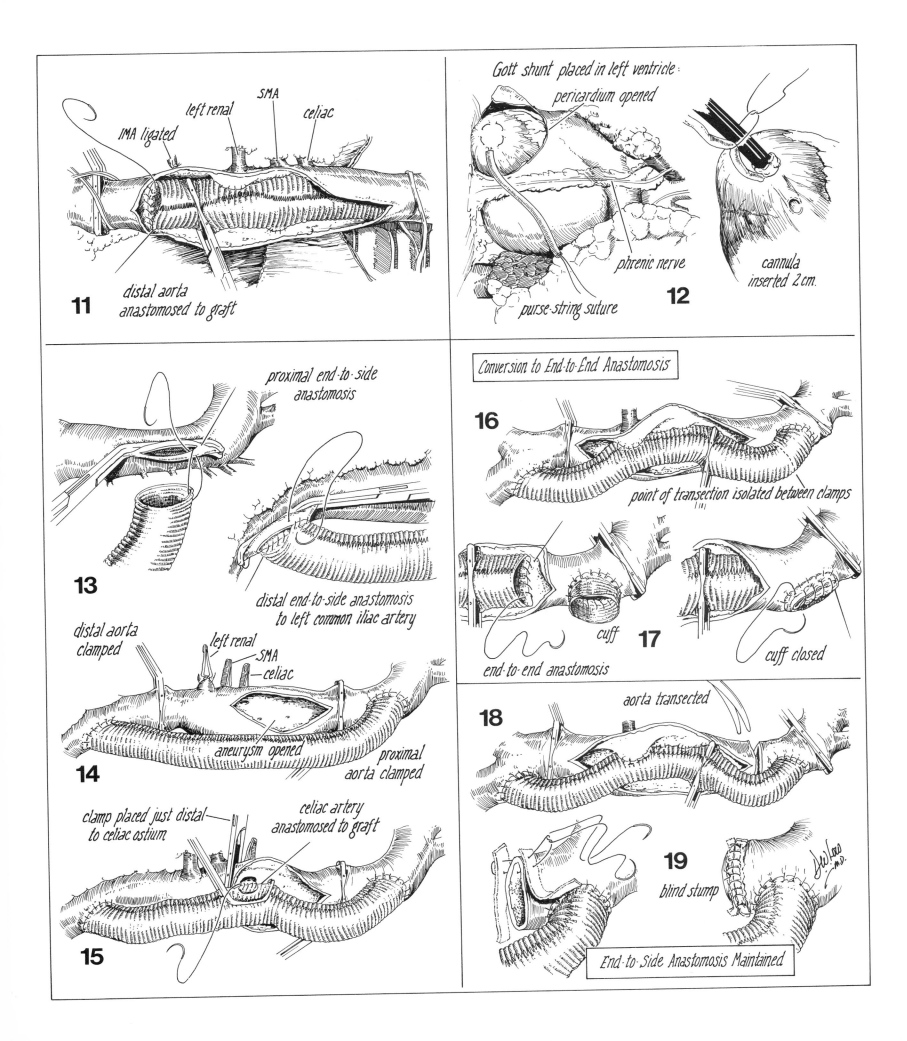

11 IMA ligated — left renal — SMA — celiac

distal aorta anastomosed to graft

12 Gott shunt placed in left ventricle: pericardium opened — phrenic nerve — cannula inserted 2 cm. — purse-string suture

13 proximal end-to-side anastomosis

distal end-to-side anastomosis to left common iliac artery

14 distal aorta clamped — left renal — SMA — celiac — aneurysm opened — proximal aorta clamped

15 clamp placed just distal to celiac ostium — celiac artery anastomosed to graft

Conversion to End-to-End Anastomosis

16 point of transection isolated between clamps

17 cuff — cuff closed — end-to-end anastomosis

18 aorta transected

19 blind stump

End-to-Side Anastomosis Maintained

Transaortic Insertion, Intra-Aortic Balloon

This procedure is used to wean occasional patients from cardiopulmonary bypass when aorto-iliac occlusive disease precludes insertion of the balloon from either groin.

1 A side-biting Cooley, Satinsky, or similar clamp is placed on the ascending aorta and a longitudinal incision is made in the aorta within the clamp.

2 Either a No. 12 preclotted woven Dacron graft or a No. 12 PFTE graft is sutured to the aortotomy with a continuous 4-0 monofilament suture. Teflon felt strips may be used if the aortic wall is thin or friable.

3 With the graft occluded, the side-biting clamp is released to test the anastomosis.

4 A stab wound is made in the upper abdomen below the midline sternotomy and the distal end of the prosthetic graft is brought through the stab wound and trimmed so that the prosthetic graft lies comfortably in the anterior mediastinum.

5 The intra-aortic balloon is measured and marked with a ligature to indicate when the balloon will be in proper position just beyond the origin of the left subclavian artery. The balloon catheter is passed through the stab wound into the mediastinum and then passed into the free end of the prosthetic graft. As the perfusion flow rate is slowed, the occluding clamp is released and the balloon advanced into the ascending aorta, arch, and proximal descending thoracic aorta to the marking ligature.

6 The graft is tied tightly around the balloon washer, which has been advanced along the balloon catheter to the end of the prosthetic graft. Full perfusion flow is resumed; a second umbilical tape ligature is tied tightly around the graft and balloon washer.

7 The end of the graft is brought into the stab wound and sutured to the subcutaneous tissue with a single suture. The skin is closed around the balloon catheter with interrupted sutures so that no portion of the graft protrudes from the wound.

BALLOON REMOVAL

8 Removal of the transaortic intra-aortic balloon is done in the operating room with a sterile thoracotomy instrument tray available. Local anesthesia is injected in the skin around the balloon catheter after the entire anterior chest is prepped and draped. The balloon is manually deflated with a 50 ml syringe; the balloon catheter is then clamped and transected. With two or three hemostats on the edges of the prosthetic graft, the umbilical tapes and ligatures around the balloon washer are cut.

9 The balloon is rapidly withdrawn; the prosthetic graft is clamped, trimmed, ligated and oversewn. The end is then pushed through the stab wound into the mediastinum and the skin of the stab wound is closed.

In two patients, subcutaneous infection at the exit site necessitated administration of general anesthesia and repeat median sternotomy to remove the entire prosthesis. Withdrawal has never caused recognized bleeding in our experience. Retention of the thrombosed graft attached to the ascending aorta has not, to our knowledge, caused any complications.

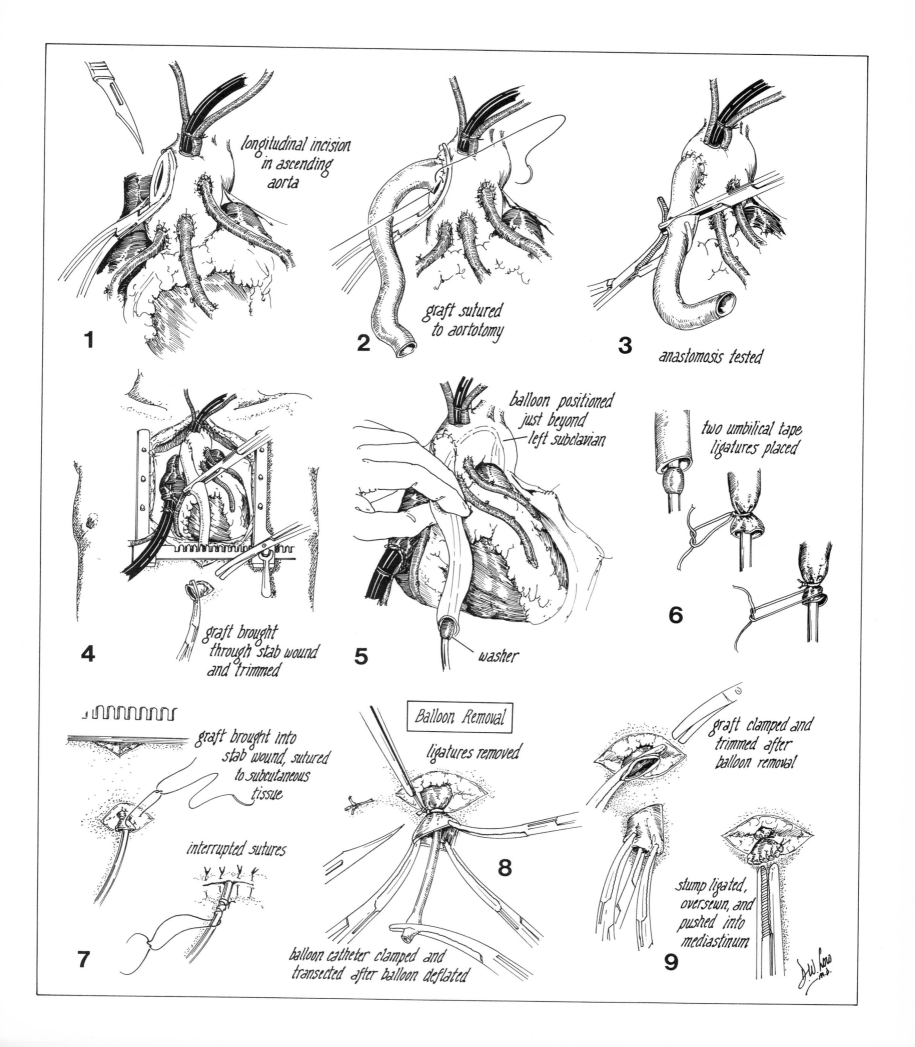

1 longitudinal incision in ascending aorta

2 graft sutured to aortotomy

3 anastomosis tested

4 graft brought through stab wound and trimmed

5 balloon positioned just beyond left subclavian

washer

6 two umbilical tape ligatures placed

7 graft brought into stab wound, sutured to subcutaneous tissue

interrupted sutures

8 Balloon Removal

ligatures removed

balloon catheter clamped and transected after balloon deflated

9 graft clamped and trimmed after balloon removal

stump ligated, oversewn, and pushed into mediastinum

Section 4

Congenital Cardiothoracic Surgery

Thoracic and Vascular Procedures

PECTUS EXCAVATUM

Pectus excavatum is a developmental malformation of the sternum and the costal cartilages characterized by posterior angulation of the inferior portion of the manubrium and its cartilaginous attachments to the thoracic cage. Usually patients are free of physiologic symptoms; psychosocial concerns predominate. There does not seem to be any ideal age for reconstructive surgery, although the techniques described here are technically simplified in the young.

1 The malformation is a three-dimensional posterior angulation and concavity of the manubrium and associated costal chondral attachments.

2 A short subcostal incision exposes the ligamentous attachments of the xyphisternum, which are then divided.

3 The sternum and costal cartilages are exposed anteriorly and posteriorly by blunt dissection.

4 The cartilages are divided laterally near the bony ribs with a bevel incision using electrocautery.

5 The inferior sternum is elevated anteriorly, exposing the posterior surface of the angulated manubrium and a sternal osteotomy of the posterior table is fashioned at the site of angulation.

6 The sternum is elevated anteriorly with the sternal costal cartilages placed anterior to those of the ribs.

7 The anterior table of the manubrium is incised centrally if necessary and bone or cartilaginous grafts are placed in the trough.

8 These are secured with stainless steel wire reinforcing sutures for stabilization of reconstructed angulation. Nonabsorbable sutures placed to stabilize the costal cartilages are then secured.

9 The wound is closed in layers, including subcuticular cutaneous closure.

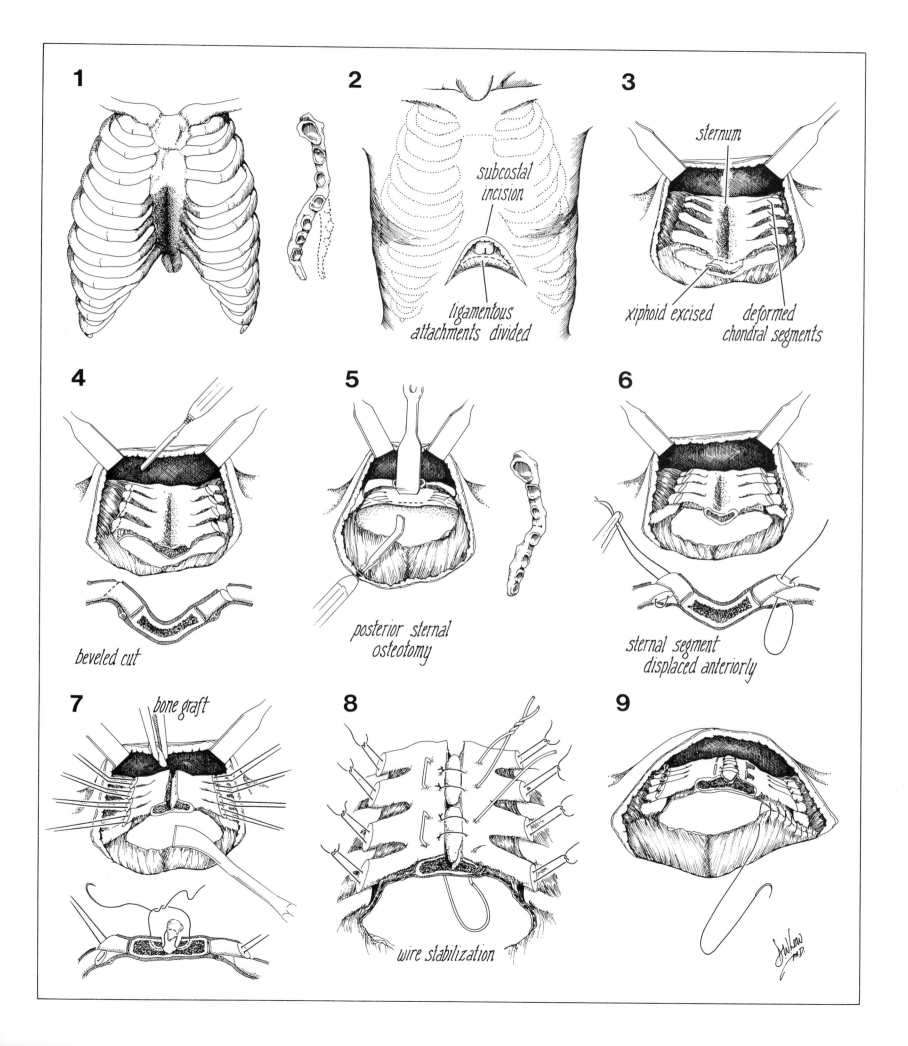

1

2

subcostal
incision

ligamentous
attachments divided

3

sternum

xiphoid excised

deformed
chondral segments

4

beveled cut

5

posterior sternal
osteotomy

6

sternal segment
displaced anteriorly

7

bone graft

8

wire stabilization

9

COARCTATION OF THE AORTA

Coarctation of the aorta was one of the first cardiovascular congenital malformations for which reparative surgical techniques were developed. Presentation may be in the neonatal period, with symptoms of severe congestive heart failure or even circulatory collapse, or the condition may be recognized only later in life by physical findings of diminished femoral pulses, upper extremity hypertension, and characteristic auscultatory findings. The timing of surgery can be dictated by symptoms in the neonatal period or planned electively in the asymptomatic child. There is a belief that delaying surgery beyond the first decade of life may increase the risk of persistent hypertension following repair.

Finally, coarctation of the aorta is not uncommonly associated with intracardiac malformations such as ventricular septal defect, which influence the timing and nature of surgical correction. The purpose of reparative surgery is to avoid complications associated with hypertension. It also avoids rupture of Beri aneurysms, occasionally associated with coarctation of the aorta, bacterial endocarditis and mycotic aneurysm, and the consequences of chronic pressure overload of the left ventricle. The classical technique was resection with end-to-end anastomosis of the aorta. When it's applied in the neonatal period there appears to be an appreciable incidence of restrictive anastomosis following growth and development of the child. Patch annuloplasty techniques, using the left subclavian artery in particular, are felt to diminish the occurrence of persistent pressure gradients between the ascending and thoracic aorta.

(1) Exposure through a fourth intercostal space lateral thoracotomy incision and the coarctation is usually readily identified by incising the parietal pleura over the thoracic aorta coarctation and left subclavan artery.

(2) Incision and end-to-end anastomosis may be accomplished by crossclamping the aorta controlling superior intercostal vessels and dividing the ligamentum arteriosus, with suture closure if necessary.

(3) The coarcted segment is excised in such a fashion as to achieve a similar circumference of proximal and distal transsected aorta.

(4) A running suture line may be placed posteriorly with interrupted anterior row, with a view to promotion of satisfactory growth and development of the repaired aorta.

Patch Angioplasty

(5) Patch angioplasty is structured with a longitudinal incision across the area of the coarctation of the aorta. The obstructing membrane may be partially excised, with care to avoid late aneurysmal formation.

Subclavian Patch Angioplasty

(6) Subclavian flap angioplasty is accomplished following ligation and division of the subclavian artery and of the ductus arteriosus if patent.

(7) An incision is carried down the left subclavian artery onto the thoracic aorta.

(8) The flap of subclavian tissue is laid across the narrowed aorta.

(9) This is sutured with a running monofilament suture.

(10) Care should be taken to extend the incision down the thoracic aorta far beyond the coarcted segment.

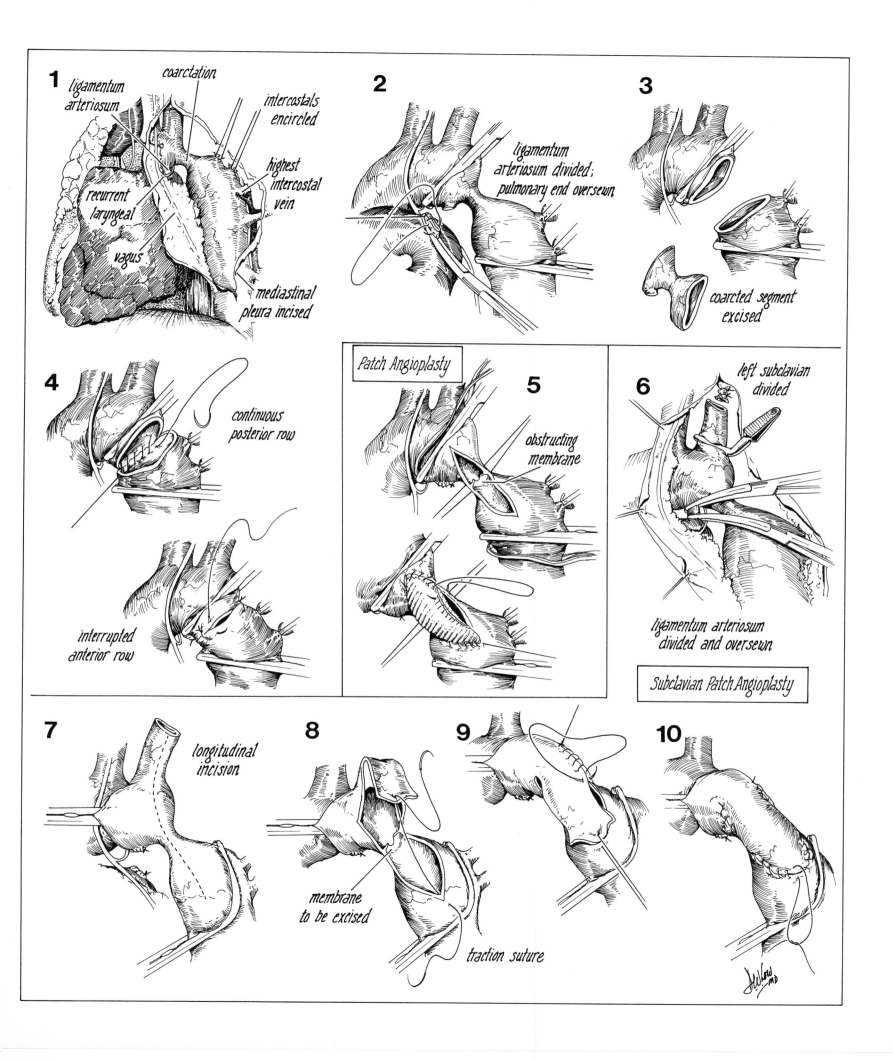

1 ligamentum arteriosum · coarctation · intercostals encircled · highest intercostal vein · recurrent laryngeal · vagus · mediastinal pleura incised

2 ligamentum arteriosum divided; pulmonary end oversewn

3 coarcted segment excised

4 continuous posterior row · interrupted anterior row

Patch Angioplasty

5 obstructing membrane

6 left subclavian divided · ligamentum arteriosum divided and oversewn

Subclavian Patch Angioplasty

7 longitudinal incision

8 membrane to be excised · traction suture

9

10

PULMONARY ARTERIAL SLING WITH ASSOCIATED TRACHEOBRONCHIAL HYPOPLASIA

In neonates with respiratory distress, the findings may be a pulmonary arterial sling with a left pulmonary artery arising from the right pulmonary artery coursing posteriorly to the trachea with associated tracheobronchial developmental abnormalities. These children present principally with ventilatory symptoms, often requiring emergency surgical intervention. Finally, isolated tracheobronchial developmental abnormalities may be managed in a similar fashion even in the absence of pulmonary arterial sling.

(1) Through a midline sternotomy, the mediastinal structures are exposed and the patient is placed on cardiopulmonary bypass.

(2) Between the aorta and the subclavian artery, the anomalous left pulmonary artery is dissected and exposed and the ligamentum arteriosus is divided.

(3) The left pulmonary artery is excised with an arterial button from the right pulmonary artery and released posteriorly from the trachea. An incision in the main pulmonary artery is carried to the left for reimplantation of the left pulmonary artery.

(4) Reanastomosis of the left pulmonary artery is fashioned to the left and anterior to the trachea, with the pulmonary arteriotomy to the right closed primarily or with patch material to avoid stricture of the right pulmonary artery.

(5) The trachea is mobilized to the thoracic inlet and the bronchi are exposed. The peritracheal fascia is incised inferiorly for mobilization of the distal tracheobronchial tree.

(6) When the stenotic segment is short, it may be excised completely with reapproximation of the trachea, using running suture technique posteriorly and interrupted sutures anteriorly.

(7) When the tracheal abnormality consists of concentric rings over a long segment, pericardial patch augmentation of the distal trachea is readily accomplished through a midline sternotomy on cardiopulmonary bypass.

(8) The pericardium is sutured over the incised distal trachea, which is dilated to ensure a uniform distal tracheal circumference.

(9) When the bronchi are similarly involved, a carinal pericardial patch may be used with extension into both right and left bronchi.

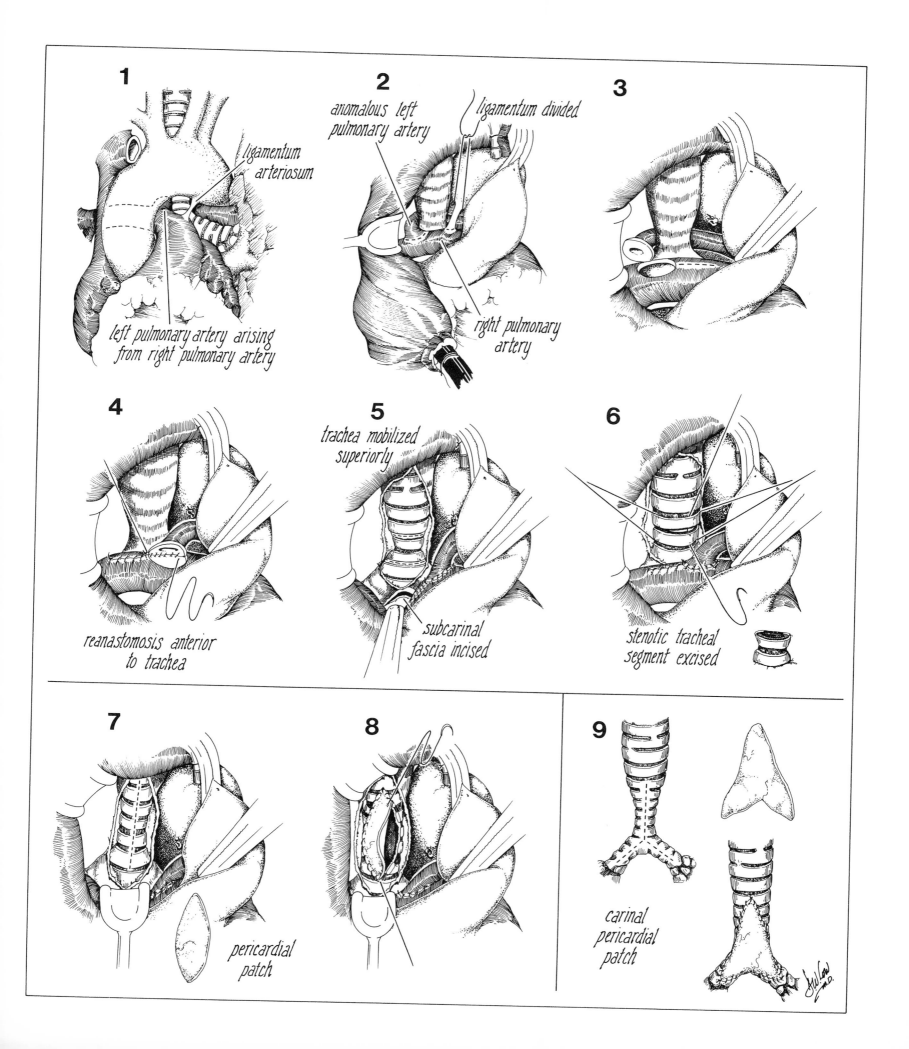

1 ligamentum arteriosum
left pulmonary artery arising from right pulmonary artery

2 anomalous left pulmonary artery · ligamentum divided
right pulmonary artery

3

4 reanastomosis anterior to trachea

5 trachea mobilized superiorly · subcarinal fascia incised

6 stenotic tracheal segment excised

7 pericardial patch

8

9 carinal pericardial patch

PALLIATIVE SHUNT PROCEDURES

In patients with right-sided obstructive lesions and consequent hypoxemia and/or dependence on patency of the ductus arteriosus, systemic arterial to pulmonary artery or systemic venous to pulmonary arterial shunts may be employed for palliation. When a shunt procedure is being performed independent of other reconstructive surgery, our preference is a Blalock-Taussig shunt of the classical type or a modification using interposition of a tube graft between the innominate artery and the right pulmonary artery. In older patients, with whom there is concern about the adverse effects of increased volume load associated with systemic to pulmonary arterial shunts, a Glenn shunt may be used. Most recently, the application of a Glenn shunt has had more limited indications because, in the usual circumstances where a Glenn shunt would be used, a modification of Fontan's procedure may be preferentially indicated.

Blalock-Taussig Shunt

1 In patients with a left aortic arch, a right thoracotomy incision in the fourth intercostal space is used to expose the innominate artery and the right subclavian artery. Initial dissection should be for exposure of the right pulmonary artery to assess the structural feasibility of the Blalock-Taussig shunt.

2 The azygous vein is doubly ligated and divided and the parietal pleura over the subclavian artery is incised, exposing the branch vessels of the left subclavian artery. The branch vessels are doubly ligated and divided.

3 The distal subclavian artery is doubly ligated and divided and brought through the loop of the recurrent laryngeal

nerve. Dissection is carried far into the right carotid artery to produce appropriate length without tension for the subclavian artery-pulmonary arterial anastomosis.

4 The right subclavian artery is clamped proximally and the distal end is amputated for the end-to-side anastomosis on the right pulmonary artery proximal to the visualized upper lobe branch. The posterior suture line is completed with running prolene suture. In small infants, the anterior portion may be completed with interrupted sutures.

5 A modification of this systemic to pulmonary arterial shunt may be by interposition of a tube graft between the innominate artery and the right pulmonary artery. The size is chosen to match the size of the patient (usually 4 mm in neonates). This procedure is generally less mutilating to the arterial structures and may minimize distorting the right pulmonary artery, particularly in the very young.

Glenn Shunt

6 The Glenn shunt is initiated by exposing the azygous vein and ligating the proximal right pulmonary artery.

7 The azygous vein is ligated and explanted from the right superior vena cava.

8 The right pulmonary artery is then amputated and anastomosed end-to-side into the superior vena cava at the level of the azygous vein.

9 The ligation of the junction of the right superior vena cava and right atrium creates obligatory flow from the superior vena cava to the right pulmonary artery.

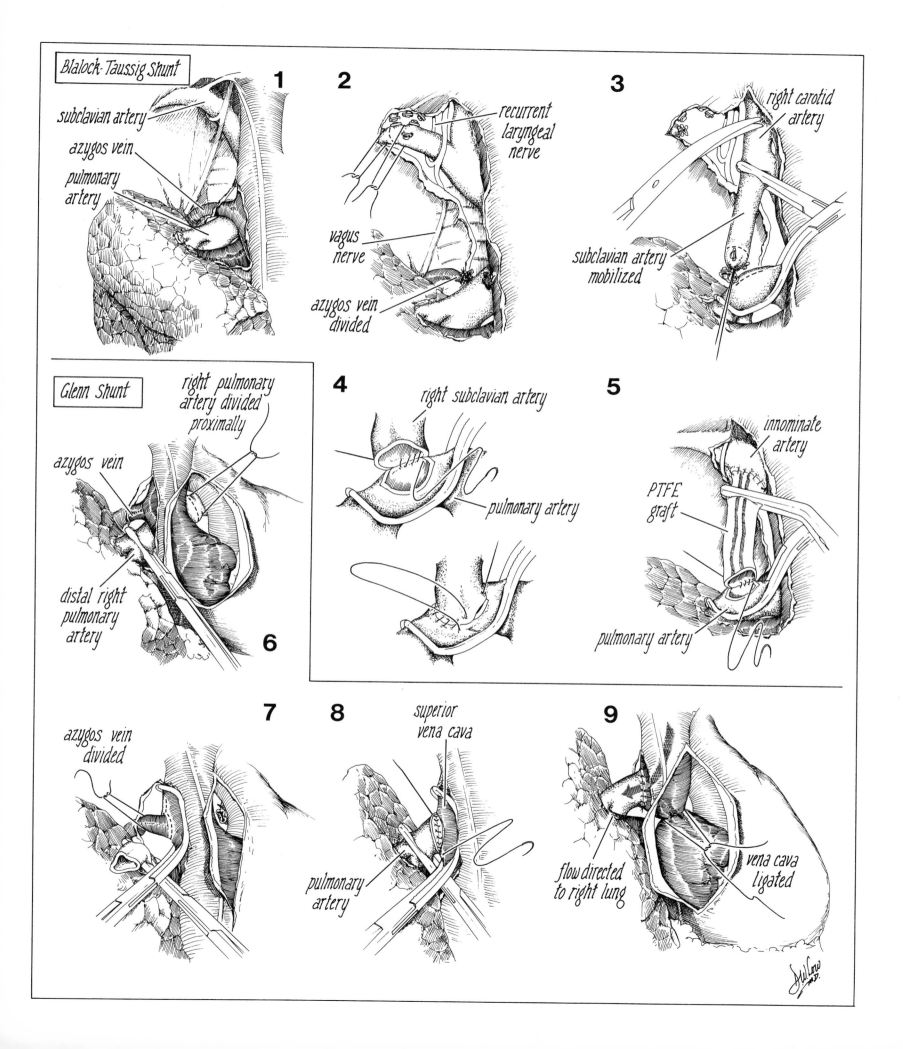

Blalock-Taussig Shunt

1
subclavian artery
azygos vein
pulmonary artery

2
recurrent laryngeal nerve
vagus nerve
azygos vein divided

3
right carotid artery
subclavian artery mobilized

Glenn Shunt

6
right pulmonary artery divided proximally
azygos vein
distal right pulmonary artery

4
right subclavian artery
pulmonary artery

5
innominate artery
PTFE graft
pulmonary artery

7
azygos vein divided

8
superior vena cava
pulmonary artery

9
flow directed to right lung
vena cava ligated

ANOMALOUS ORIGIN OF THE LEFT CORONARY
ARTERY FROM THE PULMONARY ARTERY

The anomalous origin of the left coronary artery has a roughly bimodal presentation. In the very young with few collaterals between the right and left coronary arterial system, profound left ventricular dysfunction, often accompanied by mitral regurgitation, ensues in the first weeks of life as the pulmonary vascular resistance naturally decreases. In those with more extensive collaterals between the right and left coronary systems, presentation is often later in life as a consequence of left-to-right shunt occasionally accompanied by signs of "coronary arterial steal." The coronary artery origin is variable, arising from the left lateral wall of the main pulmonary artery in most, posterior near the confluence of the right and left pulmonary arteries in some, and occasionally arising from the proximal right pulmonary artery posteriorly. Several different approaches to surgical management have been used, including ligation of the proximal left coronary artery, ligation and systemic-to-left-coronary-artery anastomosis using left subclavian artery or various forms of grafts and direct reimplantation of the coronary artery into the ascending aorta. More recently, a means of establishing a two-coronary arterial system by intrapulmonary tunneling of systemic arterial flow has been introduced. This has the advantage of being applicable to all anatomic forms of anomalous coronary origin and can be readily and rapidly performed in patients of all ages, including moribund neonates.

1 After placement on cardiopulmonary bypass and application of deep hypothermia and circulatory arrest in the infant, a pulmonary arteriotomy is performed.

2 The ostium of the anomalous left coronary artery is readily visualized through the incision.

3 A small aortopulmonary window is then created in the wall of the adjacent aorta and main pulmonary artery just distal to the semilunar valve apparatus.

4 Either free-hand excision or arterial punch techniques can be used to create 3 to 4 mm diameter holes in adjacent great vessels.

5 The aortopulmonary window is constructed by anastomosis of the perimeter of holes in the great vessels using monofilament continuous suture technique.

6 The aortopulmonary window is now the transferred ostium of the left coronary artery.

7 A patch of graft material, usually polytetrafluoroethylene (Teflon or PTFE) is sutured along the posterior wall of the pulmonary artery to create a tunnel across the posterior aspect of the main pulmonary artery trunk.

8 Creation of the baffle tunnel effectively connects the systemic arterial circulation with the left coronary artery.

9 The pulmonary arteriotomy is closed with a gusseting patch to augment anterior outflow from the right ventricle to the branch pulmonary arteries.

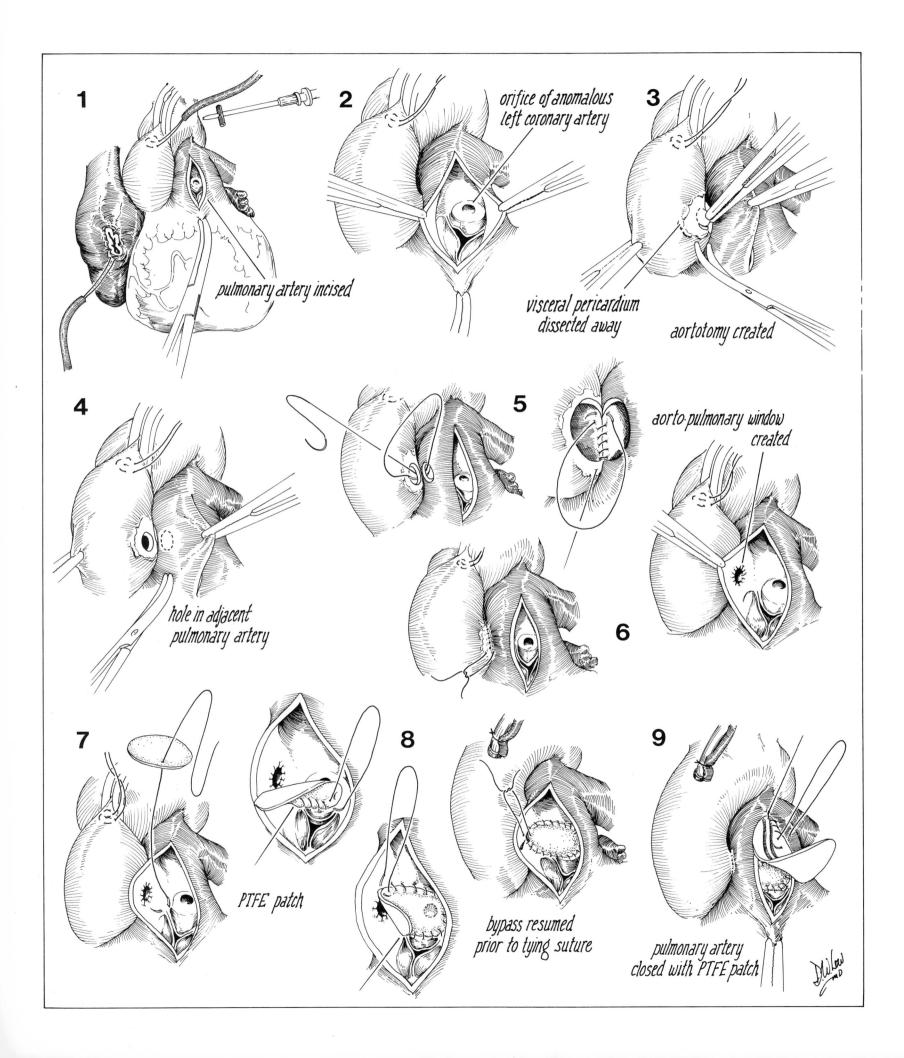

1 pulmonary artery incised

2 orifice of anomalous left coronary artery / visceral pericardium dissected away

3 aortotomy created

4 hole in adjacent pulmonary artery

5 aorto-pulmonary window created

6

7 PTFE patch

8 bypass resumed prior to tying suture

9 pulmonary artery closed with PTFE patch

Surgery for Right-Sided Obstructive Lesions

PULMONARY ATRESIA WITH INTACT VENTRICULAR SEPTUM

Pulmonary atresia with intact ventricular septum presents as cyanosis in the neonatal period with an obligatory shunt of systemic venous return to an interatrial communication to the left atrium. Pulmonary arterial blood flow depends on patency of the ductus arteriosus. Although the branch pulmonary arteries are nearly normally developed in most patients with pulmonary atresia and intact ventricular septum, the structures of the right ventricle and tricuspid valve are highly variable. In one extreme, the right ventricle may be only mildly hypoplastic, and this condition is almost always accompanied by significant tricuspid regurgitation. More commonly, the right ventricle is significantly hypoplastic, and at the other extreme, the right ventricle is diminutive and hypertensive, and contains multiple large sinusoidal communications between the right ventricle and coronary arterial system. In the uncommon patient with such marked hypoplasia and sinusoids, palliation may include creation of systemic to pulmonary arterial oversewing of the tricuspid valve orifice. In many, however, the following form of palliation can potentially lead to a two ventricular system. In patients with the larger right ventricular cavities, this palliation has proved to be a one-stage reparative procedure.

1 The characteristic external features seen through a midline sternotomy are a patent ductus arteriosus, arterial truck with the outline of the right ventricular size appreciated by the boundaries of the atrial ventricular junction to the right, and anterior descending coronary artery to the left.

2 A right atrial purse-string suture is placed in the atrial appendage for retraction and exposure.

3 The distal main pulmonary artery is crossclamped and an incision is made in the proximal main pulmonary artery to the valved plate. This incision is carried onto the right ventricular infundibular free wall, incising only the epicardium. A gusset of patch material is secured on the left lateral aspect of this incision with running monofilament suture.

4 The suture line is left incomplete on the right inferior aspect of the incision.

5 One or two sutures (interrupted) are placed in preparation for crossing the valve plate and augmenting the infundibulum of the right ventricular outflow.

6 With or without a brief period of systemic venous inflow occlusion, a No.11 blade is used to cross the valve plate and infundibulum communicating the right ventricular sinus with the main pulmonary artery. The interrupted sutures on the patch are then drawn tight for hemostasis and the running suture line is completed.

7 A systemic-to-pulmonary artery shunt is necessary in all patients in the early postoperative period to avoid destabilizing hypoxemia. This can be accomplished by infiltration of the ductus arteriosus with 6% formalin solution injected below the adventitia circumferentially around the ductus arteriosus through a 25 gauge needle. A drop of methylene blue may be added to the formalin solution to aid in the visualization of the infiltrated region. Such a systemic-to-pulmonary arterial shunt is usually temporary, lasting from several weeks to a few months. In patients with a large right ventricular sinus, closure of the shunt is only occasionally accompanied by increasing hypoxemia.

Pulmonary Stenosis

8 Patients with critical pulmonary arterial stenosis as opposed to pulmonary atresia can most effectively be managed by pulmonary valvotomy during a period of inflow occlusion. A straight side-biting clamp is placed on the main pulmonary arterial trunk and an incision is made in the anterior pulmonary artery. The superior and inferior ends are secured with monofilament sutures and lateral retraction sutures are placed.

9 The superior and inferior vena cavae are temporarily occluded and the partially occluding clamp is removed, exposing a typical pearly gray thickened pulmonary valve with a small central orifice. The commissures are identified and incised and a portion of one leaflet is excised to ensure decompression of the right ventricle.

110

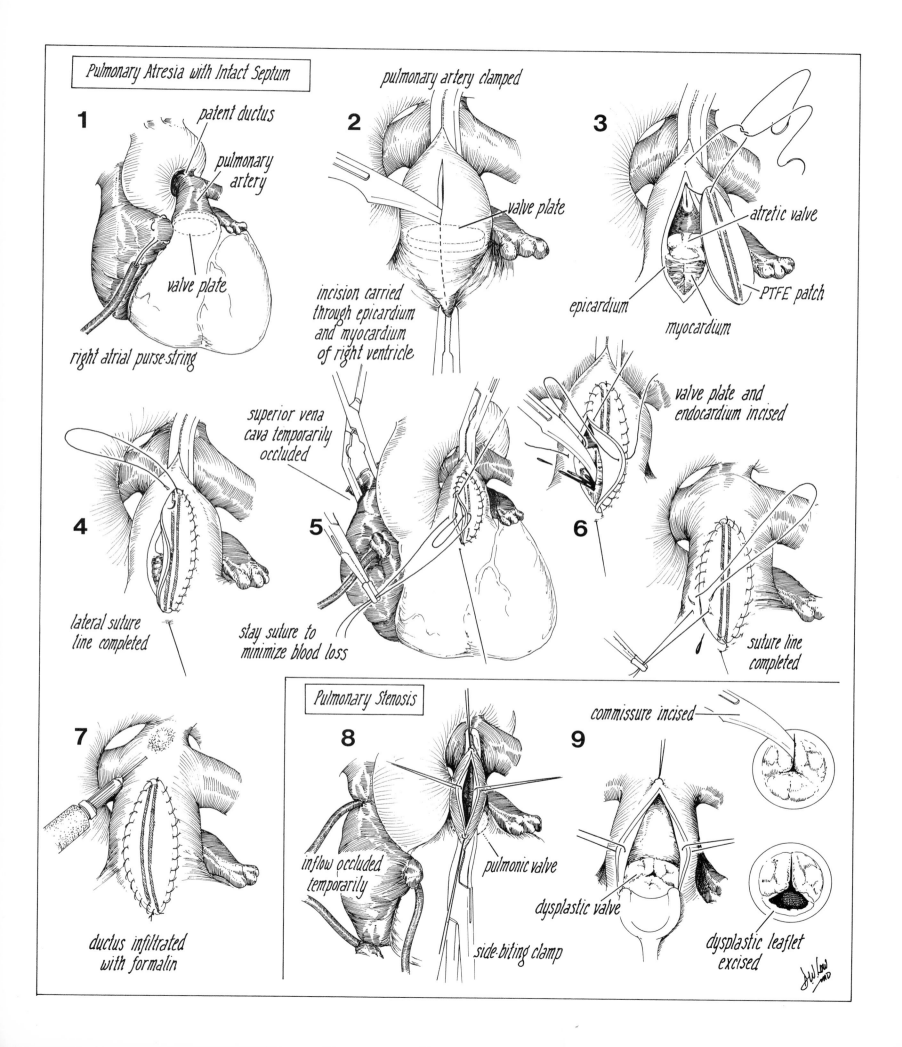

Pulmonary Atresia with Intact Septum

1 patent ductus
pulmonary artery
valve plate
right atrial purse-string

2 pulmonary artery clamped
valve plate
incision carried through epicardium and myocardium of right ventricle

3 atretic valve
PTFE patch
epicardium
myocardium

4 lateral suture line completed

5 superior vena cava temporarily occluded
stay suture to minimize blood loss

6 valve plate and endocardium incised
suture line completed

7 ductus infiltrated with formalin

Pulmonary Stenosis

8 inflow occluded temporarily
pulmonic valve
side-biting clamp

9 commissure incised
dysplastic valve
dysplastic leaflet excised

TETRALOGY OF FALLOT

Tetralogy of Fallot is the second or third most common congenital cardiac malformation that occurs in the first year of life. Although this constellation is described as four components including ventricular septal defect, right ventricular outflow tract obstruction, partial deviation of the aorta over the right ventricle, and right ventricular hypertrophy, it results from a single developmental abnormality. The infundibular septum normally extends into the Y of the anterior superior and posterior inferior limbs of the septal band, creating an intact ventricular septum. In tetralogy of Fallot, the infundibular septum is malaligned with the septal band and true trabecular septum. It is positioned anteriorly extending into the right ventricular outflow tract. Consequently, there is a large malalignment type of ventricular septal defect. The infundibulum of the right ventricle is narrow and obstructive, with consequential abnormal development of the pulmonary annulus and main pulmonary artery. Because of infundibular septum is positioned more anteriorly than normal, the root of the aorta is partially associated with the right ventricle. Chronic pressure load on the right ventricle causes right ventricular hypertrophy. Indications for repair include progressive cyanosis and hypercyanotic episodes. The role of the size of the branch pulmonary arteries and the effect of pulmonary regurgitation after transannular right ventricular outflow tract augmentation on outcome has not yet been clearly defined. Primary reparative surgery, however, is feasible and efficacious in the first year of life, and most patients probably benefit from early primary repair. The anomalous origin of the anterior descending coronary artery from the right coronary artery is considered a relative contraindication to early repair because a bridging conduit may be necessary to treat the right ventricular outflow tract obstruction.

1 Cardiopulmonary bypass is established by arterial infusion in the ascending aorta and a single venous cannula in the right atrial appendage. The main pulmonary artery of the patient with tetralogy of Fallot is foreshortened and takes a horizontal anterior posterior course. Consequently, the left pulmonary artery must angulate sharply around the reflection of the pericardium as it enters the left thorax. This angulated segment may be stenotic, requiring patch augmentation. The pericardium should be dissected from the left pulmonary artery at this point.

2 The atrial septum should be examined for the presence of an associated atrial septal defect. This defect, if present, may be repaired through an atriotomy with primary suture closure or a patch.

3 Most patients exhibit hypoplasia of the pulmonary annulus, infundibulum, and main pulmonary artery. A transannular incision into the infundibulum of the right ventricle is made, with the position of the anterior descending coronary artery and right coronary artery, carefully noted. Often hypertrophied muscle bands attach laterally to the anteriorly malaligned infundibular septum.

4 Exposure of the ventricular septal defect is facilitated by incising muscle bands if present, partially releasing the infundibular septum.

5 The ventricular septal defect may be closed through the infundibulotomy with a woven cloth patch, using a running monofilament continuous suture technique. The suture is begun at the level of the papillary muscle of the conus.

6 The suture line is carried in a clockwise fashion initially through the inferiormost aspect of the ventricular septal defect rim. It is in this region between the papillary muscle of the conus and tricuspid valve that the conduction system runs in the septal crest. Sutures are placed on the right aspect of the ventricular septum away from the septal crest in an effort to avoid injuring the conduction system in this region.

7 The remainder of the patch is closed with deep, secure bites in muscle laterally.

8 Patch closure is completed by deep bites into the extent of the infundibular septum. This maneuver partially deviates the infundibular septum, somewhat posteriorly.

9 The reconstruction is completed by augmentation of the right ventricular outflow tract with a patch of PTFE or pericardium.

10 When stenosis of the branch of the left pulmonary artery is present, the incision is carried across the stenotic region onto the left pulmonary artery and augmented with a single right ventricular outflow tract gusset.

11 When there is minimal infundibular and pulmonary annular hypoplasia, a horizontal incision in the right ventricular outflow tract may be used to gain exposure for closing the ventricular septal defect and releasing lateral anomalous muscle bundles. This incision is closed with a continuous horizontal mattress suture completed by an epicardial layer of over-and-over continuous suture.

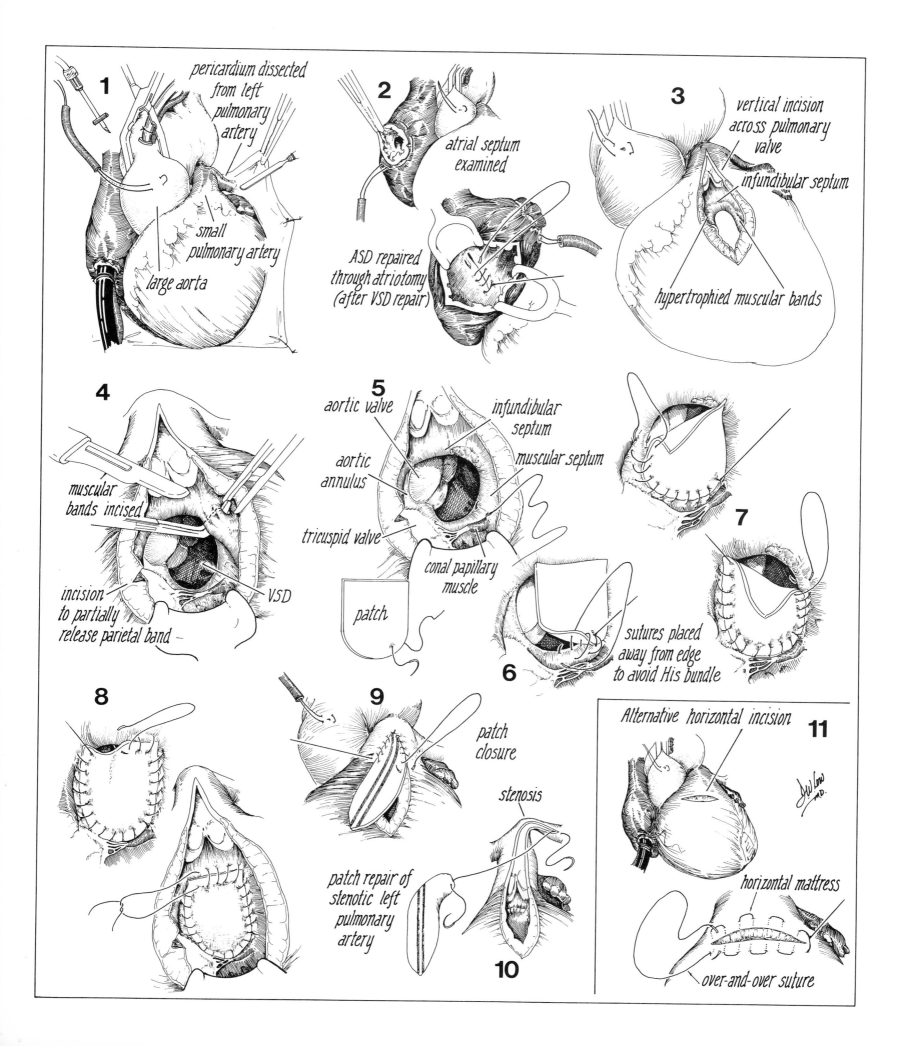

1 pericardium dissected from left pulmonary artery

small pulmonary artery

large aorta

2 atrial septum examined

ASD repaired through atriotomy (after VSD repair)

3 vertical incision across pulmonary valve

infundibular septum

hypertrophied muscular bands

4 muscular bands incised

incision to partially release parietal band

VSD

5 aortic valve

infundibular septum

aortic annulus

muscular septum

tricuspid valve

conal papillary muscle

patch

6 sutures placed away from edge to avoid His bundle

7

8

9 patch closure

patch repair of stenotic left pulmonary artery

stenosis

10

11 Alternative horizontal incision

horizontal mattress

over-and-over suture

TETRALOGY OF FALLOT WITH PULMONARY ATRESIA

Often termed pulmonary atresia with ventricular septal defect, this anatomic malformation is best understood as tetralogy of Fallot with pulmonary atresia. As previously discussed, tetralogy of Fallot is simply anterior malalignment of the infundibular septum with respect to the true trabeculated septum, resulting in ventricular septal defect, right ventricular outflow tract obstruction, partial association of the aorta with the right ventricle, and right ventricular hypertrophy. In the most severe form of right ventricular outflow tract obstruction, pulmonary atresia occurs. If atresia occurs during early gestation, primitive systemic-to-pulmonary collaterals persist and the central pulmonary artery architecture is absent. If pulmonary atresia occurs late during gestation or after birth, all elements of central pulmonary artery architecture may be present. The later the development of pulmonary atresia, the fewer systemic-to-pulmonary-arterial collaterals are present. When no central pulmonary arteries are present, a process of identification of the pulmonary arterial architecture by cardiac catheterization and recruitment of these arteries to a central confluent structure is necessary to eventually separate the pulmonary and systemic circulations. This may be performed in one or multiple stages. In a staged approach, shunts are substituted for collaterals and the collateral vessels are occluded either surgically or with coil embolization at cardiac catheterization.

The trend is toward earlier repair of tetralogy of Fallot with pulmonary atresia. But a previous strategy in patients with central pulmonary arteries has been a systemic-to-pulmonary-arterial shunt early in life to augment pulmonary blood flow, followed later by interposition of a conduit between the right ventricle and branch pulmonary arteries when no main pulmonary artery exists. Illustrated here is a special circumstance in which a child was treated with a Waterston shunt early in life.

① The external anatomy is characterized by a large aortic trunk, which has been chronically carrying both systemic and pulmonary flow. Posteriorly, there is an anastomosis between the right pulmonary artery and the ascending aorta. Often this connection kinks the branch pulmonary arteries as the child grows, causing preferential flow to the right pulmonary artery and consequential relative hypoplasia of the left pulmonary artery. The ventricular septal defect is of the malalignment type. Its characteristics have been previously described.

② The distal ascending aorta is cannulated for arterial infusion. The cannulation is at the junction of the innominate artery. Atrial cannulation can be with either double isolated cannulation of the vena cavae or a single cannula in the right atrial appendage. A period of circulatory arrest or low flow is useful because the collateral flow returning in the open pulmonary arteries can be large. The Waterston shunt after the patient goes on cardiopulmonary bypass is easily occluded by a vascular clamp.

③ The Waterston shunt is best closed by excision from the posterior aspect of the aorta. The defect in the ascending aorta can be closed primarily with running monofilament suture. Primary oversewing of the shunt often leaves hemodynamically significant distortion of the pulmonary arteries underneath the aorta and should be avoided.

④ The branch pulmonary arteries are opened wide posteriorly for augmentation to eliminate stenosis.

⑤ A right ventriculotomy is made to expose the ventricular septal defect and for interposition of a conduit between the right ventricle and pulmonary arteries. Five percent of patients have an anterior descending coronary artery arising from the right, and the infundibulotomy is made to avoid it when present. The ventricular septal defect is closed with a cloth patch using a running monofilament suture technique as previously described for repair of tetralogy of Fallot.

⑥ A conduit is then placed between the infundibulotomy and the incision in the branch pulmonary arteries. A conduit 16 mm in diameter or larger is sufficient to decompress the right ventricle in an adult with no other hemodynamic residua such as a persistent left-to-right shunt. Such a conduit can be placed in children weighing as little as 10 to 12 kg. There are many conduit materials from which to choose. In the past, a popular conduit was a Dacron tube graft containing a porcine aortic valve. This type of conduit seems particularly prone to insidious progressive obstruction with time, by both calcification of the porcine valve and accumulation of organized fibrin and thrombus. A valved conduit is probably not necessary in most patients, and a smooth wall tube of PTFE has provided excellent long-term results with an extremely low incidence of late stenosis. Illustrated here is the placement of an aortic homograft, which has the advantage of allowing hemostatic suture lines and the additional hypothetic advantage of a valve. Placing the homograft with the anterior mitral leaflet anteriorly allows shaping of the aortic arch of the graft as a gusset for the augmentation of the incised central pulmonary arteries. The insertion is begun with a running monofilament suture technique at the distal anastomosis.

⑦ The proximal anastomosis may be completed in a simple fashion with running monofilament suture, using the trimmed portion of the anterior leaflet of the mitral valve to augment the right ventriculotomy inferiorly. Some surgeons find it useful to buttress this anastomosis with felt strips or pledgets, and use a composite hooded structure of this anastomosis.

⑧ When the cine angiogram reveals an infundibulum extending to the base of the heart, there is almost always a main pulmonary artery segment with atresia of the valve plate. When this occurs, a conduit may not be necessary, and the right ventricular outflow tract can be gusseted as in tetralogy of Fallot with pulmonary stenosis. This approach has been used to extend the use of primary repair of tetralogy of Fallot and pulmonary atresia to the very young. The incision in the right ventricular outflow tract is carried across the valve plate into the main pulmonary artery and toward the left pulmonary artery.

⑨ After closure of the ventricular septal defect, the right ventricular outflow tract and main pulmonary artery are gusseted with a patch of pericardium, pulmonary homograft, or PTFE using a running monofilament suture technique.

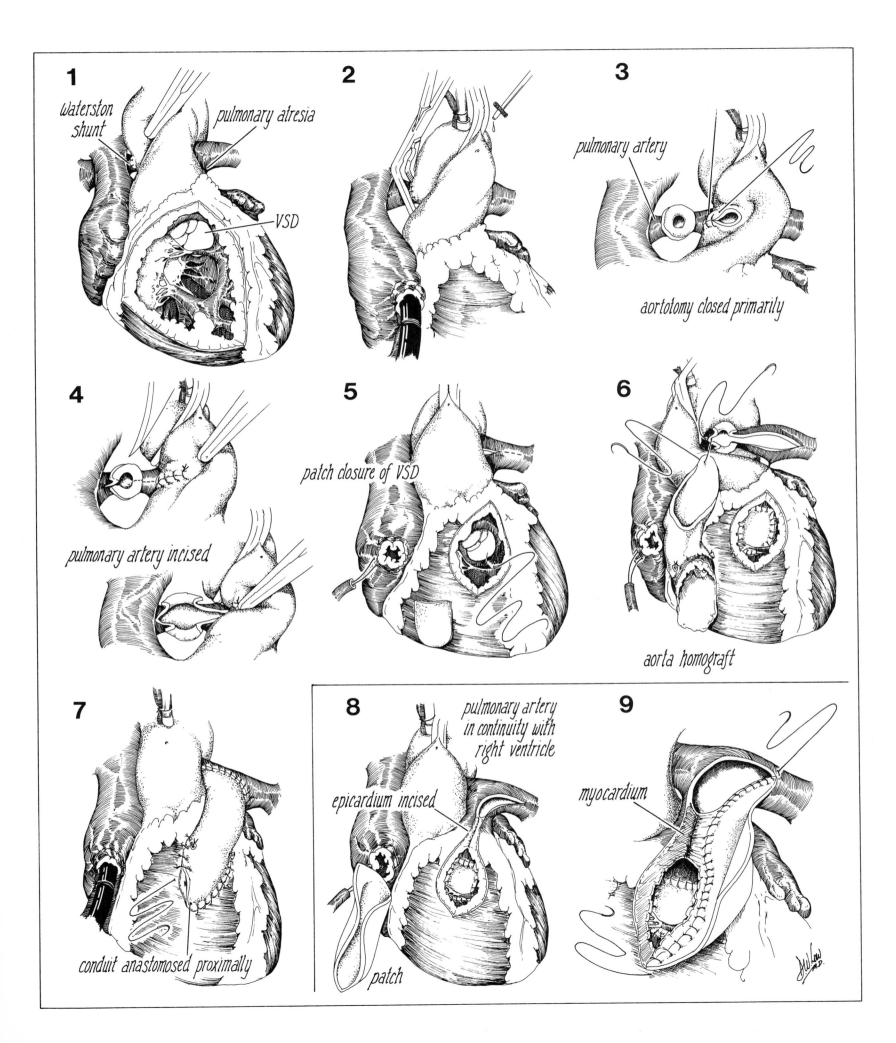

1 waterston shunt · pulmonary atresia · VSD

2

3 pulmonary artery · aortotomy closed primarily

4 pulmonary artery incised

5 patch closure of VSD

6 aorta homograft

7 conduit anastomosed proximally

8 pulmonary artery in continuity with right ventricle · epicardium incised · patch

9 myocardium

Surgery for Left-Sided Obstructive Lesions

CRITICAL AORTIC STENOSIS

Critical aortic stenosis of the neonate is a malformation of the aortic valve that causes left ventricular pressure overload and decompensation. The systemic circulation depends on patency of the ductus arteriosus. The size of the left ventricle is variable. It can be large and dilated in patients with coexisting mitral regurgitation, normal in size, or in some patients markedly hypoplastic. An end diastolic volume of 20 ml/M^2 or less should be managed as hypoplastic left heart syndrome. Echocardiography is usually sufficient for planning management. Cardiac catheterization may be counterproductive in these critically ill neonates, and pressure gradients are misleading in those with severe left ventricular failure. The aim of surgical intervention is to gain some increase in size of the aortic orifice without creating aortic regurgitation. The aortic valves are typically immature, thick, and pearly gray in appearance with a small central orifice and otherwise poorly defined valve architecture. Therefore, blunt valvotomy alone can be performed rapidly with little manipulation of the heart and resultant life-saving decompression of the left ventricle.

Valvulotomy Without Bypass

1 Through a midline sternotomy, the ascending aorta is exposed. Manipulation of the heart should be kept to a minimum because the heart is irritable and ventricular fibrillation easily ensues.

2 A purse-string suture is placed in the ascending aorta near the sinuses of Valsalva. Through a small stab incision controlled with the suture tourniquet on the ascending aorta, access to the stenotic valve is achieved.

3 A small clamp (mosquito hemostat) is placed through the small aortotomy into the orifices of the stenotic valve and blunt valvotomy is achieved. A small increase in orifice size can be effective and avoids lethal aortic regurgitation.

Alternative Valvulotomy with Bypass

4 Alternatively, a valvulotomy can be performed using cardiopulmonary bypass.

5 Cannulation is through the atrial appendage for venous return and the distal ascending aorta for arterial infusion.

6 Although some believe that venting the left side is important, in our experience it has been totally unnecessary.

7 Crossclamping of the aorta and infusion of cardioplegia solution may give the best exposure of the aortic valve.

8 Rarely is one able to identify easily the commissurae of the aortic valve in the neonate. As a child ages, the valve matures, allowing more structural definition. Often, in the symptomatic neonate, the valve has the appearance of being more unicuspid than bicuspid.

9 Occasionally, the excrescences of valved tissue prohibit movement of the leaflets, causing persistent obstruction even in the face of open commissurae. Extraneous tissue may be excised, with the caution that this tissue is extremely friable in the neonate and aortic regurgitation may be lethal.

116

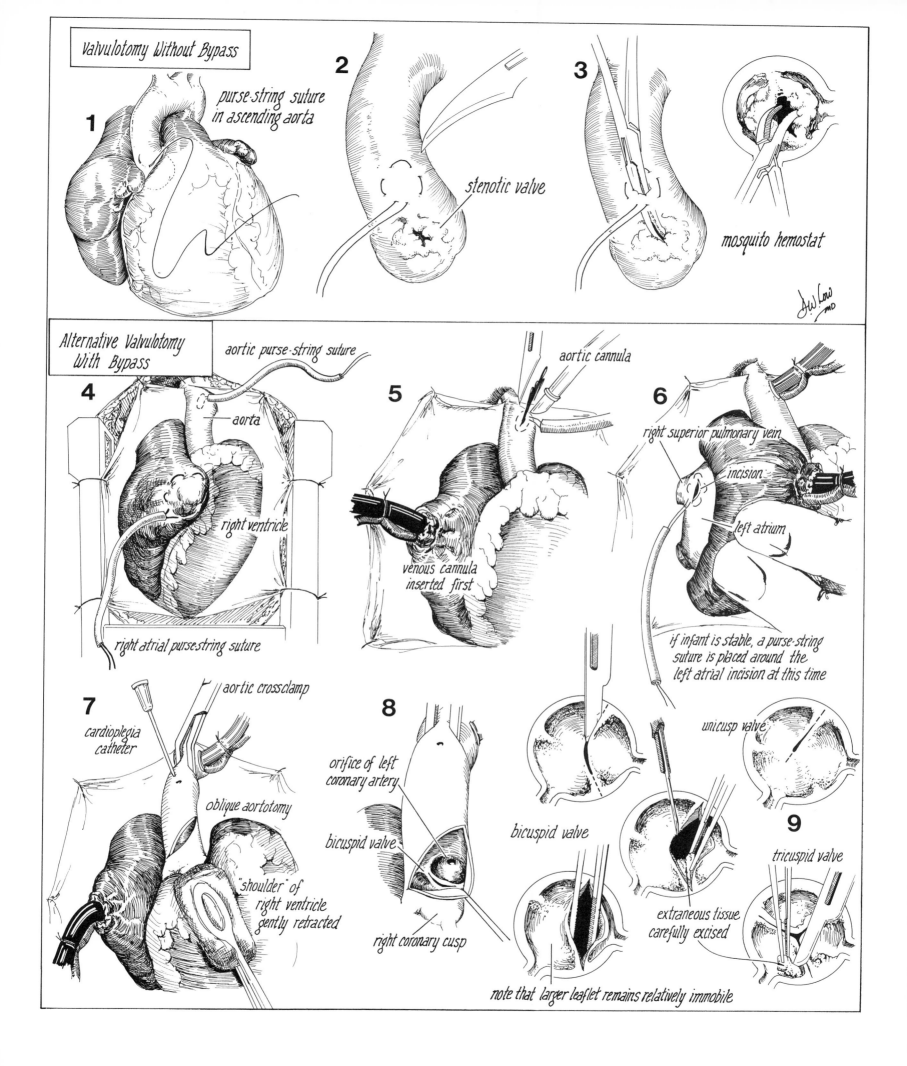

Valvulotomy Without Bypass

1

2 purse-string suture in ascending aorta

stenotic valve

3 mosquito hemostat

J.W. Low MD

Alternative Valvulotomy With Bypass

aortic purse-string suture

4 aorta

right ventricle

right atrial purse-string suture

5 aortic cannula

venous cannula inserted first

6 right superior pulmonary vein

incision

left atrium

if infant is stable, a purse-string suture is placed around the left atrial incision at this time

7 aortic crossclamp

cardioplegia catheter

oblique aortotomy

"shoulder" of right ventricle gently retracted

8 orifice of left coronary artery

bicuspid valve

right coronary cusp

bicuspid valve

unicusp valve

9 tricuspid valve

extraneous tissue carefully excised

note that larger leaflet remains relatively immobile

VALVULAR AORTIC STENOSIS

Valvular aortic stenosis in an older infant or child is generally secondary to abnormal structural development of the leaflets with varying degrees of fusion of the commissurae. In the most common variety, a bicuspid valve is seen with one somewhat larger leaflet containing a raphe, suggesting arrested development of a tricuspid valve. Less commonly, the stenosis is secondary to commissural fusion of a tricuspid valve or, most rarely, a unicuspid valve. Significant decompression on the left ventricle can be expected at least temporarily by aortic valvotomy alone in most patients with bicuspid or tricuspid valvar stenosis. The unicuspid valve is much more awkward to manage by valvotomy and may necessitate valve replacement even early in life.

It is important in the strategy of aortic valvotomy to relieve obstruction as much as possible while minimizing the potential for aortic valve regurgitation. The timing of surgical intervention should be directed by the goal of preserving good left ventricular function. Sudden death can occur from aortic valve stenosis in children, almost always in those who have developed ST-T wave changes on their electrocardiogram. Among patients with ST and T wave changes, approximately half revert to a more normal repolarization pattern on the electrocardiogram after aortic valvotomy.

① Cardiopulmonary bypass is established by placement of a single venous cannula in the right atrial appendage and cannulation for arterial infusion at the level of the branching of the innominate artery.

② Although venting the left ventricle has been considered an important component of such surgery in the past, the left ventricle can easily be decompressed during bypass and kept free of blood during valvotomy by placing suction in the main pulmonary artery.

③ After crossclamping of the aorta, cardioplegia solution may be infused into the ascending aorta. An aortotomy above the valve is carried into the noncoronary sinus of Valsalva. A traction suture may or may not be useful.

④ The most common variety of valvular stenosis is secondary to a bicuspid valve with fused commissurae, which may be incised with sharp dissection using a No. 15 or preferably No. 11 blade. Thickening of the valve leaflets with the presence of excrescences at the edge may further limit flow from the left ventricle, and efforts have been made to further decompress the left ventricle by sculpting the valved leaflets themselves. One should avoid trying to make a tricuspid valve from a clearly bicuspid valve because this usually destabilizes one leaflet, creating aortic regurgitation.

⑤ The schemes of valvotomy for the tricuspid and unicuspid valves are similar for the bicuspid valve.

⑥ When aortic valve regurgitation coexists with stenosis, cardioplegia may be infused directly into the coronary arteries after aortic valvotomy. Or, if repeat doses are deemed necessary, the illustrated technique may be used.

⑦ A simple over-and-over running suture technique is almost always satisfactory in closing the aortotomy. Alternatively, a running mattress suture technique followed by reinforcement with an over-and-over technique can be used.

⑧ Left ventricular pressure may be monitored by insertion of a needle through the right ventricular free wall into the left ventricle across the ventricular septum. The technique of placing a catheter into the left ventricle through the ascending aorta and pulling back across the valve into the ascending aorta gives the surgeon a more informative pullback gradient.

⑨ Pacing wires are placed now only when there has been a period of complete heart block in the operating room. This is rare in the management of valvular aortic stenosis, but may occur in association with ventricular septal defect closure or tricuspid valve replacement, or in patients with L-loop.

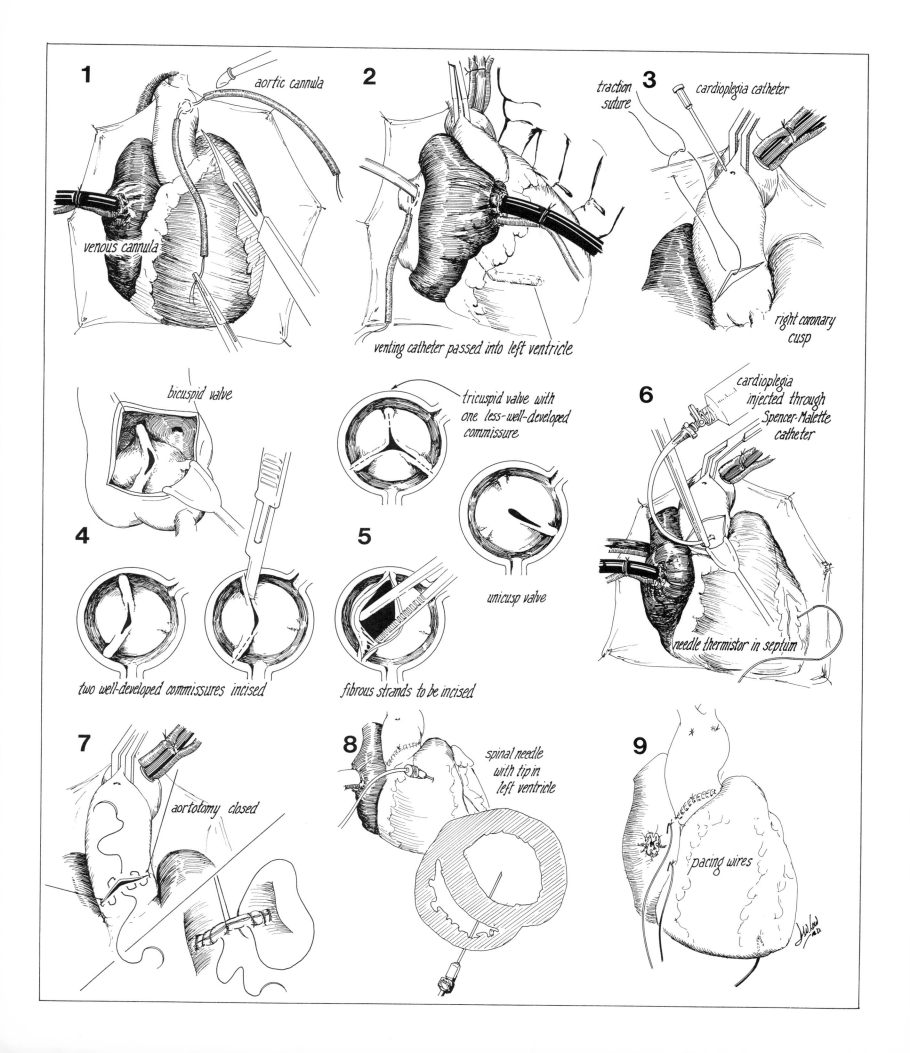

1 aortic cannula

venous cannula

2 venting catheter passed into left ventricle

3 traction suture

cardioplegia catheter

right coronary cusp

bicuspid valve

tricuspid valve with one less-well-developed commissure

6 cardioplegia injected through Spencer-Malette catheter

needle thermistor in septum

4 two well-developed commissures incised

5 fibrous strands to be incised

unicusp valve

7 aortotomy closed

8 spinal needle with tip in left ventricle

9 pacing wires

SUPRAVALVULAR AORTIC STENOSIS

Supravalvular aortic stenosis is an uncommon form of aortic stenosis often associated with Williams syndrome. This syndrome is characterized by elfin facies and hypocalcemia, usually early in life, along with the supravalvular aortic stenosis. The lesion consists of a thickened aortic wall just above the commissurae of the valve with an internal shelf that is most prominent posteriorly.

(1)   Cannulation for cardiopulmonary bypass is identical to that for valvular aortic stenosis. Externally, the supravalvular narrowing in the aorta can be seen as an hourglass configuration of the aorta.

(2)   A vent may be left in the left ventricle, but more satisfactory management is possible with pulmonary arterial suction. A longitudinal incision is made in the aorta, across the narrowing anteriorly, and carried into the noncoronary sinus of Valsalva.

(3)   A posterior shelf, characteristic and readily visible in this type of stenosis, can cause narrowing of the inlet to the left coronary sinus of Valsalva by close approximation of the commissurae of the aortic valve. Such a narrowed inlet can ultimately cause left coronary arterial obstruction. On cineangiography, there is characteristically a large left main coronary artery.

(4)   Some of the membrane or shelf may be excised.

(5)   In excising the tissue, it should be emphasized that the majority of distortion is a posterior shelf with involvement of the inlet to the left sinus of Valsalva. If the architecture is sufficiently restored by aortotomy and excision of intima posteriorly, a simple diamond-shaped gusset can be used to augment the narrowed waste of the aorta laterally.

(6)   Occasionally, the inlet to the right sinus of Valsalva is involved, and a Y-shaped incision may be carried into the right sinus of Valsalva. In this circumstance, some surgeons excise a pie-shaped portion of aortic wall as an expedient means of excising the fibrous membrane anteriorly.

(7)   Such an incision is gusseted with a Y-shaped pantaloon patch cut to fit the incision.

(8)   Some surgeons feel that a Teflon felt strip buttresses the suture line, but in most patients this is unnecessary.

(9)   Air is vented on removal of the aortic crossclamp.

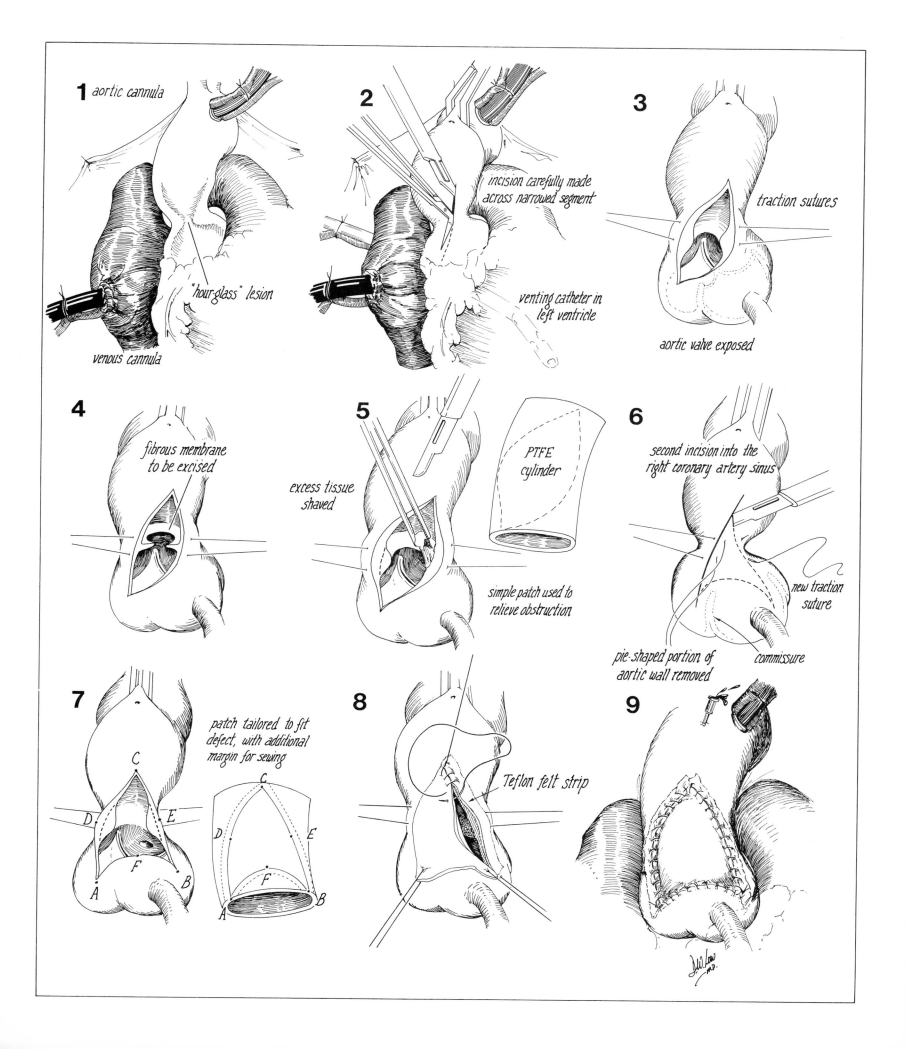

1 aortic cannula

venous cannula

"hour-glass" lesion

2 incision carefully made across narrowed segment

venting catheter in left ventricle

3 traction sutures

aortic valve exposed

4 fibrous membrane to be excised

5 excess tissue shaved

PTFE cylinder

simple patch used to relieve obstruction

6 second incision into the right coronary artery sinus

new traction suture

pie-shaped portion of aortic wall removed

commissure

7 patch tailored to fit defect, with additional margin for sewing

C

D E

F

A B

C

D E

F

A B

8 Teflon felt strip

9

SUBAORTIC STENOSIS

Subaortic stenosis can occur from discrete fibrous obstruction of the left ventricular outflow tract, which may be a delicate membranous structure with central perforation or more extensive long-segment fibrosis of the left ventricular outflow tract extending onto the aortic valve. This is an acquired process, virtually never observed in the newborn but observed in the infant and child. It is progressive, and involvement of the aortic valve occurs relatively late in the process, causing aortic valve regurgitation. It may develop as an accompaniment of a ventricular septal defect that closes naturally or is surgically closed.

Sharp incision with a surgical knife has been described as treatment, but most often a smooth plane of endocardium can be found below the fibrous tissue. Once in the proper plane, the fibrous tissue can often be stripped off the endocardium by blunt dissection and removed from the aortic valve as well. With this combination of sharp and blunt excision, aortic regurgitation is most often reversible, and when smooth endocardium remains, recurrence is rare. Long-segment or tunnel-like left ventricular outflow tract obstruction, particularly when accompanied by aortic annular hypoplasia and aortic valvular stenosis, is treatable by the Konno procedure. The operation allows enlargement of the aortic annulus for placement of a large prosthetic valve to treat aortic valvular stenosis and annular hypoplasia as well as enlargement of the left ventricular outflow tract by ventricular septal augmentation. When annular hypoplasia or aortic valvular stenosis does not coexist, modification of Konno's procedure with preservation of the annulus but also with septal augmentation may be efficacious. Outflow tract obstruction accompanying IHSS is treatable by septal myomectomy, mitral valve replacement, or pericardial patch augmentation of the anterior leaflet of the mitral valve.

1   In pathologic specimens, subaortic fibrous obstruction can be seen to encompass the immediate subaortic region circumferentially with fibrous tissue, involving the anterior leaflet of the mitral valve and extending up onto the aortic valve leaflets.

2   Obstruction results from both the fibrous encroachment on the outflow cross-sectional area and the confining enlargement of the left ventricular outflow by a "napkin ring" effect.

3   Through an aortotomy, the fibrous obstruction can be readily visualized and removal of tissue begun by obtaining the appropriate plane of dissection with sharp dissection. To aid excision of the tissue, a skin hook may be used to stabilize a segment of fibrous ring for incision with a sharp No.11 blade.

4   In the proper plane, tissue may be bluntly teased off the anterior leaflet of the mitral valve with a skin hook or forceps for retraction.

5   The tissue often extends up onto the leaflets of the aortic valve, and blunt dissection advantageously relieves the aortic leaflets to reverse aortic valve regurgitation.

6   Similarly, the tissue can be removed from the septal surface with a combination of blunt and sharp dissection exposing normal endocardium. Leaving normal endocardium may attenuate recurrence.

Modified Konno Operation

7   The modified Konno operation can be used to augment a hypoplastic aortic root by carrying an aortotomy down between the right and left coronary ostia through the annulus of the aortic valve into the ventricular septum. A right ventriculotomy in the infundibulum is made to better expose the extent of the ventricular septal augmentation. An elongated diamond-shaped Dacron patch can be sutured into the ventricular septum with running or interrupted sutures to the level of the aortic annulus. A large prosthetic valve can usually be placed, securing the anteriormost rim of the prosthetic sewing ring to the midportion of the Dacron gusset.

8   Completion of augmentation of left ventricular outflow is accomplished by augmenting the aortotomy with the superior half of the Dacron augmentation patch.

9   Closure of the ventriculotomy with a pericardial patch extending up around the Dacron patch on the ascending aorta minimizes the postoperative bleeding from the Dacron graft by allowing drainage from the Dacron gusset suture line to flow into the infundibulum and pulmonary artery.

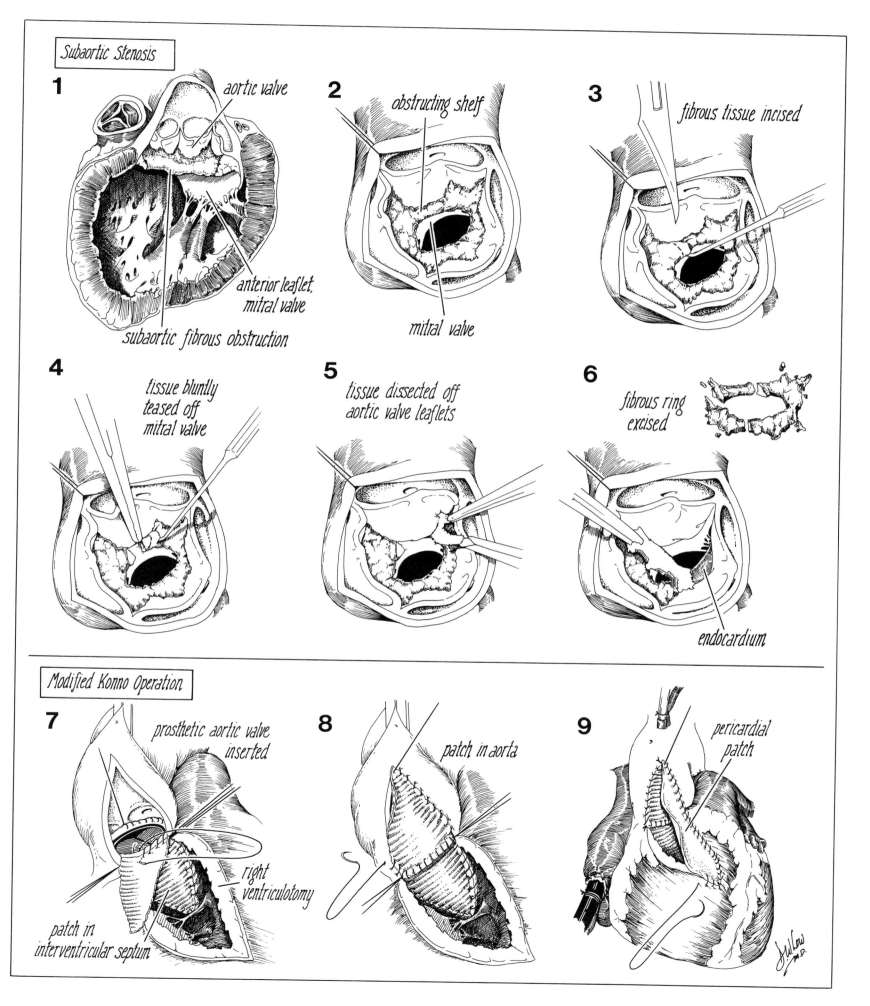

Subaortic Stenosis

1 aortic valve
subaortic fibrous obstruction
anterior leaflet, mitral valve

2 obstructing shelf
mitral valve

3 fibrous tissue incised

4 tissue bluntly teased off mitral valve

5 tissue dissected off aortic valve leaflets

6 fibrous ring excised
endocardium

Modified Konno Operation

7 prosthetic aortic valve inserted
right ventriculotomy
patch in interventricular septum

8 patch in aorta

9 pericardial patch

APICAL AORTIC CONDUIT

Complex left ventricular outflow tract and aortic root obstruction, particularly following multiple operations or in the very young, can be treated by interposition of a valved conduit between the apex of the left ventricular and thoracic aorta. When aortic regurgitation is not present, these complex obstructions are easily managed by conduit interposition without cardiopulmonary bypass.

1 For ease of conduit placement and replacement, a sixth intercostal space left lateral thoracotomy incision is made, exposing the contents of the lower left thorax. Following superior retraction of the lung, the parietal pleura over the distal thoracic aorta is incised, exposing the aorta.

2 A side-biting clamp is placed on the thoracic aorta and the distal anastomosis of a prosthetic-valved Dacron conduit of appropriate size is established with a running monofilament suture line. Bleeding is minimal in the absence of heparinization, and a controlling occluding clamp is placed on the very distal aspect of the valved conduit after removal of the aortic clamp.

3 An incision in the pericardium anterior to the phrenic nerve exposes the apex of the left ventricle. The apex is readily identified by the anatomical boundary of the anterior and posterior descending coronary arteries and easily recognized by palpation with an index finger. Four felt pledgeted, buttressed, double-armed sutures are placed in four quadrants of the apex of the left ventricle in preparation for securing the apical conduit stent.

4 A stab incision is made in the left ventricular apex and a balloon-tipped Foley catheter is inserted. The balloon is inflated and the catheter is withdrawn to interface the balloon snugly with the endocardial surface of the left ventricle. This maneuver keeps the papillary muscles away from the apical ventriculotomy and provides hemostatic control.

5 An appropriate-sized cork borer, the same size as the lumen of the apical stent, is then threaded over the balloon-tipped catheter and a core of apical muscle is gently excised by twirling the cork borer against gentle retraction on the Foley catheter.

6 The cork borer is then removed from the catheter and replaced by the apical stent, which is inserted into the apical incision. The stent is positioned so that the Dacron tube will face posteriorly and to the left for anastomosis with the valved conduit.

7 The four stay sutures are then placed through the sewing ring of the apical stent as bleeding is controlled with balloon occlusion of the tip of the stent. Although it is unnecessary in most cases, the stent may be further secured to the myocardium with a running suture technique.

8 The balloon-tipped catheter is deflated and removed as the Dacron portion of the apical stent is occluded with a vascular clamp.

9 The simple reconstruction is completed by anastomosis of the apical stent to the Dacron-valved conduit with a running monofilament suture, and de-airing is accomplished with removal of the distal and subsequently proximal clamps.

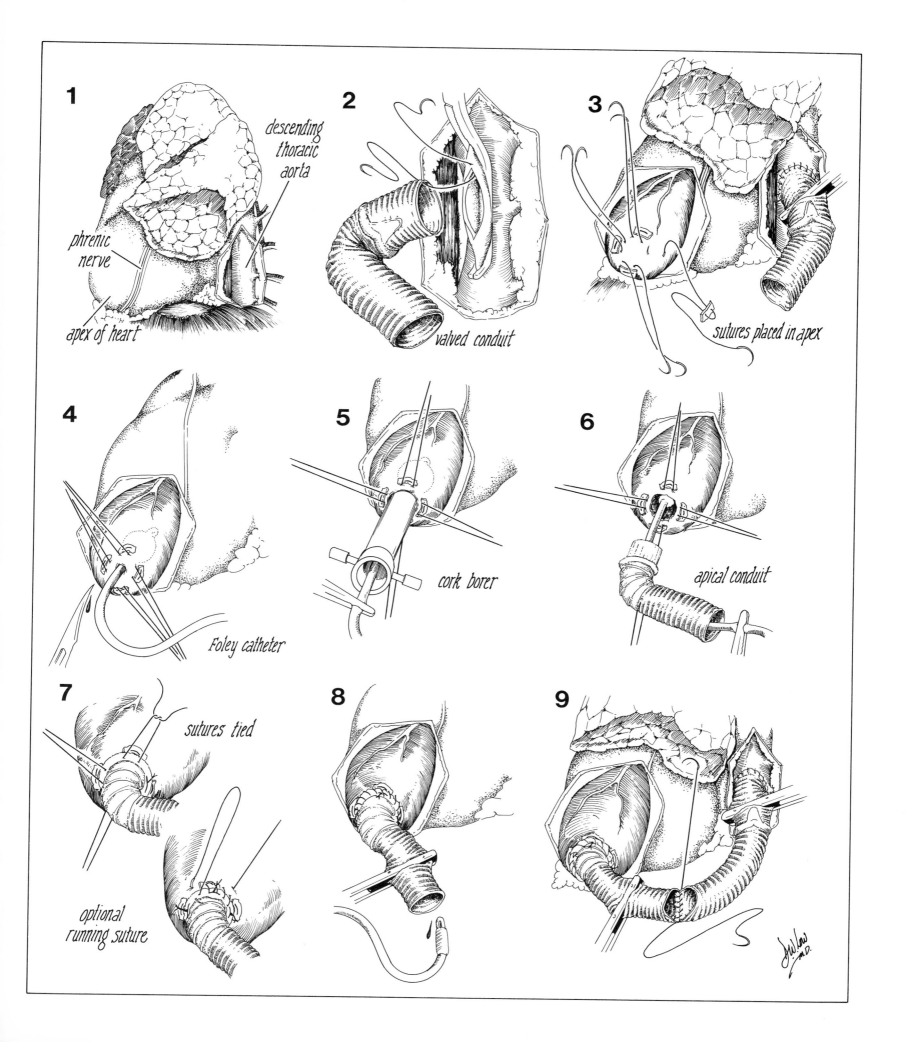

1
phrenic nerve
descending thoracic aorta
apex of heart

2
valved conduit

3
sutures placed in apex

4
Foley catheter

5
cork borer

6
apical conduit

7
sutures tied
optional running suture

8

9

HYPOPLASTIC LEFT HEART SYNDROME

Hypoplastic left heart syndrome is the most common form of congenital cardiac malformation in which there is only one ventricle. In principle, extensive physiologic repair can be achieved by application of Fontan's procedure. At birth, the pulmonary vascular resistance is naturally elevated, nearly systemic, precluding an early Fontan procedure, yet the child has a systemic circulation dependent on patency of the ductus arteriosus. Therefore, a staged surgical strategy is necessary. Initial palliation is designed to associate the right ventricle to the aorta, regulate pulmonary blood flow, and avoid pulmonary venous hypertension by excision of the atrial septum. All children should be managed preoperatively by continuous infusion of the prostaglandin E1 to maintain patency of the ductus arteriosus. Any metabolic acidosis is treated by sodium bicarbonate infusion. Catecholamine infusion is rarely necessary and may be counterproductive. Hyperventilation or ventilation with a high FiO_2 should be avoided preoperatively.

1 Most infants with hypoplastic left heart syndrome have aortic valve atresia, and as a consequence, flow in the aortic arch and ascending aorta is retrograde. The ascending aorta is diminutive (1 to 3 mm in diameter) carrying only flow to the coronary vascular bed. Cardiopulmonary bypass is instituted by cannulation of the large main pulmonary artery trunk and a single venous cannula is placed in the right atrial appendage. The branch pulmonary arteries are occluded with tourniquets during core cooling on cardiopulmonary bypass, and the brachycephalic vessels are isolated.

2 The circulation is arrested, the brachycephalic vessels are occluded, and the cannulae for cardiopulmonary bypass are removed. Through a right atrial appendage cannulation site, the septum primum is visualized and resected. The main pulmonary artery is then divided at the origin of the right and left pulmonary artery branches.

3 The distal main pulmonary artery is oversewn, using a patch to avoid late occurrence of discontinuity between the right and left pulmonary artery branches. The ductus arteriosus is ligated and divided.

4 An incision is carried into the thoracic aorta for 1 to 1 1/2 cm and retrograde on the aortic arch and ascending aorta to the level of the proximal transsected main pulmonary artery. This wide aortotomy is generated to enlarge the ascending aorta and aortic arch to a normal size and configuration.

5 The patch material used for this gusset can be made from pulmonary homograft. The gusset is begun far into the thoracic aorta to avoid late development of coarctation of the aorta and right ventricular hypertension.

6 A 4 mm tube graft is interposed between the aortic arch and the branch pulmonary arteries to provide appropriate pulmonary blood flow.

7 The gusset is sutured to the ascending aorta to within 5 mm of the proximal incision.

8 The reconstruction is completed by anastomosis of the proximal main pulmonary artery to the ascending aorta and pulmonary homograft. In those with the most diminutive ascending aortas, measuring 1 to 2 mm in diameter, multiple interrupted sutures avoids purse-stringing the aortic root, which can compromise coronary perfusion.

9 The main pulmonary artery is sutured in a running continuous suture technique to the pulmonary homograft, completing the neo-aorta.

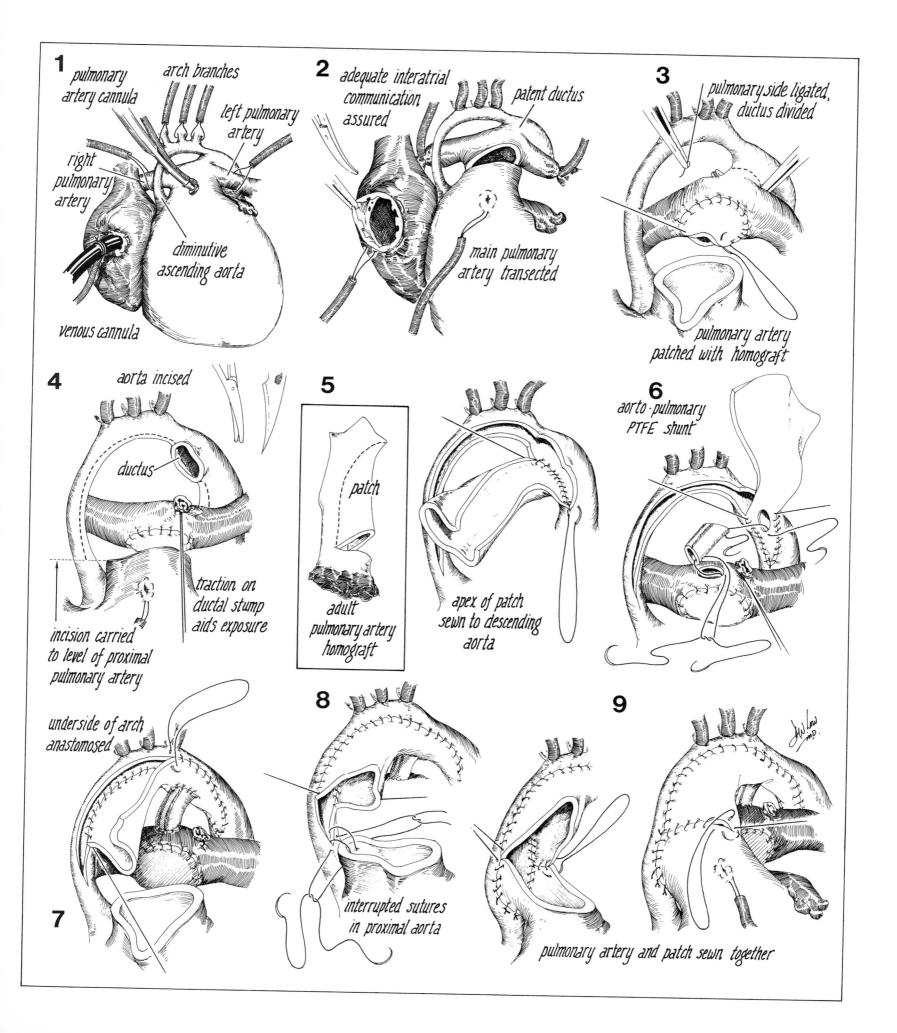

1
pulmonary artery cannula
arch branches
left pulmonary artery
right pulmonary artery
diminutive ascending aorta
venous cannula

2 adequate interatrial communication assured
patent ductus
main pulmonary artery transected

3 pulmonary side ligated, ductus divided
pulmonary artery patched with homograft

4 aorta incised
ductus
traction on ductal stump aids exposure
incision carried to level of proximal pulmonary artery

5
patch
adult pulmonary artery homograft
apex of patch sewn to descending aorta

6 aorto-pulmonary PTFE shunt

7 underside of arch anastomosed

8 interrupted sutures in proximal aorta

9 pulmonary artery and patch sewn together

HYPOPLASTIC LEFT HEART SYNDROME—MODIFIED
FONTAN PROCEDURE

When a child with hypoplastic left heart syndrome is at approximately 18 months of age, a modified Fontan procedure is performed to complete staged reconstructive surgery with a view to preserving right ventricular function.

(10) Cardiopulmonary bypass is instituted and the patient is cooled to 20° C. During this time, the central shunt is occluded and the branch pulmonary arteries are exposed posterior to the aorta.

(11) The pulmonary artery is incised anteriorly to the left upper lobe branch and right upper lobe branch. The central pulmonary artery architecture is augmented with a patch of pulmonary homograft material to avoid distortion of the central pulmonary arteries.

(12) This augmentation gusset is secured with running monofilament suture.

(13) An incision is made in the right atrium from the sulcus terminalis to the insertion of the eustachian valve inferiorly on the right lateral free wall of the right atrium. A separate incision is made superiorly in the dome of the atrium and extended into the right superior vena cava posteriorly to the adjacent incision in the right pulmonary artery.

(14) The right pulmonary artery and right atrium are sutured to form the floor of the systemic venous connection to the pulmonary arteries.

(15) Half of a cylindric tube graft is sutured in the right atrium along the right lateral free wall to baffle the systemic venous return from the inferior vena cava to the anastomosis to the right pulmonary artery superiorly.

(16) Thus, this interatrial systemic venous channel is formed in part with the right atrial free wall to accommodate growth and in part with the baffle.

(17) The pulmonary homograft gusseting the central pulmonary arteries is sutured to the right atrium and right superior vena cava, completing the roof of the anastomosis between the systemic venous channel and the right pulmonary artery.

(18) Thus, systemic venous return is baffled to the right pulmonary artery and pulmonary venous return enters the diminutive left atrium and passes through the widened interatrial communication to the right atrium, which acts as a pulmonary venous reservoir and fills the right ventricle.

(19) An alternative approach is to place an intra-atrial tube graft, channeling superior vena caval return to the superior aspect of the right atrium. Interatrial tube grafts may be useful in applying Fontan's procedure to complex congenital cardiac malformations in which the systemic and pulmonary venous connections are complicated.

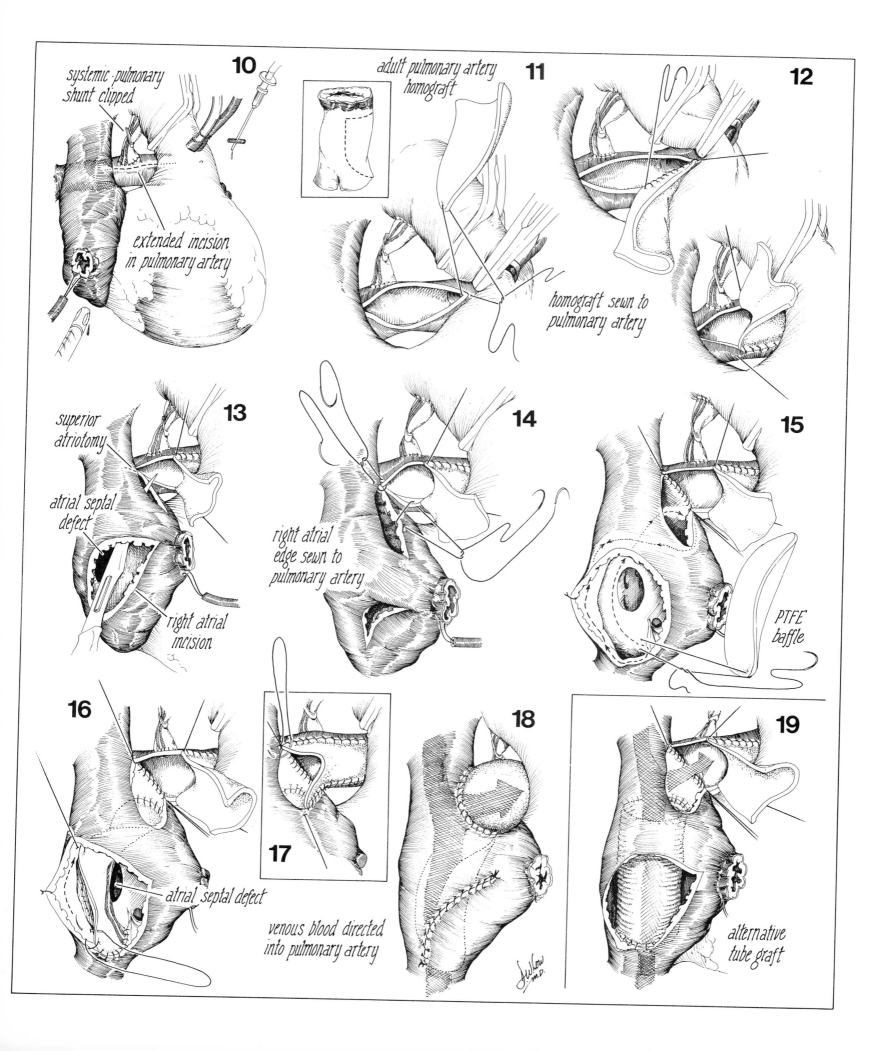

10 systemic-pulmonary shunt clipped

extended incision in pulmonary artery

11 adult pulmonary artery homograft

12 homograft sewn to pulmonary artery

13 superior atriotomy

atrial septal defect

right atrial incision

14 right atrial edge sewn to pulmonary artery

15 PTFE baffle

16 atrial septal defect

17

18 venous blood directed into pulmonary artery

19 alternative tube graft

Surgery for Malformations Resulting in Left-To-Right or Right-To-Left Shunts

ATRIAL SEPTAL DEFECT OF THE SECUNDUM TYPE

Excluding defects of the common atrium, there are three types of atrial septal defect: ostium primum, ostium secundum, and sinus venosus. The secundum type is a consequence of abnormal development of the septum primum. The deficiency may occur superiorly, causing a defect that appears to be a large foramen ovale, because the length of the septum primum is insufficient to abut with the superior limbic band. The septum primum may be totally absent, and the inferior vena cava inflow runs directly across the floor of the atrium toward the mitral valve. Moreover, there may also be multiple fenestrations of the septum primum.

In an isolated atrial septal defect, the compliance of the right ventricle is much greater than that of the left ventricle, and during ventricular diastole, flow across the interatrial communication is from left to right, causing pulmonary overcirculation and volume load on the right ventricle. In isolated atrial septal defect, if physical findings and echocardiography are characteristic, they may be relied on for preoperative diagnostic information. There is generally a right ventricular heave, an accentuated P2 that is widely split and often fixed. A systolic murmur in the region of the pulmonary valve is characteristic, and when the Qp:Qs is greater than 2, a diastolic rumble can often be heard. The electrocardiogram characteristically demonstrates a long PR interval and RSR[1] waveform in the early precordial leads. Right axis deviation distinguishes an atrial septal defect of the ostium secundum type from one of the ostium primum type in 95% of cases.

Children are usually asymptomatic of atrial septal defect. Occasionally an infant develops severe congestive heart failure and fails to thrive. Even in the absence of symptoms, atrial septal defects should probably be closed because of the potential for late development of arrhythmias, right ventricular dysfunction, pulmonary vascular obstructive disease, or paroxysmal embolus in adulthood.

1 Although a midline sternotomy incision is the most conventional means of exposing an atrial septal defect, this defect can be readily managed through a right thoracotomy incision in the fourth intercostal space. Exposure of the heart is through an incision in the pericardium anterior to the phrenic nerve after posterior retraction of the lung.

2 Cannulation for cardiopulmonary bypass is by arterial infusion in the ascending aorta and venous cannulae placed in the superior and inferior vena cava through incisions in the right atrial appendage and inferior vena caval-right atrial junction controlled with purse-string sutures.

3 Cardiopulmonary bypass is initiated and the venous cannulae threaded just into the distal vena cavae. Venous drainage is isolated from the right atrium with suture tourniquets around the cavae. The aorta can then be crossclamped and cardioplegia solution infused in the proximal aortic root. An incision in the right atrium then exposes the atrial septum.

4 Exploration of the internal anatomy of the atrium confirms the level of systemic and pulmonary venous drainage in atrial septal anatomy.

5 The secundum type of defect characteristically has a superior boundary composed of the superior limbic band.

6 When the atrial septal defect is oval in configuration and the lateral borders are easily juxtaposed without tension, the defect can be closed, primarily with a running suture technique. The suture line should be begun inferiorly and finished superiorly to minimize entrapment of air in the left atrial side.

7 The anesthesiologist can assist in evacuating air from the left side by inflating the lung with a Valsalva maneuver while the final throw of the suture is pulled tight.

8 When the atrial septal defect is large, round in configuration, or has walls that are not easily brought together without tension, closure is accomplished with a patch. The material used is probably not important here, but is either pericardium or a thin sheet of Teflon. Again, the patch is secured inferiorly first with running suture technique, and air is evacuated from the left atrium in a fashion similar to that used in primary suture closure.

9 The aortic crossclamp is removed with air venting through the cardioplegia cannulation site. The atriotomy is closed using a running monofilament suture technique and the caval tourniquets are released just before completion of this suture line to evacuate air from the right atrium. This surgical procedure is completed during a period of moderate hypothermia (rectal temperature approximately 32° C. When the patient has been rewarmed to 36 or 37° C, cardiopulmonary bypass is discontinued, and decannulation is accomplished.

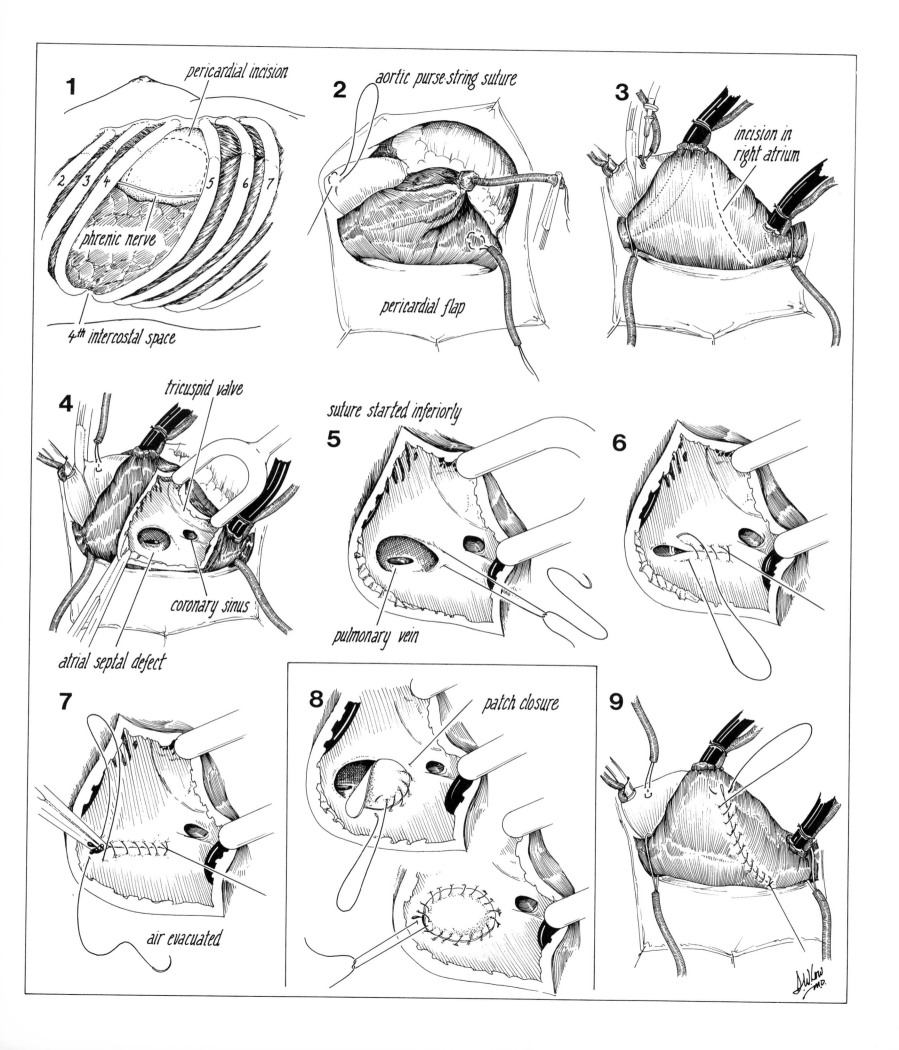

1 pericardial incision
phrenic nerve
4th intercostal space

2 aortic purse-string suture
pericardial flap

3 incision in right atrium

4 tricuspid valve
coronary sinus
atrial septal defect

5 suture started inferiorly
pulmonary vein

6

7 air evacuated

8 patch closure

9

ATRIAL SEPTAL DEFECT OF THE OSTIUM PRIMUM TYPE

An atrial septal defect of the ostium primum type is a form of abnormal development of the atrial ventricular canal. Although there is no ventricular septal defect in this malformation, deficiency of the atrioventricular canal causes displacement of the plane of the atrioventricular valves inferiorly and to the left. As a consequence, the distance between the plane of the mitral valve and the apex of the left ventricle is shorter than the distance from the aortic valve to the apex of the left ventricle where these distances are equivalent in the normal heart. The septum primum is present, at least in part, in the majority. There may be a patent foramen ovale. Characteristic in electrocardiograms of patients with a septum primum atrial septal defect is a counterclockwise loop with left-axis deviation as a consequence of deficiency of the atrioventricular canal.

1 Cannulation for total cardiopulmonary bypass is similar to that for exposure of an atrial septal defect of the secundum type. The incision can be identical or perhaps more conveniently placed posteriorly.

2 Retraction of the anterior free wall of the right atrium exposes the ostium primum atrial septal defect. Almost always there is a cleft in the anterior leaflet of the left atrioventricular valve. It is felt that this valve develops with three dominant leaflets as opposed to two in the normal heart.

3 In circumstances where there is atrioventricular valve regurgitation, this "cleft" may be approximated by several interrupted monofilament sutures. When regurgitation is not present, there is some controversy about the efficacy of approximation of the valve leaflets to prevent potential future development of regurgitation.

4 The atrial septal defect is closed with an appropriate-sized patch. In this case, pericardium again can be used. A smooth type of patch material is chosen to minimize the possibility of hemolysis if mild to moderate mitral regurgitation is present postoperatively.

5 It is convenient to begin a continuous suture technique at the central portion of the mitral and tricuspid valve confluence. The suture line can be carried inferiorly, remaining in atrioventricular valve tissue until one is beyond the coronary sinus, and thus away from the course of the conduction tissue.

6 The patch is then secured superiorly and concluded in the atrial septum.

7 A left atrial pressure monitoring catheter may be placed in the left atrium through a small incision at the junction of the superior right pulmonary vein and atrium and sutured in place.

8 The atriotomy is closed with a continuous monofilament suture technique.

9 Although mitral insufficiency may be assessed by palpation in the larger patent, left atrial pressure, pressure waveform, and echocardiography are the most reliable means of determining the presence and significance of mitral regurgitation in most patients early in the postoperative period.

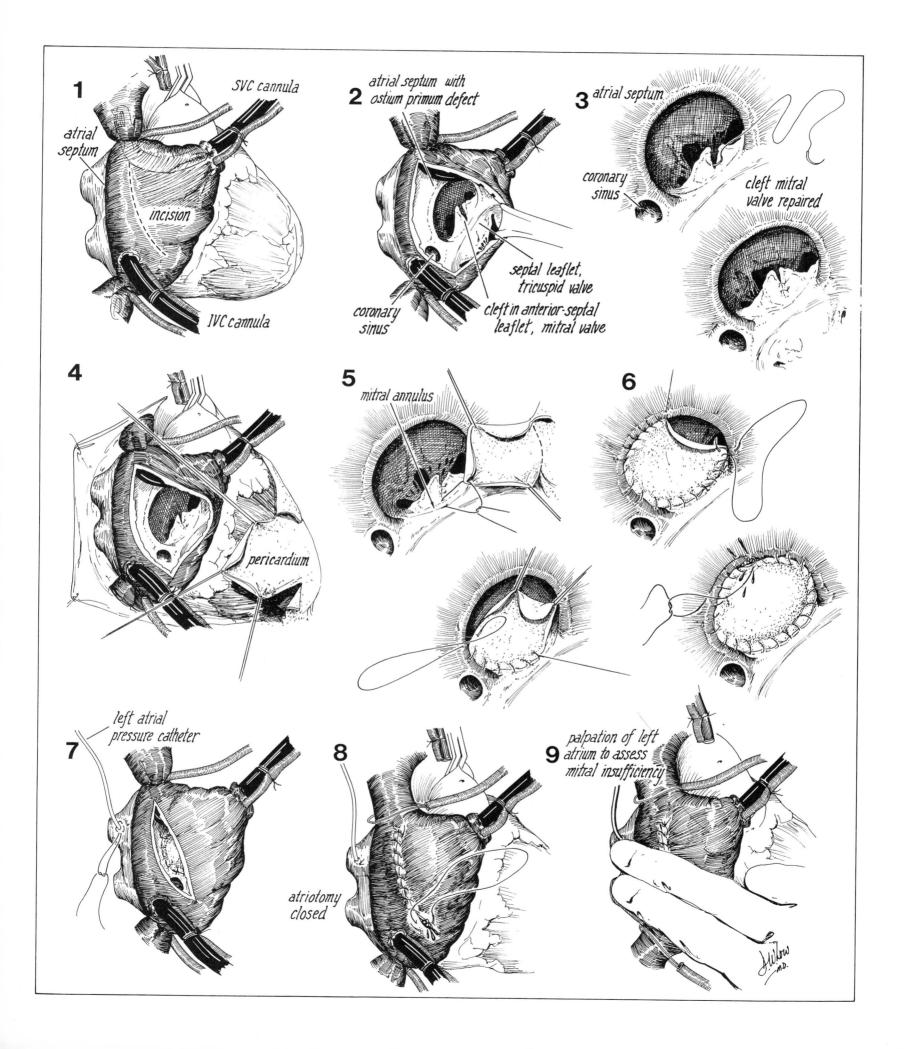

1   SVC cannula   atrial septum   incision   IVC cannula

2   atrial septum with ostium primum defect   septal leaflet, tricuspid valve   coronary sinus   cleft in anterior-septal leaflet, mitral valve

3   atrial septum   coronary sinus   cleft mitral valve repaired

4   pericardium

5   mitral annulus

6

7   left atrial pressure catheter

8   atriotomy closed

9   palpation of left atrium to assess mitral insufficiency

SINUS VENOSUS ATRIAL SEPTAL DEFECT

The sinus venosus type of atrial septal defect is less common than the secundum or ostium primum type and occurs in about 5% of patients with atrial septal defects. It is usually superior and associated with absence of the right lateral superior limbic band. There is often anomalous pulmonary venous connection of the right pulmonary veins with superior vena cava and right atrium in the region of the sinus venosus defect.

(1) The anomalous connection of the upper lobe pulmonary veins is often recognizable from the outside of the heart.

(2) Closure of the atrial septal defect includes the pulmonary veins on the left atrial aspect of the newly reconstructed atrial septum. Satisfactory exposure can most often be accomplished by cannulation of the superior vena cava through the right atrial appendage in the usual fashion. Alternatively, the superior vena caval snare can be placed superior to the entrance of the pulmonary veins and a purse-string suture placed in the superior vena cava. A right-angled cannula may facilitate this form of cannulation.

(3) An incision is made in the right atrium to expose the sinus venosus defect after acquisition of total cardiopulmonary bypass aortic crossclamping and infusion of cold cardioplegic solution.

(4) The atrial septal defect is superior and to the right of the septum primum.

(5) To facilitate association of the upper lobe pulmonary veins to the left atrium, the atrial septal defect can be enlarged inferiorly by excision of the atrial septum.

(6) The atrial septal defect is closed with patch material, which may be pericardium.

(7) A running suture technique is satisfactory.

(8) Pulmonary venous blood is thus shunted to the left atrium underneath the atrial septal defect patch.

(9) The atriotomy can be closed primarily, or the inferior aspect of the right superior vena cava can be enlarged with a patch to ensure unobstructed drainage of both the pulmonary veins and the superior vena cava.

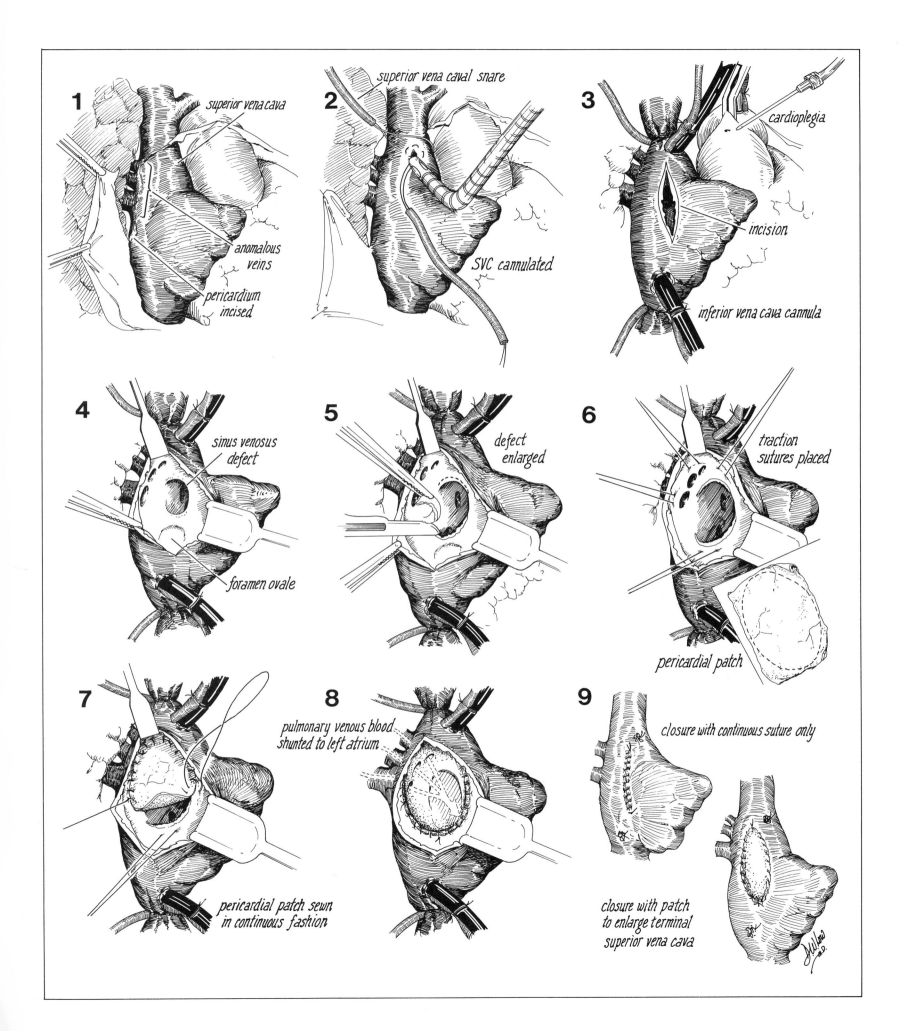

1
superior vena cava
anomalous veins
pericardium incised

2
superior vena caval snare
SVC cannulated

3
cardioplegia
incision
inferior vena cava cannula

4
sinus venosus defect
foramen ovale

5
defect enlarged

6
traction sutures placed
pericardial patch

7
pericardial patch sewn in continuous fashion

8
pulmonary venous blood shunted to left atrium

9
closure with continuous suture only
closure with patch to enlarge terminal superior vena cava

COMPLETE COMMON ATRIOVENTRICULAR CANAL DEFECT

Complete common atrioventricular canal defect is caused by a deficiency in the canal septum and development of atrioventricular valves. The consequences are a ventricular septal defect, usually large; an atrial septal defect; and associated abnormal development of the atrioventricular valves. Rastelli and colleagues described three distinct anatomic types, defined by the structure of the superior cushion elements of the atrioventricular valves. These discrete types actually form a continuum in developmental abnormality of the valves. Rastelli type A is partial or complete division of the superior cushion elements with chordal attachments of these leaflets to the septal crest. Type B is an extremely rare type with valve leaflets similar in structure to type A but with chordae passing from the left AV valve component to a papillary muscle associated with the right ventricle usually in the ventricular septum. Type C is an undivided free-floating superior leaflet with no chordal attachments to the ventricular septum.

Forty-five to 50% of patients with trisomy-21 (Down's syndrome) have a cardiac malformation, which is usually an atrioventricular canal defect. The next most common defects in patients with trisomy-21 are ventricular septal defect and tetralogy of Fallot. Most often, the ventricular septal defect associated with complete common atrioventricular canal is large, and babies with this defect often have nearly systemic pulmonary arterial pressure, fail to thrive, and require surgical management in the first year of life. When mitral regurgitation coexists, congestive heart failure is exacerbated.

(1) Rastelli types A, B, and C of atrioventricular valve anatomy are illustrated.

(2) Repair in type A may be accomplished with a single patch with suspension of the AV valve leaflets to the patch or, alternatively, two separate patches, one for the ventricular septal defect and one for the atrial septal defect. When a single patch is used to repair type A, complete common atrioventricular canal defect, separation of the mitral and tricuspid portion of the superior leaflets may be completed.

(3) Although some surgeons prefer interrupted sutures, ventricular septal defect component is usually closed by continuous suture in the rightward aspect of the ventricular septum. The septal crest is avoided inferiorly to remain distant from the conduction system.

(4) The two septal components of the left atrioventricular valve may be approximated centrally if regurgitation is assessed by injection of saline into the left ventricle. In the absence of regurgitation, approximation is not necessary.

(5) The atrioventricular valve leaflets are attached to the patch with a running suture technique and secured with a few interrupted pledgeted sutures.

(6) Following assessment of the competence of the left atrioventricular valve and appropriate restructuring, the atrial septal defect component is closed with continuous monofilament sutures.

(7) Again, the conduction system is avoided by anchoring the atrial septal defect patch in atrioventricular valve tissue until one is beyond the coronary sinus ostium. Alternatively, the atrial septal defect patch may be fashioned or secured around the coronary sinus so that the coronary sinus drainage is diverted to the left atrium.

(8) Rastelli Type B atrioventricular canal defect can be managed by incising appropriate chordae or, alternatively, placing the ventricular septal defect patch around the right-sided papillary muscle.

(9) Rastelli type C atrioventricular canal defect can be managed with a single- or double-patch technique. When a single-patch technique is used, the superior cushion element is incised, borrowing somewhat from the tricuspid valve portion to restructure the mitral valve.

(10) When mitral regurgitation is severe and AV valve tissue is insufficient to reconstruct a competent mitral valve, valve replacement is indicated.

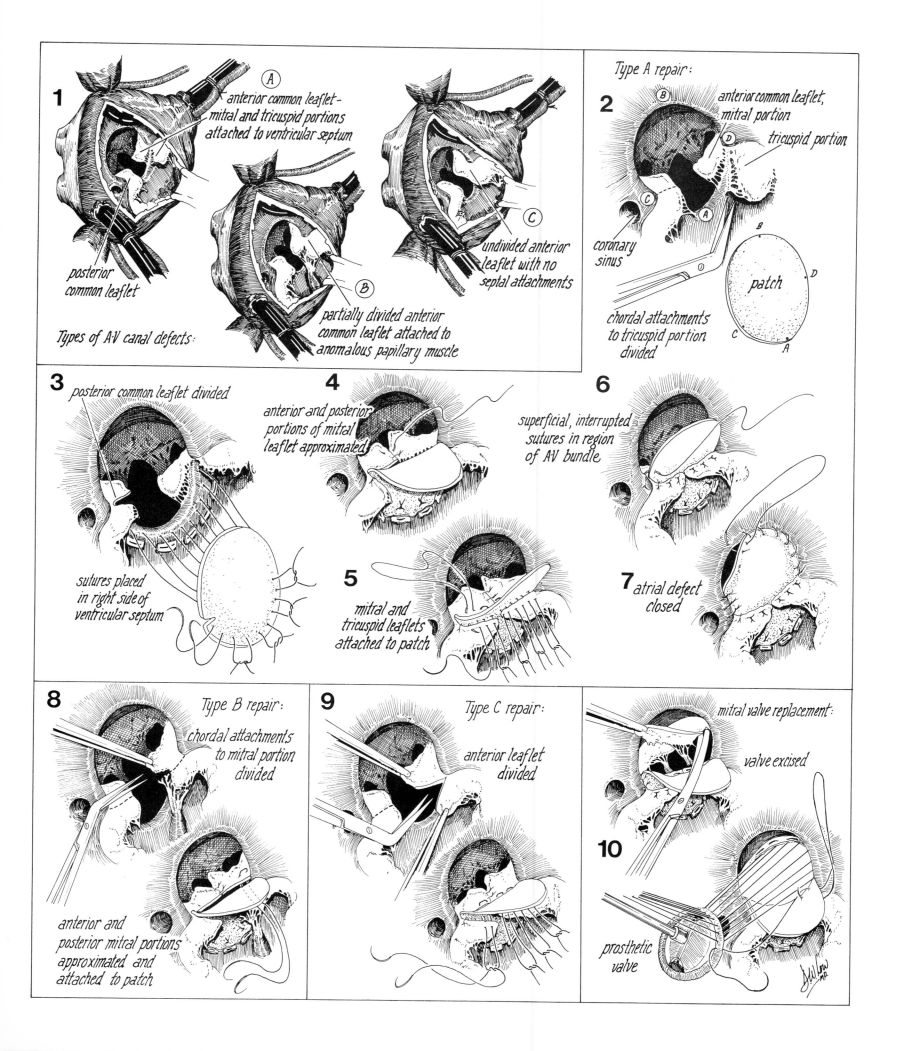

MUSTARD'S OPERATION

Transposition of the great arteries {S,D,D} is the second or third most common congenital cardiac malformation presenting in the first year of life. Anatomically, transposition of the great arteries is simply the aorta arising from the anatomical right ventricle and the pulmonary artery arising from the anatomical left ventricle. In situs solitus with dextro-loop, the systemic venous return is pumped by the right ventricle back to the body while pulmonary venous return goes to the lungs. After birth, admixture of systemic and pulmonary blood must occur to provide sufficient oxygenation for survival. This takes place in the newborn period by way of the patent ductus arteriosus and foramen ovale. In the early 1960s, a convenient and satisfactory means of palliation of children with transposition of the great arteries was developed by William Rashkind and colleagues using a balloon-tipped catheter to disrupt the septum primum of the atrial septum.

Definitive surgical management was initially directed at transposing the two great arteries. Initial successful treatment, however, was reported by Ake Senning. He baffled systemic venous return to the left ventricle using a series of flaps of atrium and septum. This atrial inversion strategy was simplified by Mustard. This contribution became a widely accepted means of definitive management of transposition of the great arteries (TGA) in the 1960s and early 1970s.

Approximately 25% of patients with TGA {S,D,D} have an associated ventricular septal defect. Those with an intact ventricular septum should probably undergo definitive surgery in the first year of life to avoid the possible development of abnormalities associated with chronic cyanosis and development of pulmonary vascular obstructive disease.

1 During a period of circulatory arrest, an incision in the right atrium is begun in the atrial appendage and extended posteriorly between the right upper and lower lobe veins.

2 The tricuspid valve, mitral valve, and pulmonary veins are thus readily exposed. It is important that the superior limbic band be excised because it may form a ridge supporting the systemic venous baffle that will lead to obstruction if left in place.

3 The inlet to the left atrial appendage is easily visualized and is used as a landmark for the placement of the systemic venous baffle.

4 A patch of cloth is cut in the shape of trousers. Insertion of the baffle is begun in the posterior midportion of the mitral valve with a continuous monofilament suture technique.

5 The suture line is run superiorly between the pulmonary veins and the left atrial appendage toward the right lateral aspect of the inlet of the right superior vena cava with the right atrium.

6 Inferiorly, the suture line is directed toward the right lateral aspect of the inlet of the inferior vena cava.

7 A separate suture is placed in the central portion of the baffle and the juncture of the mitral and tricuspid valves centrally. This running suture line inferiorly and superiorly around the caval inlets completes the systemic venous channel.

8 This interatrial baffle directs systemic venous blood into the mitral valve.

9 The right atriotomy, which is between the right upper and right lower lobe pulmonary veins, is augmented with a patch of pericardium to avoid pulmonary venous obstruction. Pulmonary venous return then enters the heart posteriorly and flows around the baffle into the native right atrium and the tricuspid valve.

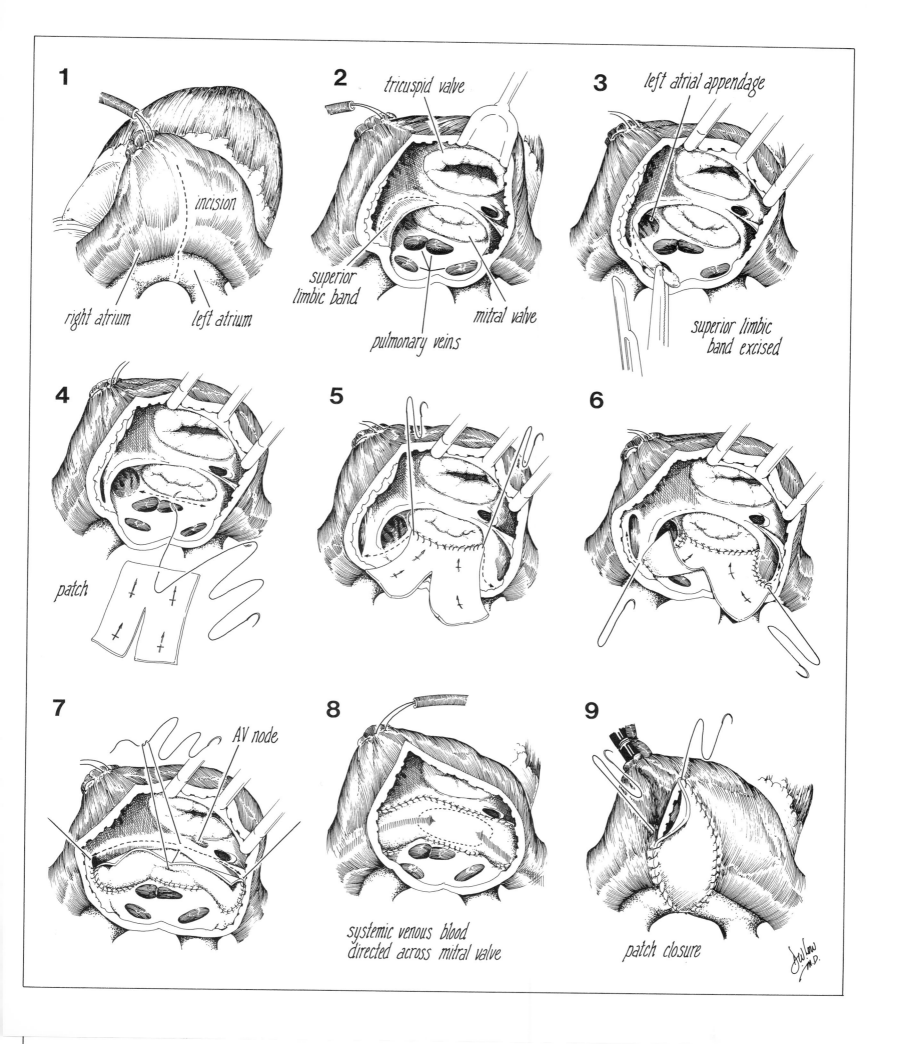

1
incision
right atrium
left atrium

2
tricuspid valve
superior limbic band
pulmonary veins
mitral valve

3
left atrial appendage
superior limbic band excised

4
patch

5

6

7
AV node

8
systemic venous blood directed across mitral valve

9
patch closure

INTERRUPTED AORTIC ARCH

Interrupted aortic arch can occur with normally related great arteries or transposition of the great arteries. It is almost always accompanied by a defect in the interventricular septum. The conoventricular type of ventricular septal defect is most common in normally related great arteries, but the defect may also be of the malalignment type with posterior deviation of the infundibular septum. The interruption can occur between the ductus arteriosus and the left subclavian artery (type A), between the left carotid and left subclavian artery (type B), or rarely between the innominate and left carotid artery (type C). A major portion of the systemic circulation depends on patency of the ductus arteriosus. The ascending aorta is usually diminutive compared to the main pulmonary artery, ductus arteriosus, and thoracic aortic continuum. Although, in the past, several means of palliating or reconstructing the aorta with tube graft interposition combined with pulmonary artery banding or closure of the ventricular septal defect were advanced, the current preference is primary reparative surgery in the neonatal period through a midline sternotomy by direct anastomosis of the ascending aorta and thoracic aorta combined with closure of the ventricular septal defect. If severe subaortic obstruction of the long segment type caused by posterior malalignment of the infundibular septum is present, aortic reconstruction must include anastomosis of the proximal main pulmonary artery to the ascending aorta. Closure of the malalignment ventricular septal defect is then carried around the pulmonary annulus and a tube graft is interposed between the infundibulum of the right ventricle and the distal main pulmonary artery. Severe subaortic obstruction in the newborn is uncommon, however, and simple ventricular septal defect closure at the time of aortic arch reconstruction usually gives the most satisfactory results.

1 The ventricular septal defect is usually of the conoventricular type and is readily identified in the region of the tricuspid valve annulus superiorly at the level of the papillary muscle of the conus. This is readily visualized through a standard right atriotomy.

2 Primary repair is most readily accomplished with a period of deep hypothermia and circulatory arrest. Arterial infusion can most often be satisfactorily obtained by infusion through the main pulmonary artery with occlusion of the branch pulmonary arteries during the cooling phase, or, occasionally, two aortic cannulae may be used; one in the ascending aorta and one in the main pulmonary artery and attached by a Y connector to a single arterial infusion cannula from the pump oxygenator.

3 Before circulatory arrest, the branch vessels of the aortic arch are occluded with suture tourniquets. The ductus arteriosus is ligated and transected at its entrance into the isthmus and thoracic aorta. An incision is made in the ascending aorta into the left carotid artery and carried into the left subclavian artery in this example of type B interrupted aortic arch. Aortic arch reconstruction is accomplished by running suture anastomosis of the incisions in the proximal and distal aorta root and branch vessel.

4 With sufficient tissue, the reconstruction can be completed with a primary anastomosis using running monofilament suture.

5 With absence of aortic arch tissue, the inferior anterior aspect of the anastomosis can be augmented with patch material with a view to achieving a uniform size of ascending aorta, aortic arch, and thoracic aorta. A tissue-type patch material helps to facilitate hemostasis in the suture line postoperatively.

Interrupted Arch with Transposition

6 When an interrupted arch accompanies transposition of the great arteries, there is often a malalignment type of ventricular septal defect. In this case, the infundibular septum is malaligned anteriorly, causing significant subaortic obstruction. The only comprehensive means of managing this constellation are by arterial switch repair of transposition of the great arteries, reconstruction of the interrupted aortic arch, patch closure of the malalignment ventricular septal defect, and patch augmentation of the right ventricular outflow tract. In this anatomical malformation, cardiopulmonary bypass can be established by either single or double arterial cannulae technique.

7 The ascending aorta and main pulmonary artery are divided in the usual fashion for an arterial switch procedure and the ductus arteriosus is ligated and divided. The ascending aorta is incised laterally up into the left carotid artery and an incision in the thoracic aorta and left subclavian artery is made as in the repair of interrupted aortic arch. Because of the large discrepancy in size between the ascending aorta and the main pulmonary artery, the aortic arch and ascending aorta are gusseted with a patch of pulmonary homograft material. The branch coronary arteries are excised from the posterior aspect of the ascending aorta and transplanted into the proximal main pulmonary artery as in the arterial switch procedure. The left carotid and left subclavian artery are anastomosed side to side and the underside of the new aortic arch and ascending aorta are gusseted with a patch of pulmonary homograft using a running monofilament suture technique. The size of the gusset is chosen to create a new ascending aorta and aortic arch of uniform size from proximal main pulmonary artery to thoracic aorta.

8 The branch pulmonary arteries, brought anterior to the distal ascending aorta, and the proximal main pulmonary artery distal ascending aorta are anastomosed, creating the new ascending aorta arising from the left ventricle and giving rise to the transplanted coronary arteries. Because of the subaortic stenosis and infundibular narrowing, an incision is carried anteriorly in the proximal native ascending aorta across the annulus into the infundibulum of the right ventricle, exposing the ventricular septal defect.

9 Through the infundibulotomy, the ventricular septal defect is readily visualized and closed with a patch, in this case using a running monofilament suture technique. The defects in the aorta, secondary to coronary artery excision, are patch-closed. The posterior aspect of the anastomosis between the proximal native ascending aorta and main pulmonary artery is begun and the entire right ventricular outflow tract is now augmented with a patch of pulmonary homograft placed anteriorly, using a running monofilament suture technique. When an atrial septal defect coexists, this is closed, completing the reconstruction of this complex, uncommon, but not rare congenital cardiac malformation.

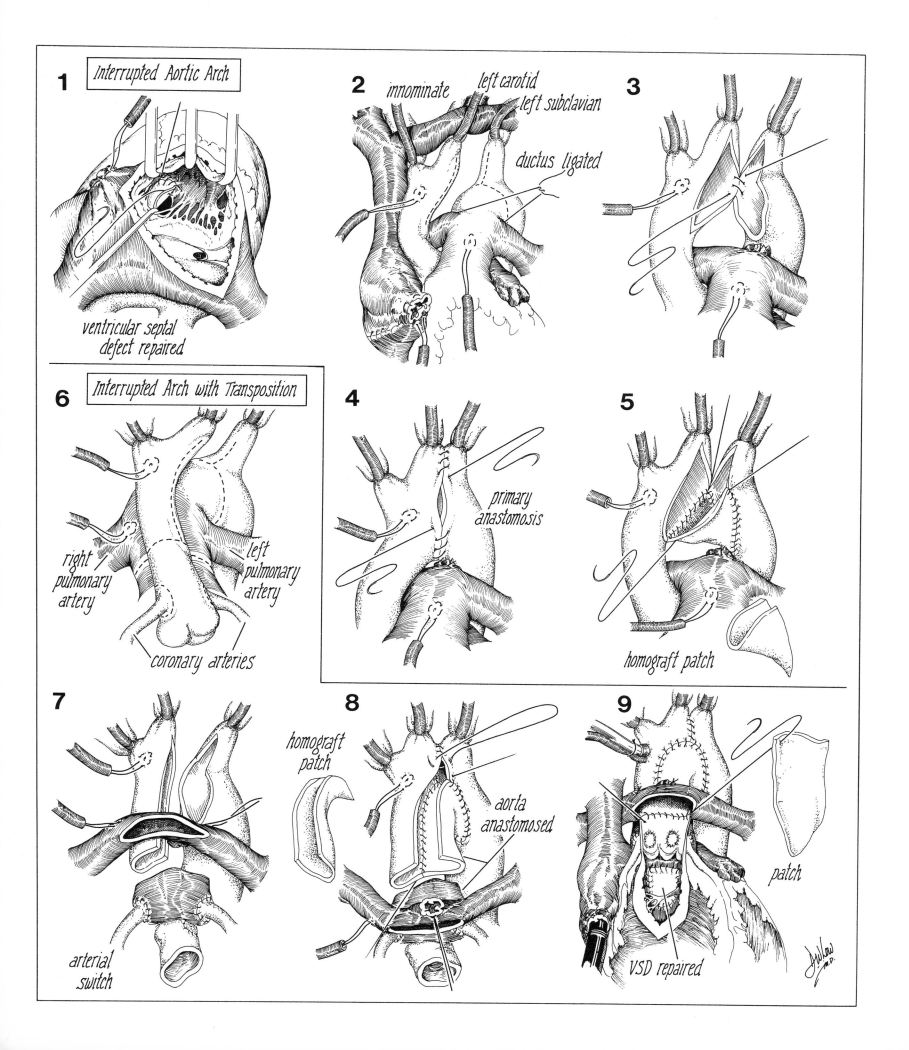

1 Interrupted Aortic Arch

ventricular septal defect repaired

2 innominate left carotid left subclavian

ductus ligated

3

6 Interrupted Arch with Transposition

right pulmonary artery

left pulmonary artery

coronary arteries

4 primary anastomosis

5 homograft patch

7 arterial switch

8 homograft patch

aorta anastomosed

9 homograft patch

patch

VSD repaired

TOTAL ANOMALOUS PULMONARY VENOUS CONNECTION

Total anomalous pulmonary venous connection (TAPVC) almost always presents in the newborn period with symptoms of cyanosis and/or tachypnea. The connection between the pulmonary veins and the systemic veins can be stenotic. The degree of obstruction varies from patient to patient. The symptoms and physiologic abnormality are variable, and this variation is largely a consequence of the variation in pulmonary venous obstruction. The challenge for the neonatologist and cardiologist is to appropriately distinguish the symptomatic neonate with TAPVC from the more common newborn with lung disease or persistent fetal circulation.

Simplistically, there are four anatomic patterns. The most common is drainage to a connection of pulmonary veins to a central common vein that is horizontal and posterior to the left atrium. There is a persistent left superior vena cava, allowing pulmonary venous return to the innominate vein and right superior vena cava. A less common pattern is connection of the central pulmonary venous confluence to the coronary sinus in the absence of a left superior vena cava. The pulmonary venous connection is usually only mildly stenotic. Infradiaphragmatic drainage is characterized by a pulmonary venous confluence that is vertical posterior to the left atrium with a venous communication passing through the diaphragm to the portal system. The incidence and degree of venous obstruction of this type is greatest. Finally, combinations of pulmonary venous communications with the systemic veins of what is known as the mixed type are possible.

Occasionally there is little or no pulmonary venous obstruction, usually in the supracardiac or intracardiac type of drainage. In this circumstance, the general physiology is similar to that of an atrial septal defect, with few symptoms, and may go unrecognized early in life. More commonly, some degree of pulmonary venous obstruction is present, with reactive elevation of pulmonary vascular resistance. The chest film reveals the characteristic stippled or reticular pattern of pulmonary venous obstruction. When venous obstruction is severe, most commonly in the infradiaphragmatic of type drainage, there may be associated significant right-to-left shunting through the ductus arteriosus. Patients with pulmonary hypertension will fail to thrive, and delaying surgical intervention is not efficacious. Total anomalous pulmonary venous connection should be repaired when the abnormality is recognized, even in the newborn period.

It is thought that the embryologic cause of total anomalous pulmonary venous connection is a failure of fusion of the posterior venous confluence with the inferior/superior aspect of the cardiac loop that forms the atrium. The lungs develop as evaginations from the foregut and the pulmonary veins coalesce as a lake of venous structures posterior to the developing heart. Initially, drainage from this venous confluence is through the primitive cardinal veins superiorly and the vitelline veins inferiorly. With fusion of this venous coalescence posterior to the developing heart, the cardinal vitelline venous system involutes and the posterior aspect of the developing atrium is completed. With failure of fusion, one or more primitive venous systems persist.

Supracardiac Drainage

(1) The strategy of repair of total anomalous pulmonary venous connection is to connect the pulmonary venous system with the left atrium and ligate anomalous connections to the systemic veins. Cardiopulmonary bypass is established by arterial cannulation of the ascending aorta and a single venous cannula in the atrial appendage. A period of hypothermic total circulatory arrest provides ideal conditions for establishing a patulous anastomosis. The left superior vena cava is ligated between the innominate vein and the pulmonary veins. If a connection between the left superior vena cava and the coronary sinus persists, this too should be ligated.

(2) Exposure of the pulmonary venous confluence is best achieved by anterior retraction of the right atrium with exposure of the veins from the right lateral aspect of the mediastinum. An incision is made in the pulmonary venous trunk and adjacent posterior left atrium to achieve the longest, widest anastomosis.

(3) The leftmost lateral aspect of the anastomosis is accomplished with a running monofilament suture technique.

(4) The rightmost aspect of the anastomosis is completed by interrupted sutures.

Cardiac Drainage to Coronary Sinus

(5) The cardiac drainage pattern is common pulmonary vein connection to the coronary sinus. This is most conveniently repaired by exposing the coronary sinus and atrial septum through a right atriotomy. With one limb of scissors placed in the coronary sinus, a common incision is made in the coronary sinus septum and the septum primum.

(6) This incision exposes the left atrium to the large coronary sinus.

(7) Because the pulmonary venous connection to the coronary sinus is unobstructed in most patients, normal pulmonary venous drainage to the left atrium can be achieved by closing the newly created atrial septal defect and coronary sinus ostium with a single patch. The remaining defect in the coronary sinus septum allows common drainage of pulmonary veins and cardiac veins to the left atrium.

Infradiaphragmatic Drainage

(8) The least common pattern is the infracardiac type. Illustrated here is the vertical rather than the horizontal confluence of the pulmonary veins posterior to the left atrium. The vein passing through the diaphragm is ligated at that level and divided.

(9) A fishmouth incision is made in the pulmonary venous confluence and an adjacent vertical incision is made in the left atrium posteriorly to achieve the most patulous anastomosis possible.

(10) Again, the leftmost lateral aspect of the anastomosis may be accomplished with running monofilament suture and the rightmost portion of the anastomosis completed with interrupted sutures.

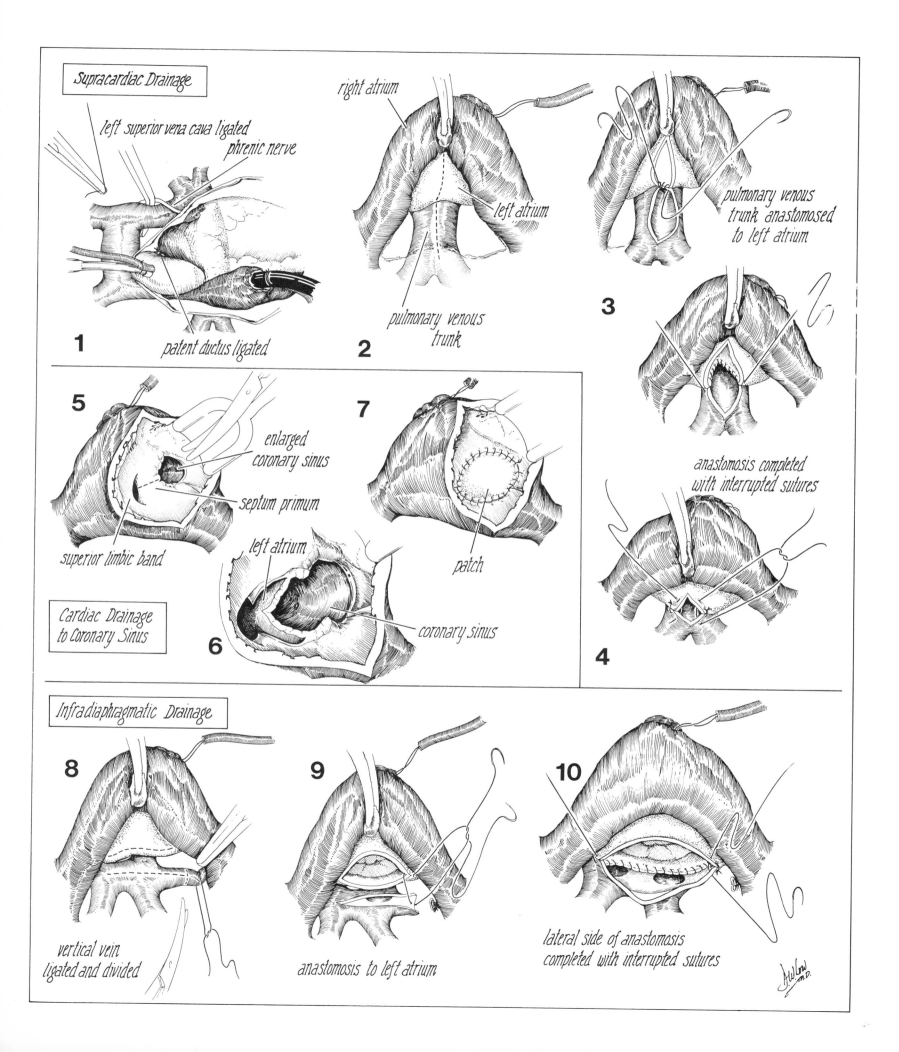

Supracardiac Drainage

1

left superior vena cava ligated
phrenic nerve

patent ductus ligated

2

right atrium

left atrium

pulmonary venous trunk

3

pulmonary venous trunk anastomosed to left atrium

anastomosis completed with interrupted sutures

4

Cardiac Drainage to Coronary Sinus

5

enlarged coronary sinus

septum primum

superior limbic band

6

left atrium

coronary sinus

7

patch

Infradiaphragmatic Drainage

8

vertical vein ligated and divided

9

anastomosis to left atrium

10

lateral side of anastomosis completed with interrupted sutures

DOUBLE-OUTLET RIGHT VENTRICLE

During normal development of the conotruncus, the bulbus cordis divides into two tubular structures lying side by side over the true, primitive left ventricle. Semilunar valves separate arterial structures of the aorta and pulmonary artery superiorly from the muscular coni inferiorly. The infundibular septum in this stage is in the anterior-posterior plane separating the aortic conus from the conus of the pulmonary artery. Normally, the conus of the aorta involutes or does not grow, leaving the aortic valve in fibrous continuity with the mitral valve of the left ventricle. The conus of the pulmonary artery does grow, however, causing rotation of the infundibular septum and pulmonary artery so that the pulmonary artery resides anterior and to the left of the aorta and the infundibular septum rotates into the plane of the true trabeculated septum. In double-outlet right ventricle, the conus of the aorta does not involute but grows, and as a consequence, the infundibular septum remains close to the anterior-posterior plane. There is a muscular discontinuity between the aortic valve and the mitral valve. The aorta and main pulmonary artery lie side by side, and the aorta is mostly or completely associated with the right ventricle. As a consequence of the position of the infundibular septum, there is a large ventricular septal defect (malalignment type). Most commonly, the infundibular septum is to the left of the right ventricular outflow tract, causing some degree of subpulmonary obstruction, and the ventricular septal defect is mostly underneath the aortic valve. Occasionally, both the aortic and pulmonary arterial outflow tract are equal and the ventricular septal defect lies partly beneath the pulmonary artery and partly beneath the aorta. If the infundibular septum is to the right, the ventricular septal defect is below the pulmonary valve, creating the so-called Taussig-Bing malformation. There may be some degree of subaortic obstruction. Rarely, the infundibular septum is hypertrophied and partially fills the limbs of the septal band. There may be a muscular or inlet type of ventricular septal defect far inferior to the aortic and pulmonary valves.

Occasionally, double-outlet right ventricle is associated with unusal ventricular relations such as superior-inferior ventricular disposition, with abnormalities in the development of the viscera such as heterotaxy syndrome, or with atrioventricular valve abnormalities such as mitral atresia or complete common atrioventricular canal defect with or without malalignment of the atrioventricular canal. In the latter, associations the left or the right ventricle may by absolutely hypoplastic. In these most complex constellations, application of Fontan's procedure may be considered in the strategy of palliative and reconstructive reparative surgery.

Subaortic VSD

(1) The most common form of isolated double-outlet right ventricle is the type with a subaortic ventricular septal defect and pulmonary stenosis. This variety is reminiscent of tetralogy of Fallot physiologically.

(2) Repair is analogous to that of tetralogy of Fallot and pulmonary stenosis except that the ventricular septal defect patch needs to function as a baffle from the perimeter of the ventricular septal defect to the perimeter of the aortic valve. The baffle is placed with monofilament running suture technique beginning at the level of the papillary muscle of the conus.

(3) The baffle is sutured around the aortic valve and into the infundibular septum, separating the aortic and pulmonary valves.

(4) It is usually advisable to augment the right ventricular outflow tract to avoid obstructions posteriorly from the newly placed baffle. This gusset is sutured with running monofilament suture as it is in repair of tetralogy of Fallot.

Subpulmonary VSD—"Taussig-Bing Malformation"

(5) An uncommon variety of double-outlet right ventricle is that described by Taussig and Bing. The subpulmonary ventricular septal defect results in a physiology similar to d-transposition of the great arteries with a large ventricular septal defect. Left ventricular outflow is through the ventricular septal defect, predominantly to the pulmonary artery, while systemic venous return streams predominantly to the aorta. Through a right ventriculotomy, the ventricular septal defect can be readily visualized.

(6) An oval patch is secured with running monofilament suture around the perimeter of the ventricular septal defect and the pulmonary valve from the right ventricular aspect.

(7) Although atrial inversion surgery may be used, arterial switch is probably the most efficacious means of completing this form of reconstructive surgery. The great arteries are divided and the coronary arteries are excised with buttons of native aortic wall. The right ventricular outflow tract is gusseted with a patch, using running monofilament suture.

(8) The coronary arteries are transplanted into the proximal native main pulmonary artery with running monofilament suture. Depending on the relative position of the aorta and the main pulmonary artery, the branch pulmonary arteries may be brought anterior to the distal ascending aorta or remain posterior. The distal ascending aorta is anastomosed to the proximal main pulmonary artery, completing aortic reconstruction.

(9) Because the aorta and main pulmonary artery are side by side as opposed to the anterior-posterior position as in transposition of the great arteries, the pulmonary arterial anastomosis is best completed by partial closure of the leftward aspect of the distal main pulmonary artery and an incision in the right pulmonary artery for translocation of the distal main pulmonary arterial orifice rightward to line up with the proximal native aorta. The reconstruction is then completed by anastomosis of the native ascending aorta which will function as the right ventricular outflow trunk to the pulmonary artery with running monofilament suture. The defects in the wall of the proximal native aorta secondary to excision of the coronary arteries may be closed independently or with a single large patch of pericardium.

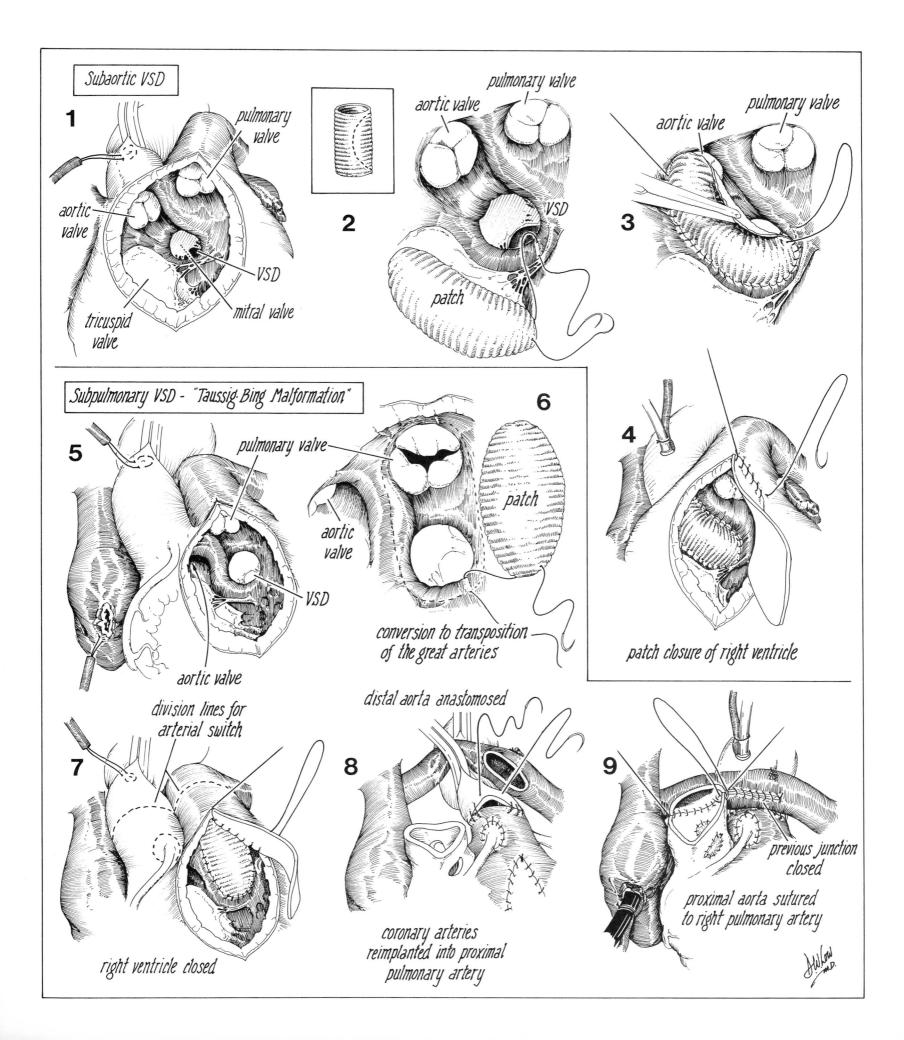

Subaortic VSD

1

pulmonary valve

aortic valve

VSD

tricuspid valve

mitral valve

2

pulmonary valve

aortic valve

VSD

patch

3

aortic valve

pulmonary valve

4

patch closure of right ventricle

Subpulmonary VSD - "Taussig-Bing Malformation"

5

pulmonary valve

VSD

aortic valve

6

aortic valve

patch

conversion to transposition of the great arteries

7

division lines for arterial switch

right ventricle closed

8

distal aorta anastomosed

coronary arteries reimplanted into proximal pulmonary artery

9

previous junction closed

proximal aorta sutured to right pulmonary artery

Doubly Committed VSD

(10) When the ventricular septal defect resides equally underneath the aortic and pulmonary valves, it is baffled to the aortic valve, thus associating the aorta with the left ventricle.

(11) An appropriately structured baffle is sutured with continuous monofilament suture beginning at the papillary muscle of the conus.

(12) The baffle runs clockwise, placing shallow bites in the right ventricular aspect of the ventricular septum to avoid the conduction system.

(13) The baffle is completed by suturing the left lateral aspect to the infundibular septum.

(14) Again, to avoid right ventricular outflow tract obstruction, the infundibulotomy is gusseted with a patch secured with running monofilament suture.

Noncommitted VSD

(15) When the ventricular septal defect is far inferior to the aortic valve, one can extend the extent of the ventricular septal defect superiorly by excising a portion of the septum.

(16) The patch must be structured as a teardrop configuration to extend inferiorly to the crest of the ventricular septum to channel flow from the left ventricle to the aortic valve through the extended ventricular septal defect.

(17) The baffle may be place underneath chordae associated with the septal leaflet of the tricuspid valve.

(18) Air is evacuated from the left ventricle and baffle as the suture securing the baffle is tied.

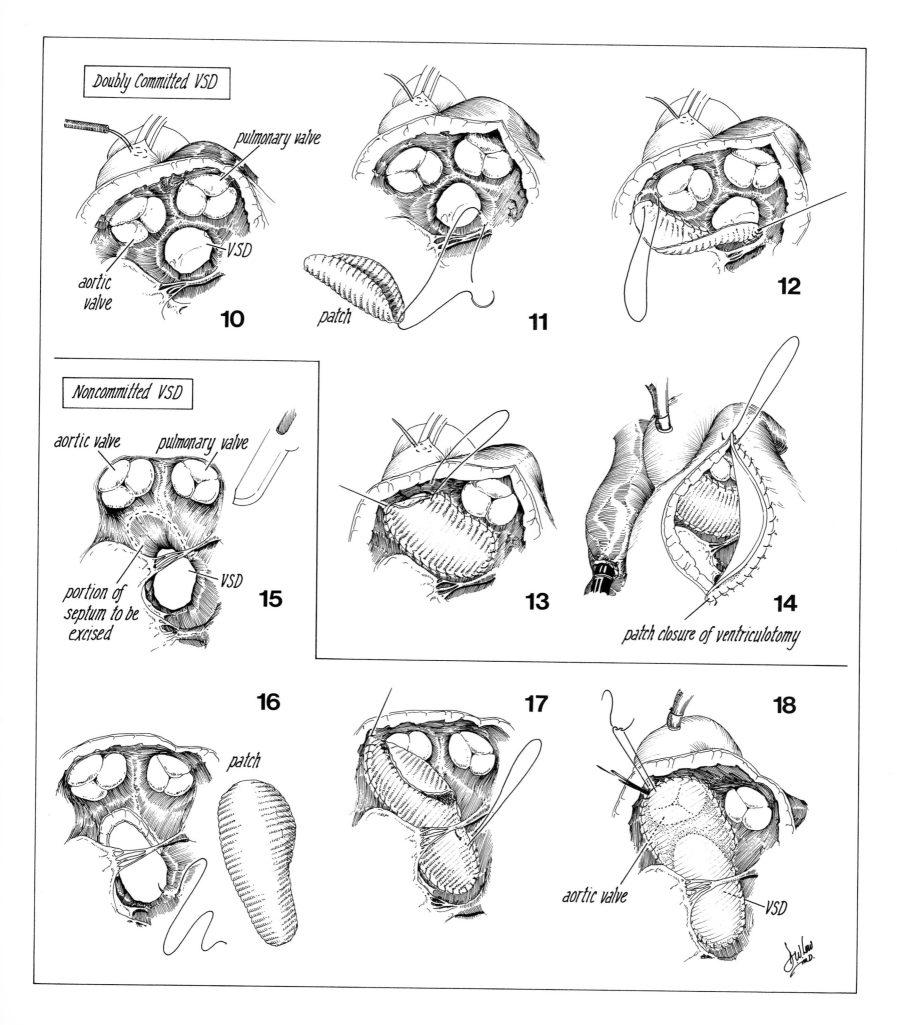

Doubly Committed VSD

pulmonary valve

aortic valve

VSD

10

patch

11

12

Noncommitted VSD

aortic valve

pulmonary valve

portion of septum to be excised

VSD

15

13

patch closure of ventriculotomy

14

16

patch

17

18

aortic valve

VSD

EPSTEIN'S ANOMALY

Epstein's anomaly is an unusual but characteristic abnormality of the development of the tricuspid valve, right ventricle, and right atrium. The principal symptom is cyanosis, a consequence of some limitation of blood flow from right atrium to main pulmonary artery, and as a consequence a right-to-left shunt at the atrial level. There may be associated hypoplasia of the right ventricular outflow tract with pulmonary stenosis or atresia. The interatrial communication is usually a large foramen ovale. When the right-to-left shunt is large, hypoxemia may be severe, causing symptoms in the newborn period. When the malformation is mild, the degree of hypoxemia is also mild and may be tolerated for years without surgical intervention. Often there is associated abnormal development of the conduction system with characteristic electrocardiographic findings of accessory atrial pathways. Indeed, some patients develop supraventricular tachycardia and even death as a consequence. This abnormality presents an awkward anatomic and physiologic association in the symptomatic neonate. The heart is generally enlarged, and simple palliation by a systemic-to-pulmonary artery shunt may not significantly alleviate physiologic embarrassment as one might otherwise expect.

(1) The characteristic findings are a displaced tricuspid valve with a septal leaflet spiralling into the right ventricle. The anterior leaflet is often not attached to normal chordae or papillary muscles, but rather attached in a veil-like fashion on the anterior free wall. The portion of right ventricle between the true fibrous annulus and the displaced tricuspid valve is thin and appears more like an atrial wall than a ventricle. The coronary sinus is in the usual position and the atrial septal defect is usually a large foramen ovale. The combined right ventricle and right atrium are markedly enlarged.

(2) In an older child, teenager, or young adult, one may treat this malformation by plicating the atrialized portion of the right ventricle with interrupted sutures through the attachments of the septal leaflet and the true annulus fibrosis.

(3) When the tricuspid valve anatomy is not severely deranged, this alone may allow closure of the interatrial communication with satisfactory repair.

Valve Replacement

(4) Often the anterior leaflet is so abnormal and obstructive to the right ventricular outflow tract that valve replacement is necessary in addition to plication.

(5) A low-profile prosthetic valve is chosen and secured inferiorly with interrupted plicating sutures.

(6) Superiorly, a running suture technique is used.

(7) When the interatrial communication is large, it should be closed with a patch.

(8) The enlarged right atrium may be reduced in size, not only by plication of the atrialized right ventricle, but also by excision of right atrial free wall.

(9) This combination of reconstructive modalities can significantly reduce the symptoms in young adults. Complete heart block is a risk with placement of the prosthetic valve. Some postulate that the risk of complete heart block can be reduced by placing the prosthesis superior to the coronary sinus.

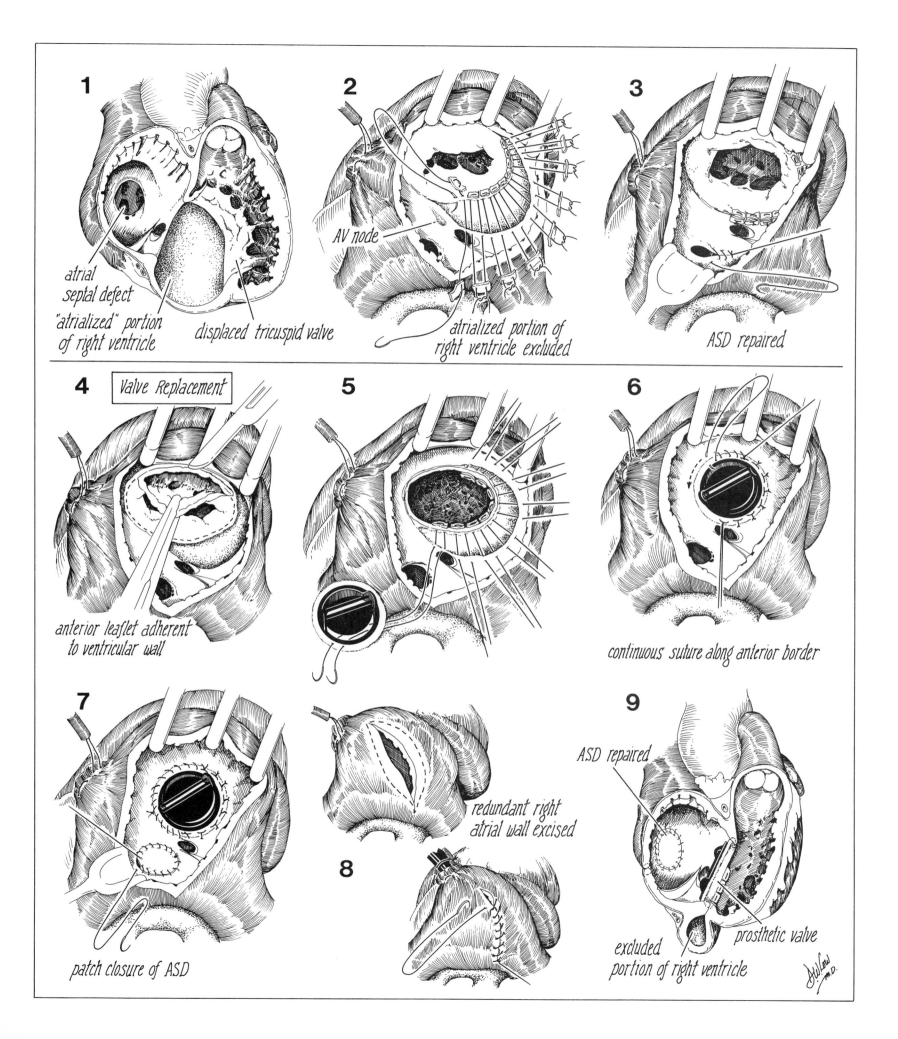

1

atrial
septal defect

"atrialized" portion
of right ventricle

displaced tricuspid valve

2

AV node

atrialized portion of
right ventricle excluded

3

ASD repaired

4 Valve Replacement

anterior leaflet adherent
to ventricular wall

5

6

continuous suture along anterior border

7

patch closure of ASD

8

redundant right
atrial wall excised

9

ASD repaired

excluded
portion of right ventricle

prosthetic valve

FONTAN'S PROCEDURE

In the late 1960s and early 1970s, Francis Fontan added to the foundations of reconstructive surgery of congenital cardiac malformations by providing principles and techniques for extensive physiologic repair of complex congenital cardiac malformations when there is only one effective ventricle. His original contributions involved the management of tricuspid atresia. The initial thrust was to recruit what was perceived as a hypertrophied right atrium in tricuspid atresia as a substitute ventricle for systemic venous return. Therefore, the original approach included placement of a valve in the inferior vena cava and interposition of a valved conduit between the right atrial appendage and pulmonary arteries or infundibulum. Physiologic and technical understanding of this mode of therapy has evolved extensively over the last decade. It is now recognized that the central features inherent in applying Fontan's procedure for reconstructive surgery of complex congenital cardiac malformations are a low pulmonary vascular resistance and low pulmonary venous pressure, implying satisfactory atrioventricular valve function and normal ventricular compliance. The age of the patient at the time of Fontan's operation is a factor only insofar as it implies the state of maturation of the pulmonary vasculature after birth or potential ventricular failure and/or acquired pulmonary vascular obstructive disease in the older palliated patient. The size of the patient is irrelevant because a large anastomosis can be made without the use of conduits. Finally, the systemic and pulmonary venous drainage pattern is important only in determining whether the systemic venous return should be baffled to the pulmonary arteries or pulmonary venous return channeled to a large atrioventricular valve.

Whereas the physiology of the systolic time period dominates the physiology of most patients following open heart surgery, it is the diastolic properties that influence the physiologic state following Fontan's reconstructive repair. Approximately 50% of patients who are otherwise hemodynamically stable and well following surgery develop significant pleural and pericardial effusions. Virtually all these effusions abate within weeks postoperatively, never to return. When effusions do recur, the patient should be reinvestigated for acquired anatomic abnormalities.

Tricuspid Atresia

(1) The original form of single ventricle managed by Fontan was tricuspid atresia. In patients with normally related great arteries, types B and C have a ventricular septal defect, some right ventricular chamber, and a main pulmonary artery. Often an infant with tricuspid atresia requires a systemic-to-pulmonary-artery shunt or occasionally a pulmonary artery band before the pulmonary vasculature is mature enough for Fontan's procedure. Cardiopulmonary bypass is instituted by cannulation of the ascending aorta and right atrial appendage. The systemic-to-pulmonary-artery shunt (in this case, a left Blalock-Taussig shunt) is closed. Any communication between the left ventricle and pulmonary arteries may be obliterated by patch closure of the ventricular septal defect, oversewing the pulmonary valve, or ligation of the proximal main pulmonary artery.

(2) In patients with type IC tricuspid atresia and a large ventricular chamber, one may consider interposition of a valved conduit between the right atrium and infundibulum of the right ventricle with a view to recruiting systolic volume and pressure work from the attenuated right ventricular chamber. Most commonly, however, the key to a good outcome is a large unobstructive and lasting communication between the systemic venous return and the pulmonary arteries. This is readily achieved by anastomosis of the superior aspect of the right atrium and right superior vena cava to the right pulmonary artery. The anastomosis between the systemic venous return and arteries is thus not subject to compression by the anterior chest wall.

(3) Through this incision, the atrial septal defect is visualized. Most often, it is closed with a patch that can be secured with a running monofilament suture technique. A large central arteriotomy is made, extending the incision to the take-off of the upper lobe branches of the right and left pulmonary arteries.

(4) The posterior aspect of the anastomosis is begun by a running monofilament suture connecting the right superior vena cava, right atrium, and right pulmonary artery.

(5) The anterior aspect of the pulmonary arteriotomy is gusseted with some form of patch material to ensure the largest possible communication between the pulmonary arteries and the systemic venous return.

(6) Cardiopulmonary bypass may be resumed during the process of gusseting the anastomosis, using a cardiotomy sucker for systemic venous return.

(7) The shunt is ligated and the ventricular pulmonary artery communication obliterated.

Single Ventricle with Transposition

(8) Another form of complex congenital cardiac malformation treatable by application of Fontan's procedure is of the single left ventricle with transposition of the great arteries {S,L,L}. A growing opinion is that virtually all children with this condition should be palliated early in life with anastomosis of the proximal main pulmonary artery to the ascending aorta, creation of pulmonary atresia, and a systemic-to-pulmonary arterial shunt. This approach allows for satisfactory oxygenation of systemic arterial perfusion to meet metabolic demands, normal maturation of the pulmonary vasculature, and most importantly, avoidance of insidious debilitating obstruction between the ventricle and aorta. When the child is between 1 and 2 years old, the Fontan's procedure may be undertaken. Shown here is patch closure of the tricuspid valve. The mitral valve is normal in size. Because of late dehiscence of the tricuspid valve patch and the risk of complete heart block, a more satisfactory alternative approach is to baffle the inferior vena caval return along the right lateral aspect of the right atrium to the anastomosis between the superior aspect of the right atrium, right superior vena cava, and right pulmonary artery. This alternative is described in more detail in the section on management of hypoplastic left heart syndrome. The incisions are in the pulmonary artery and right atrium.

(9) The anastomosis between the right atrium and the right pulmonary artery is completed by augmentation of the anterior aspect of the right pulmonary artery, right superior vena cava, and right atrium with a gusset of patch material.

166

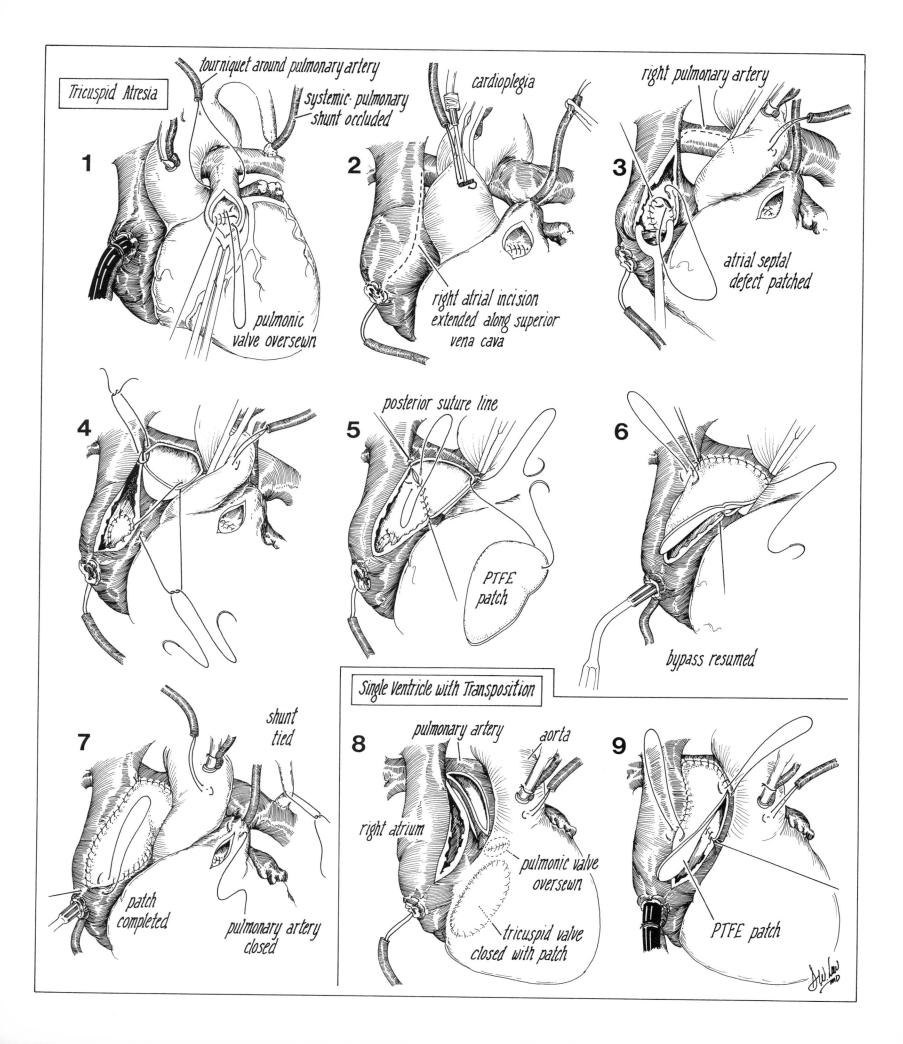

Tricuspid Atresia

1. tourniquet around pulmonary artery / systemic-pulmonary shunt occluded / pulmonic valve oversewn

2. cardioplegia / right atrial incision extended along superior vena cava

3. right pulmonary artery / atrial septal defect patched

4.

5. posterior suture line / PTFE patch

6. bypass resumed

7. shunt tied / patch completed / pulmonary artery closed

Single Ventricle with Transposition

8. pulmonary artery / aorta / right atrium / pulmonic valve oversewn / tricuspid valve closed with patch

9. PTFE patch

TRANSPOSITION OF THE GREAT ARTERIES {S,L,L AND S,D,D} WITH SUBPULMONARY STENOSIS

Congenitally corrected transposition of the great arteries occurs in two forms, situs solitus with levo-loop and situs inversus with dextro-loop. Transposition of the great arteries {S,L,L} can exist without other associated abnormalities such as ventricular septal defect or pulmonary stenosis, and patients with this condition can go unrecognized as having a heart malformation. The conduction system is abnormal and tenuous in hearts with this anatomy, and early and late development of congenital heart block can occur. Ventricular septal defect and subpulmonary stenosis are common accompaniments of congenitally corrected transposition, and surgical intervention may be required to correct or improve the physiology. Sequelae associated with reparative surgery include a relatively higher incidence of complete heart block than in hearts with dextro-looping, partly because of the unusual course of the conduction and partly because of the tenuous nature of the connections of the conduction system between the atrium and ventricles. The tricuspid valve is usually structurally abnormal, reminiscent of the valve of Epstein's anomaly, and tricuspid regurgitation can occur in some patients, particularly postoperatively.

In patients with transposition of the great arteries {S,D,D}, a common occurrence is posterior malalignment of the infundibular septum, which causes a malalignment type of ventricular septal defect and long-segment obstruction of the left ventricular outflow tract. A form of surgical management often used in this constellation is known as Rastelli's operation.

Congenitally Corrected Transposition

(1) In patients with corrected transposition, the ascending aorta is to the left and takes a long sweeping course superiorly. The left ventricle is to the right and anterior and the right ventricle posterior and to the left. In situs solitus, the atria are in their normal position. The ventricular septal defect is most often of the conoventricular type. Subpulmonary stenosis can coexist and is often tunnel-like and unresectable because of close proximity of the mitral valve to the right and right coronary artery superiorly.

(2) Closure of the ventricular septal defect can be accomplished through a right atriotomy by way of the tricuspid valve. Because the conduction system in the L-loop runs superiorly and courses in the morphologic left ventricle, closure of the ventricular septal defect to avoid complete heart block may be accomplished by a running suture technique in which the superior bites are placed through the ventricular septal defect on the morphologic right ventricular aspect of the ventricular septal defect rim.

(3) When subpulmonary stenosis is significant and unresectable, interposition of a conduit between the pulmonary artery and the anterior free wall of the left ventricle is necessary to decompress the left ventricle. When a finger is placed through the mitral valve, a portion of the free wall not occupied by papillary muscle or chordal is identifiable, and a ventriculotomy can readily be made with this guidance.

(4) A tube graft is then interposed between the ventriculotomy and an incision in the main and right pulmonary artery. Care must be taken to leave a sufficient length of the conduit to avoid compression of the right coronary artery. Various conduits can be used, but illustrated here is placement of an aortic homograft between the branch pulmonary arteries and the ventriculotomy.

(5) The distal anastomosis is completed first, with the proximal anastomosis fashioned with a running monofilament suture technique using the trimmed anterior leaflet of the mitral valve to gusset the ventriculotomy.

Rastelli's Operation

(6) In patients with transposition of the great arteries {S,D,D}, malalignment ventricular septal defect, and left ventricular outflow tract obstruction, a systemic-to-pulmonary-artery shunt has usually been created early in life to augment the pulmonary blood flow, thus palliating severe hypoxemia. This shunt is closed after institution of cardiopulmonary bypass, and with the aorta crossclamped and cardioplegia solution infused, a right infundibulotomy is made, exposing the ventricular septal defect.

(7) The malalignment ventricular septal defect is closed with a patch on the perimeter of the ventricular septal defect and aortic valve to associate left ventricular outflow with the aorta through the ventricular septal defect. A single monofilament running suture technique is begun at the papillary muscle of the conus.

(8) A pulmonary arteriotomy is made and the pulmonary valve is oversewn.

(9) A conduit is interposed between the pulmonary arteries and the infundibulotomy beginning with the distal anastomosis.

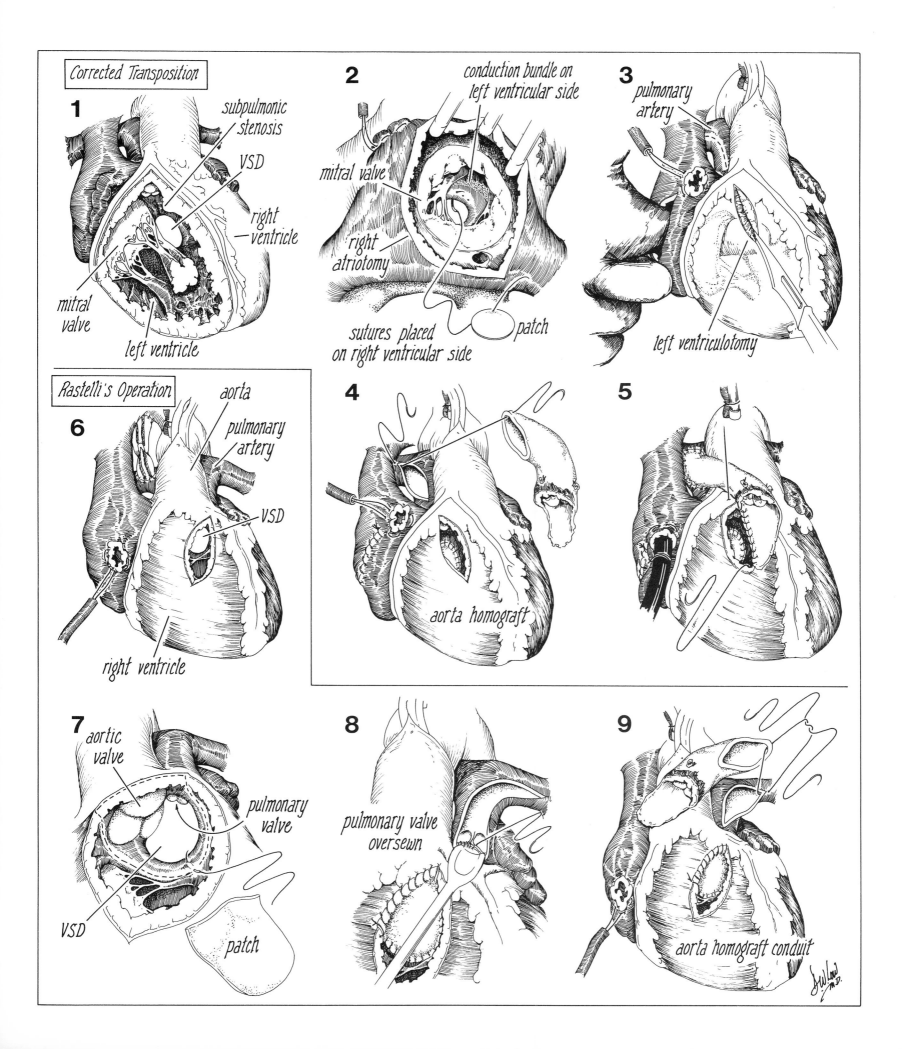

Corrected Transposition

1
subpulmonic stenosis
VSD
right ventricle
mitral valve
left ventricle

2
conduction bundle on left ventricular side
mitral valve
right atriotomy
sutures placed on right ventricular side
patch

3
pulmonary artery
left ventriculotomy

Rastelli's Operation

6
aorta
pulmonary artery
VSD
right ventricle

4
aorta homograft

5

7
aortic valve
pulmonary valve
VSD
patch

8
pulmonary valve oversewn

9
aorta homograft conduit

SEPARATION OF SINGLE VENTRICLE

Although, at present, a modified Fontan procedure appears a satisfactory form of management for single left ventricle with double inlet, an alternative approach is septation of the ventricle. Results with such surgery performed later in life suggest that a possible advantageous approach is staged septation begun in the first months of life.

(1) TGA {S,L,L} single left ventricle is a malformation with an outlet chamber to the aorta and an adjacent pulmonary valve. When there is no pulmonary obstruction, the outlet to the aorta may become increasingly obstructive with time. In true single ventricle, there are two atrioventricular valves, and in the case of equivalent right and left atrioventricular valves, septation is possible.

(2) The conduction system runs superiorly in this malformation and resides on right lateral aspect of the bulboventricular foramen.

(3) A perforated patch is sutured between the atrioventricular valves around the pulmonary artery and bulboventricular foramen with multiple widely spaced pledgeted sutures. Wide spacing of the sutures minimizes conduction system abnormalities.

(4) Perforation of the patch allows it to become organized and stiff with time during the palliated state. As the heart grows, the muscular attachments invaginate, forming part of the new septum. The suture line between the AV valves is a continuous suture technique.

(5) To avoid late subaortic obstruction, pulmonary artery banding is not performed; rather, the main pulmonary artery is transected.

(6) The distal main pulmonary artery is oversewn with a patch and the proximal main pulmonary artery is anastomosed to the ascending aorta with a running monofilament suture technique.

(7) A 4 mm tube graft is then interposed between the innominate artery and the branch pulmonary arteries to provide pulmonary blood flow in the palliated state.

(8) At 2 to 3 years of age, a ventriculotomy is preformed. The perforation in the septation patch is identified and closed with a patch.

(9) An aortic homograft conduit is interposed between the right half of the septated ventricle and the distal branch pulmonary arteries, completing staged septation.

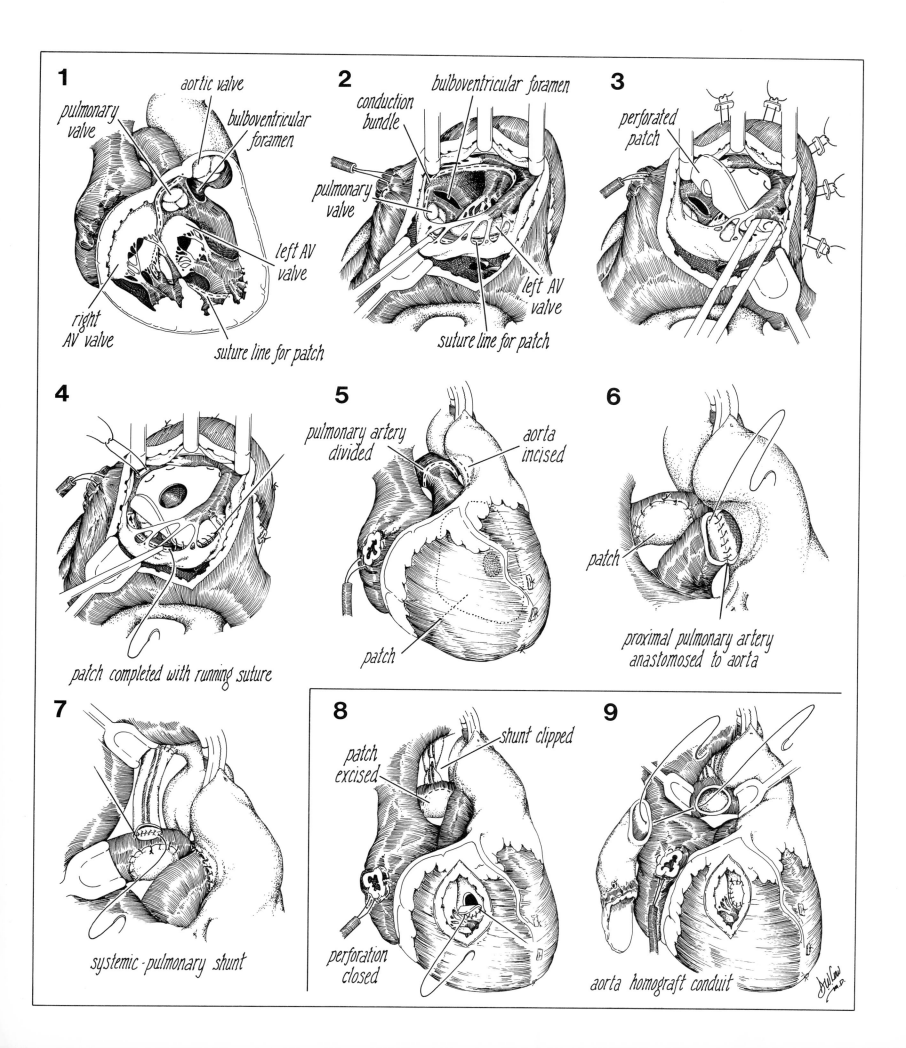

1
pulmonary valve
aortic valve
bulboventricular foramen
left AV valve
right AV valve
suture line for patch

2
conduction bundle
bulboventricular foramen
pulmonary valve
left AV valve
suture line for patch

3
perforated patch

4
patch completed with running suture

5
pulmonary artery divided
aorta incised
patch

6
patch
proximal pulmonary artery anastomosed to aorta

7
systemic-pulmonary shunt

8
patch excised
shunt clipped
perforation closed

9
aorta homograft conduit

Section 5

Pulmonary and Mediastinal Operations

Tracheostomy

1 A vertical skin incision is best for emergency tracheostomy when acute obstruction of the upper airway or lack of proper equipment prevents immediate translaryngeal intubation. Even in an emergency, a roll or small pillow should be placed under the shoulders to extend the neck. The midline incision begins 2 to 3 cm below the laryngeal notch and is 4 to 5 cm long.

2 Carefully staying in the midline, the surgeon can advance the knife to the trachea just below the cricoid cartilage. Three tracheal rings and the intervening membranes are incised in the midline. The membrane between the cricoid cartilage and upper tracheal ring is cut, but the cricoid cartilage is not divided.

3 With twisting of the knife blade and handle, the soft tissues can be separated sufficiently to allow air to enter and exit from the trachea.

4 For cosmetic reasons, a transverse incision is preferred for elective tracheostomy except in patients with short and fat or muscular necks. The operation is performed using aseptic technique with either general or local anesthesia. Prior passage of an endotracheal tube and extension of the neck facilitate the procedure. A symmetric, transverse incision, 4 to 5 cm long and centered in the midline, is made in or parallel to a natural skin crease, 2 cm superior to the clavicular heads.

5 The platysma muscle is incised in line with the incision. Upper and lower flaps are raised to expose the anterior strap muscles. The anterior jugular vein is divided and ligated. Electrocautery can be used to control subcuticular bleeding, but skin edges must not be burned.

6 The fascia investing the anterior strap muscles is divided in a vertical direction, and the left and right sternothyroid and sternohyoid muscles are retracted laterally. The isthmus of the thyroid gland is retracted cephalad after blunt dissection. The pretracheal fascia is incised by scissors or knife directly over the trachea. Small hernia retractors, held by an assistant, are used to separate the strap muscles.

7 The anterior trachea is cleared of soft tissue to facilitate identification of the cricoid and thyroid cartilages and upper tracheal rings. With a No. 10 or 12 Fr suction catheter available, a 1 cm transverse incision is made in the anterior tracheal membrane between the second and third tracheal rings, or between the first and second tracheal rings. A tracheal hook is inserted into the lower tracheal cartilage to stabilize the trachea while the lower tracheal cartilage is cut in a vertical direction at each end of the transverse incision. This creates a small tracheal flap, hinged at the inferior margin of the tracheal opening. Alternatively, a single vertical incision can be made in two adjacent tracheal rings. Secretions and blood are aspirated from the opened trachea, which is steadied by the tracheal hook in the flap.

8 After suction, the tracheostomy tube with stylet in place is carefully inserted into the tracheal opening and gently slid into position within the trachea. This should be done carefully and with direct vision because the tube can easily be passed downward in the pretracheal plane if the tracheal opening is missed. The diameter of the tracheostomy tube (usually 6 to 8 Fr for adults) should be chosen to allow easy passage into the trachea and a somewhat loose fit.

9 A plastic or metal tracheostomy tube with or without a side fenestration can be used. Large-volume, low-pressure cuffed tubes should have an external balloon connected to the cuff so that inflation pressure within the cuff can be manually monitored and adjusted to the lowest pressure needed to prevent air leak at the inspiratory pressure required for assisted ventilation. The tracheostomy tube is held in place with a tracheostomy tape around the neck. It is often wise to place a foam rubber strip around the tape at the back of the wound.

One or two monofilament sutures on either side of the tracheostomy tube are used to close skin edges. A dry, partially split sponge is inserted beneath the tracheal tape around the tracheostomy tube.

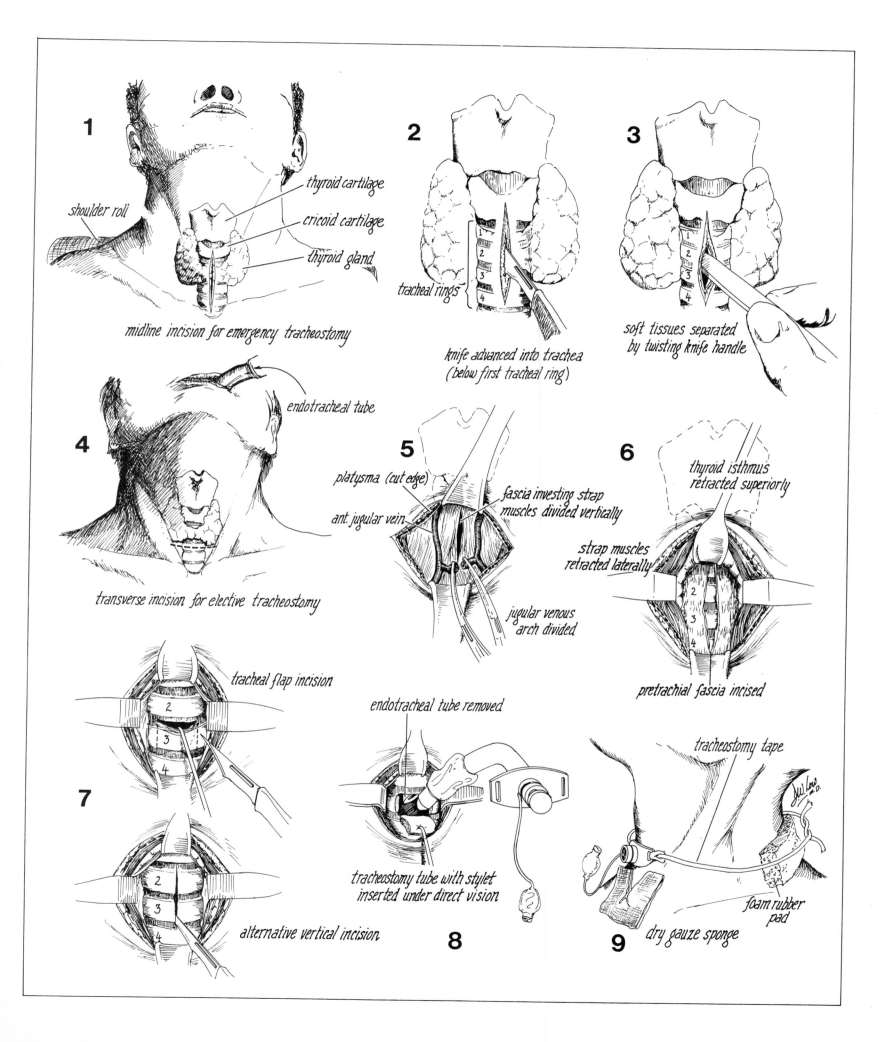

1 midline incision for emergency tracheostomy

shoulder roll

thyroid cartilage
cricoid cartilage
thyroid gland

2 knife advanced into trachea
(below first tracheal ring)

tracheal rings

3 soft tissues separated
by twisting knife handle

4 transverse incision for elective tracheostomy

endotracheal tube

5

platysma (cut edge)

ant. jugular vein

fascia investing strap
muscles divided vertically

jugular venous
arch divided

6

thyroid isthmus
retracted superiorly

strap muscles
retracted laterally

pretrachial fascia incised

7 tracheal flap incision

alternative vertical incision

8 tracheostomy tube with stylet
inserted under direct vision

endotracheal tube removed

9 dry gauze sponge

tracheostomy tape

foam rubber
pad

Pleural Biopsy

NEEDLE PLEURAL BIOPSY

A needle biopsy of the pleura is made with a Cope "hooked" needle and local anesthesia. The patient is preferably seated in an upright position, but the procedure can also be done with the patient in the supine, lateral, and prone positions.

(1) The site or sites are selected and prepped; lidocaine is injected down to and just over the top of the underlying rib.

(2) A nick is made in the skin with a No. 11 scalpel blade. The needle with sharp trocar is inserted to and over the top of the rib and advanced into the pleural space.

(3) While the patient exhales, the beveled stylet is removed and the Cope needle is inserted fully. Full insertion brings the blunt-tipped Cope needle into the pleural space beyond the sheath. The needle is rotated if necessary so that the hook is away from the rib and slightly angled. The needle is withdrawn slowly to feel the hook engage the pleura. The needle is then pulled into the sheath and withdrawn while the patient exhales. The trocar is reinserted to prevent air entry while the specimen is inspected and removed. The tract does not require suture when the sheath is removed.

OPEN PLEURAL BIOPSY

This procedure is performed under general anesthesia.

(4) With the patient in the lateral thoracotomy position, a 3 to 5 cm incision is made over the selected site. The incision is carried down to the rib or intercostal space.

(5) A segment of rib is removed if a large biopsy is required. An incision in the intercostal space is sufficient for a 1 cm by 3 to 4 mm biopsy.

(6) The elliptical incision is made using forceps or a sharp hook to hold the specimen. Slight positive pressure is maintained on the lungs to minimize entry of air into the pleural space.

(7) After the specimen is removed, a small rubber tube is left in the chest while the intercostal muscles are closed. The lungs are inflated and the tube is withdrawn as coaptation of soft tissues seals off the pleural space.

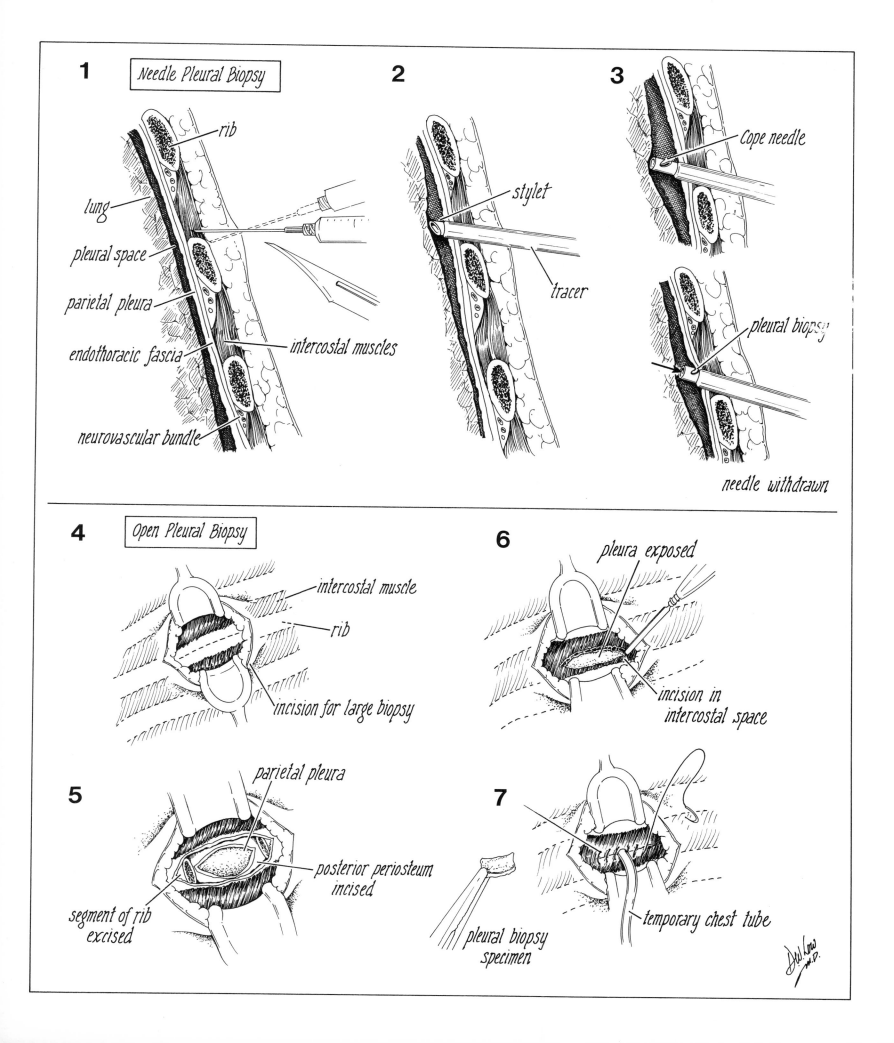

1 Needle Pleural Biopsy

rib

lung

pleural space

parietal pleura

endothoracic fascia

intercostal muscles

neurovascular bundle

2

stylet

tracer

3

Cope needle

pleural biopsy

needle withdrawn

4 Open Pleural Biopsy

intercostal muscle

rib

incision for large biopsy

5

parietal pleura

posterior periosteum incised

segment of rib excised

6

pleura exposed

incision in intercostal space

7

pleural biopsy specimen

temporary chest tube

Pulmonary Anatomy

The adult trachea is 10 to 12 cm in length from inferior cricoid cartilage to carina. Flexion or extension of the neck can push most of the trachea into the chest or pull more than two-thirds into the neck. The arterial blood supply is segmental; branches from the inferior thyroid, first intercostal, internal thoracic (mammary), and superior and middle bronchial arteries supply the trachea.

The hilum of each lung contains more than airways and pulmonary arteries and veins. The medial edge of each lower lobe is attached to mediastinal pleura by a fold of pleura named the pulmonary ligament. Phrenic nerves pass anterior to the two hila; the vagi pass posteriorly along the esophagus but provide branches to each lung. Bronchial arteries arise from the aorta and travel with the bronchi into the lung parenchyma.

(1) Segmental bronchial anatomy differs between the two lungs. On the left, the apical and posterior segmental bronchi in the upper lobe have a common origin, as do the anterior and medial basilar segmental bronchi in the lower lobe. The left main bronchus is longer than the right and is located posterior to the proximal left pulmonary artery. The left main bronchus divides into upper and lower lobe bronchi. Lingular bronchi arise from the upper lobe bronchus. The superior segmental bronchus arises well below the upper lobe bronchus. On the right, the upper and middle lobe bronchi are separate. The origins of the three upper lobe segmental bronchi are separate branches of the upper lobe bronchus. Unlike the left lung, the right superior segmental bronchus arises nearly opposite the origin of the middle lobe bronchus. The names and location of the segmental bronchi are illustrated.

(2) Mediastinal nodes draining the lung are described as tracheobronchial nodes and paratracheal nodes. Tracheobronchial nodes surround the origin of the right and left bronchi and are located beneath the tracheal bifurcation (subcarinal nodes) and at the right and left obtuse angles of the trachea and main bronchi outside the pretracheal fascia. Paratracheal nodes lie along each side of the trachea and drain into inferior cervical (scalene) nodes at the root of the neck. The right paratracheal nodes lie posterior to the superior cava and origin of the innominate artery. Generally, there are more right paratracheal nodes than left.

Intrapulmonary nodes are generally located along segmental bronchi or in bifurcations of segmental pulmonary arterial branches. Interlobar nodes are located at the origins of lobar bronchi, and hilar nodes are found along the right or left main bronchi.

(3) The right main pulmonary artery arises posterior to the medial border of the ascending aorta, passes posterior to the ascending aorta and superior vena cava, and is usually outside the pericardial cavity except at its origin. The right pulmonary artery passes *anterior* to the right upper lobe bronchus and posterior to the branches of the superior pulmonary vein into the major fissure. After giving off the middle lobe branch or branches, the artery passes posterior to the middle lobe bronchus into the lower lobe.

The origin of the left pulmonary artery is within the pericardial cavity. Beyond the pericardial reflection, the artery winds around the superior and *posterior* surfaces of the left main and upper lobe bronchi and enters the interlobar fissure caudad to the lingular bronchus. In both lungs, segmental pulmonary arteries are generally lateral or superior to corresponding segmental bronchi. Pulmonary arteries rarely cross planes between parenchymal segments.

(4) The right superior pulmonary vein is anterior and slightly inferior to the right pulmonary artery. The superior vein collects blood from both the upper and middle lobe and, unlike arteries, segmental pulmonary veins often lie in planes between parenchymal segments. The right inferior pulmonary vein is inferior and more posterior than the superior vein and is best seen by dividing the pulmonary ligament and retracting the right lower lobe anteriorly and superiorly.

The left superior pulmonary vein is also anterior to the left pulmonary artery and bronchus and receives blood from the upper lobe and lingula. The left inferior pulmonary vein is inferior to the lower lobe bronchus and, like the right, is best seen by retracting the lower lobe anteriorly and superiorly.

Pulmonary segmental arteries have the same names as the segmental bronchi. The names of the pulmonary segmental veins are not important.

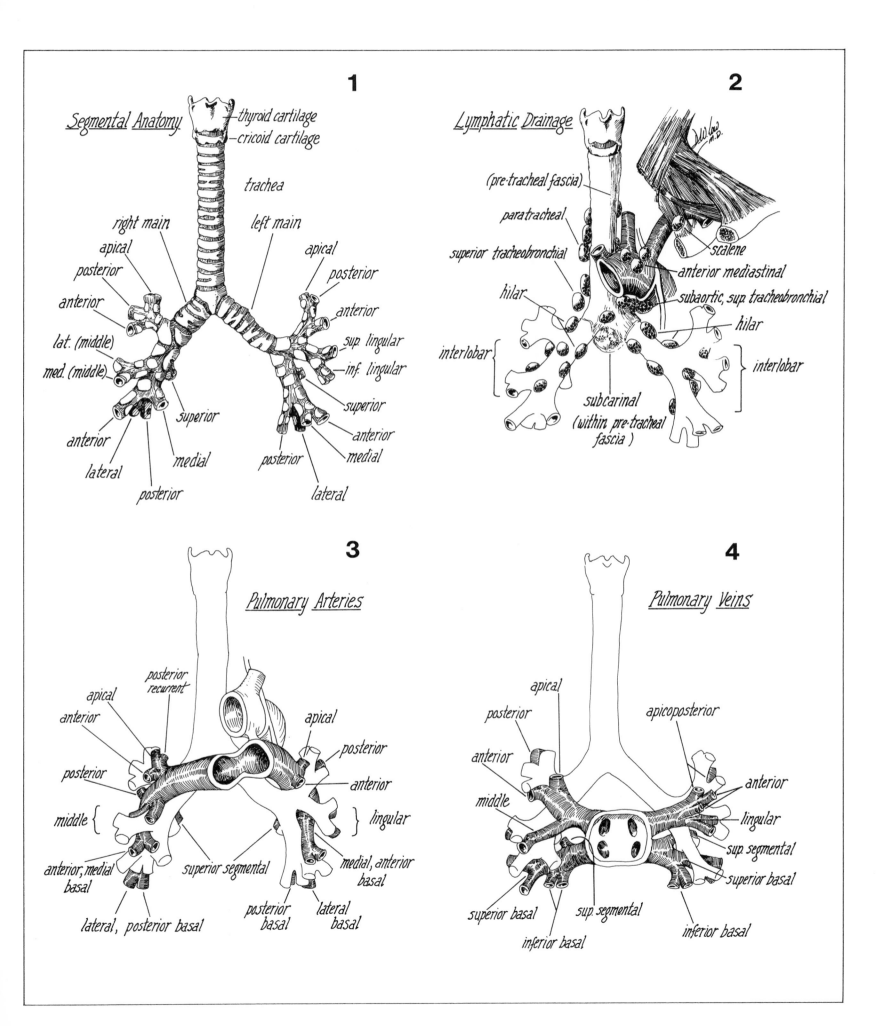

1

Segmental Anatomy

thyroid cartilage
cricoid cartilage

trachea

right main
left main

apical
apical

posterior
posterior

anterior
anterior

lat. (middle)
sup. lingular

med. (middle)
inf. lingular

superior

anterior
superior

lateral
anterior
medial

medial
posterior

posterior
lateral

2

Lymphatic Drainage

(pre-tracheal fascia)

paratracheal
scalene

superior tracheobronchial
anterior mediastinal

hilar
subaortic, sup. tracheobronchial

hilar

interlobar
interlobar

subcarinal
(within pre-tracheal fascia)

3

Pulmonary Arteries

posterior recurrent

apical
apical

anterior
posterior

posterior
anterior

middle {
} lingular

anterior, medial basal
medial, anterior basal

superior segmental

lateral, posterior basal
posterior basal
lateral basal

4

Pulmonary Veins

apical

posterior
apicoposterior

anterior
anterior

middle
lingular

sup. segmental

superior basal

superior basal
sup. segmental
inferior basal

inferior basal

Routine Pulmonary Operative Techniques

After induction of anesthesia and endotracheal intubation, the surgeon passes a fiberoptic bronchoscope to inspect the airways, if he has not previously done so. The relationship and distances between visible endotracheal tumors and the planned level of bronchial amputation are noted, as are anatomic variations in bronchial anatomy and the presence of purulent secretions. Following this brief bronchoscopic inspection, the single-lumen endotracheal tube is replaced with a Robertshaw double-lumen endotracheal tube. This tube permits collapse of the ispilateral lung during operation, facilitates dissection, allows open anastomoses of the bronchus, and permits smaller thoracotomy incisions. The double lumen tube also protects the downside ventilated lung in case purulent material or blood escapes into the airways during the dissection.

Most pulmonary resections can be performed through a lateral or posterolateral thoracotomy incision. Excision of a segment of the fifth rib provides satisfactory exposure for pneumonectomy, upper or lower lobectomy, or segmental resections. Occasionally, thoracotomy with excision of the sixth rib is preferred for lower lobe resections. If the rib is not removed, the chest is usually entered through the fourth or fifth intercostal space.

(1) The patient is positioned in a straight (90 degrees) lateral position with an arm roll under the downside axilla to protect against a brachial plexus injury. A rolled sandbag is placed along the spine and another sandbag is placed under the upper abdomen. The downside arm is extended onto an armboard; the upper arm is flexed and placed on a small pillow or folded blanket. Occasionally, the upper arm is suspended over the patient's head if a high anterior thoracotomy incision is required. The downside leg is usually flexed slightly at the hip and knees; the upside leg is extended on a pillow placed between the legs. The cautery grounding plate is placed on the posterior surface of the upside thigh. A wide band of adhesive tape is passed over the hips below the iliac crest and attached to the anterior and posterior sides of the operating table to provide further stability.

(2) Pulmonary vessels are thin-walled and often friable. Double ligation of all pulmonary arterial and venous stumps is recommended. If two encircling ligatures are used, a 3 to 4 mm segment of vessel should separate the two ligatures and another 4 to 5 mm cuff of vessel should extend beyond the last ligature. Often the second ligature is a suture ligature to ensure against slippage. If vessel length is inadequate, the divided end of a vascular stump is oversewn with a double suture line of fine nonabsorbable suture. Hemaclips are sometimes used on distal vessels (to be removed with the specimen), but not on vascular stumps.

(3) With rare exceptions, bronchi are stapled closed with a closing stapling instrument (RC-30 or RC-60, Ethicon Division, Johnson & Johnson Inc., Somerville, NJ). A transected open bronchus can also be closed with multiple interrupted sutures placed 1 mm apart 4 to 5 mm from the end of a bronchus. The sutures are placed in such a way as to invaginate the membranous bronchus into the curved cartilagenous wall.

(4) After lobar or segmental resections, two No. 28 or No. 32 chest tubes are inserted through stab wounds in the anterior and midaxillary lines below the incision. The straight tube, placed in the anterior stab wound, is positioned to remove any air that collects in the apex of the hemithorax. The angled posterior tube is placed so that blood or serum collecting in the posterior gutter near the diaphragm can be removed. Before bringing the chest tubes through the chest wall, a heavy nonabsorbable mattress suture is placed across the stab wound. This suture is wound around the chest tube to prevent premature removal and tied to close the stab wound after the chest tube is removed.

Injection of ipsilateral, intercostal nerves two interspaces above and below the thoracotomy incision with 0.25 to 0.50% long-acting anesthetic (No. 22 needle) is optional. The anesthetic is placed beneath the parietal pleura near the nerve, but away from the intercostal vessels.

Before the chest is closed, the bronchial stump is tested for leaks by inflating the residual lung to 40 cm H_2O airway pressure while the bronchial stump is submerged in warm saline. Any large leaks in the lung parenchyma are closed by pursestring or continuous absorbable sutures.

The thoracotomy incision is closed using interrupted absorbable sutures to close the intercostal muscles on either side of the resected rib. If the rib has not been resected, the intercostal muscles and pleura above the stripped rib are sutured to the undivided intercostal muscles below. A rib approximator may be used to hold the wound closed while the intercostal sutures are tied. No sutures are placed around the ribs against the intercostal nerve. The remaining muscles are sutured together using heavy absorbable continuous sutures. The subcutaneous tissue is closed with a continuous suture, and the skin is closed with a subcuticular stitch or with skin staples. A light dressing using paper tape is placed over the wound. Dry gauze is placed around the chest tubes and secured with tape.

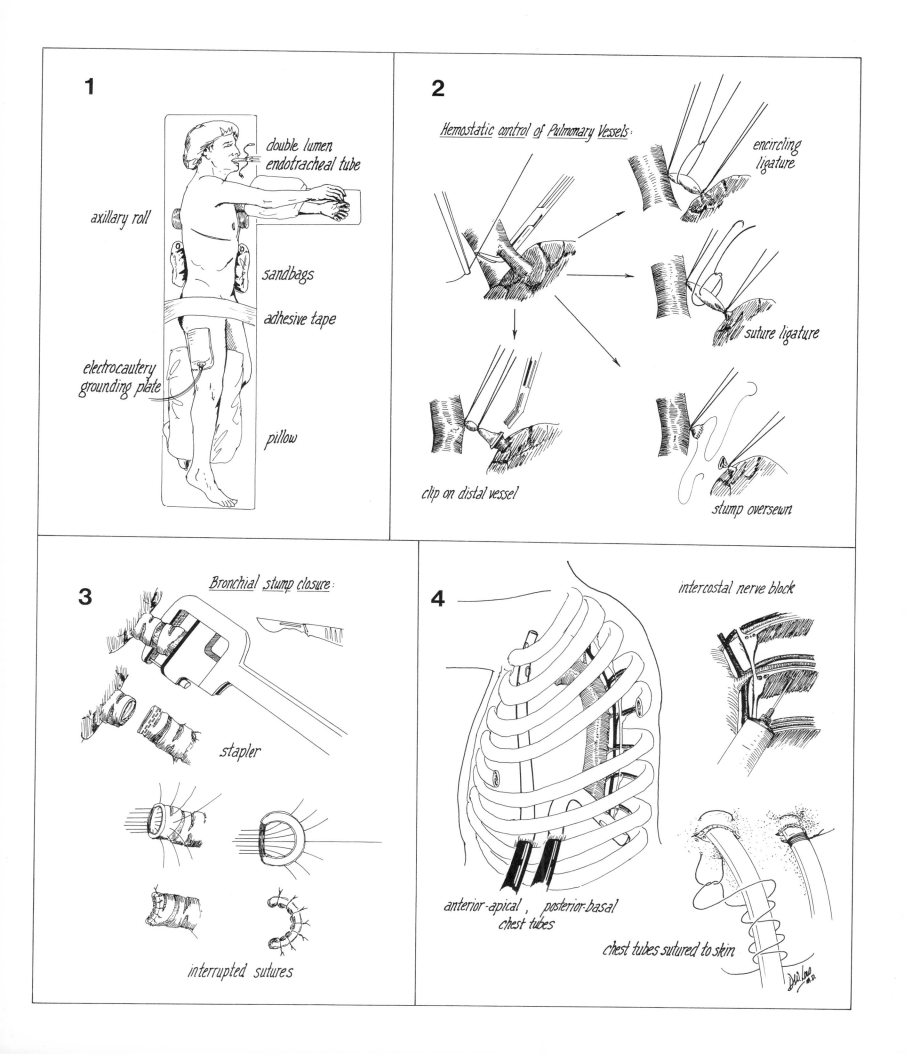

1

double lumen
endotracheal tube

axillary roll

sandbags

adhesive tape

electrocautery
grounding plate

pillow

2

Hemostatic control of Pulmonary Vessels:

encircling
ligature

suture ligature

clip on distal vessel

stump oversewn

3

Bronchial stump closure:

stapler

interrupted sutures

4

intercostal nerve block

anterior-apical, posterior-basal
chest tubes

chest tubes sutured to skin

Right Upper Lobectomy

After placement of a Robertshaw endotracheal tube, the chest is entered through a right lateral thoracotomy incision. A segment of the fifth rib is excised and pleural adhesions, if present, are taken down. The chest is explored to confirm the location of the lesion, the absence of other suspicious lesions, and the status of regional and paratracheal lymph nodes.

1 The collapsed lung is retracted posteriorly and inferiorly. The mediastinal pleura posterior to the right phrenic nerve and anterior to the right superior pulmonary veins is incised. The incision is carried cephalad to the azygos vein, which may or may not be divided. The superior margin of the right superior pulmonary vein is dissected out to expose the right main pulmonary artery posteriorly and superiorly.

2 The dissection continues around the anterior and superior margins of the pulmonary artery. Branches to the anterior and apical segments may arise separately or as a single trunk and are located anteriorly to the upper lobe bronchus. The apical and anterior pulmonary arteries are dissected out, ligated, and divided. The superior pulmonary vein is dissected out to expose approximately 1.5 cm of the first-order branches. None of the veins is ligated at this time.

3 Dissection continues in the major fissure, where the pulmonary artery is the most anterior structure. Pulmonary arterial branches to the middle lobe, superior segment of the lower lobe, and posterior segment of the upper lobe are clearly identified. The latter vessel is ligated and divided. The anterior wall of the pulmonary artery posterior to the superior pulmonary vein is dissected free of the overlying parenchyma.

4 The minor fissure, separating the upper and middle lobes, is developed using cautery to incise the visceral pleura at the fine line demarcating the two lobes. After incising the pleura, the fissure is developed by blunt dissection until the parenchyma is only 1 to 2 cm thick.

5 The lung is retracted posteriorly and the middle lobe pulmonary veins joining the right superior pulmonary vein are identified. The upper lobar venous branches are triply ligated and divided.

6 A linear cutting (PLC 50, Ethicon Division, Johnson & Johnson Inc., Somerville, NJ) stapling device is placed across the undivided parenchyma between upper and middle lobes to complete the division of the minor fissure.

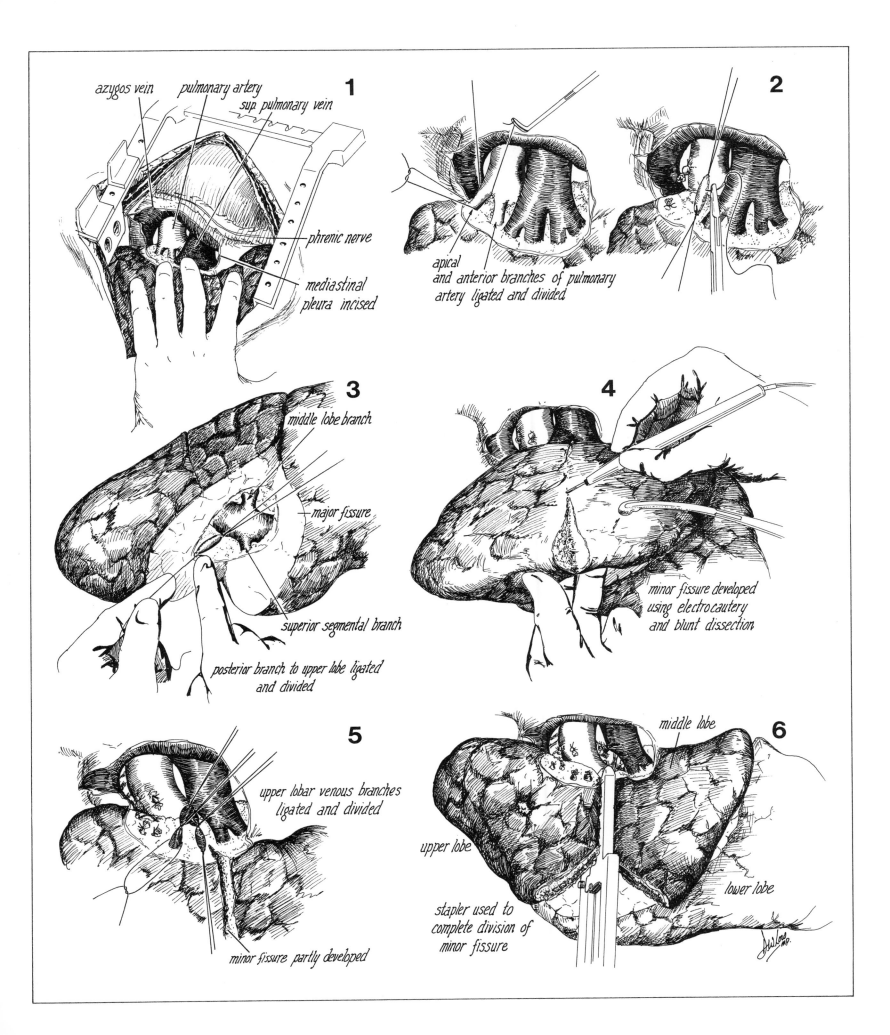

1

azygos vein

pulmonary artery

sup. pulmonary vein

phrenic nerve

mediastinal pleura incised

2

apical
and anterior branches of pulmonary
artery ligated and divided

3

middle lobe branch

major fissure

superior segmental branch

posterior branch to upper lobe ligated
and divided

4

minor fissure developed
using electrocautery
and blunt dissection

5

upper lobar venous branches
ligated and divided

minor fissure partly developed

6

middle lobe

upper lobe

lower lobe

stapler used to
complete division of
minor fissure

7 The major fissure between the upper lobe and the superior segment of lower lobe is also divided using the linear cutting stapler.

8 The pulmonary ligament is divided and the mediastinal pleura posterior to the bronchus is divided to expose the right main bronchus posterior to the pulmonary artery. Hilar lymph nodes are swept toward the specimen. The lung is then retracted anteriorly so that the right upper lobe bronchus can be dissected free of mediastinal tissue posteriorly. Bronchial vessels are either clipped or cauterized.

9 A closing stapler is placed across the upper lobe bronchus approximately 1 cm from its origin from the main bronchus. The bronchus is stapled closed (usually with short staples) and divided. It is usually not necessary to cover the bronchial stump, but a flap of posterior parietal pleura can be used for this purpose.

10 After expansion of the middle and lower lobes and testing of the bronchial closure for leaks, under warm saline one straight and one angled chest tube (No. 32) are inserted through separate stab wounds below the incision in the anterior and midaxillary lines. The tubes are positioned to remove apical air and fluid that accumulate posteriorly near the diaphragm.

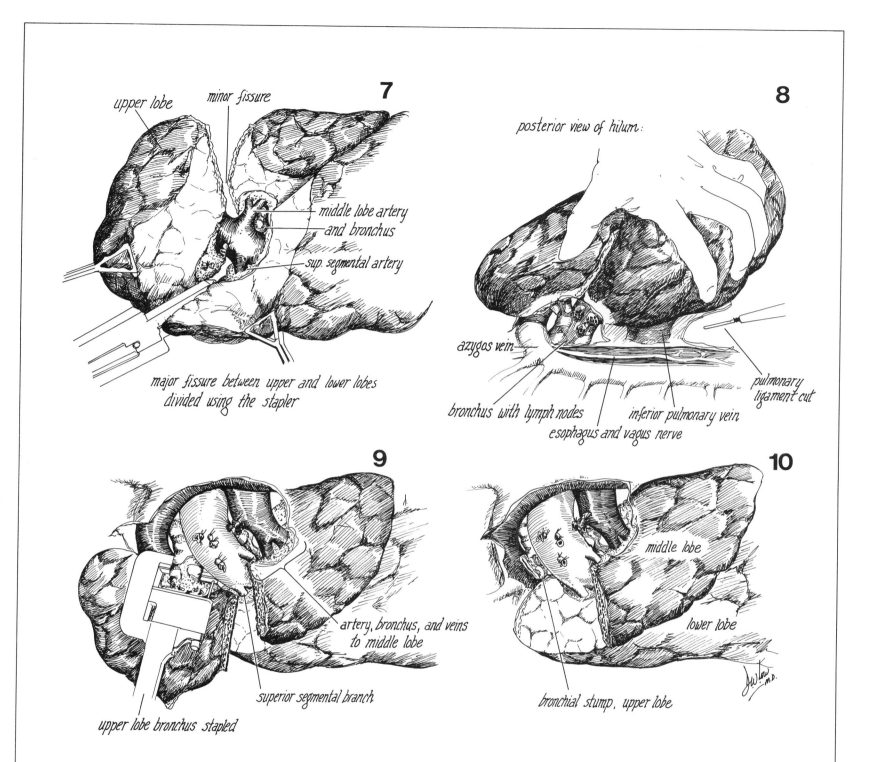

7

upper lobe

minor fissure

middle lobe artery
and bronchus

sup. segmental artery

major fissure between upper and lower lobes
divided using the stapler

8

posterior view of hilum:

azygos vein

bronchus with lymph nodes

esophagus and vagus nerve

inferior pulmonary vein

pulmonary
ligament cut

9

artery, bronchus, and veins
to middle lobe

superior segmental branch

upper lobe bronchus stapled

10

middle lobe

lower lobe

bronchial stump, upper lobe

Right Middle Lobectomy, Right Upper and Middle Lobectomy

Resection of the right middle lobe for benign or selected malignant lesions conserves lung tissue and therefore lung function. The operation is the reciprocal of right upper lobectomy and is performed through a right lateral thoracotomy incision. A Robertshaw endotracheal tube is used.

1 The junction of the major and minor fissures is most easily detected with the right lung inflated. After the visceral pleura and areolar tissue over the pulmonary artery at the fissural junction are incised, the right lung is allowed to collapse. The interlobar portion of the pulmonary artery is dissected to expose the middle lobar pulmonary artery or arteries, and the artery to the superior segment of the lower lobe.

2 The middle lobar pulmonary artery or arteries are dissected out and encircled with a 3-0 nonabsorbable ligature. The vessels are not tied at this time. The middle lobe bronchus can be palpated posterior to the middle lobe artery.

3 The lung is retracted posteriorly and the mediastinal pleura over the superior pulmonary vein is incised. First-order branches of the superior pulmonary vein are dissected out.

4 The minor fissure is usually incomplete and occasionally may not be present at all. Before vessels are ligated and divided, the fissure is partially developed by identifying the fine line demarcating the junction of the upper and lower lobes. The visceral pleura at this line is incised with the cautery, and the minor fissure is partially developed by blunt dissection. After partial development of the minor fissure, positive identification of the middle lobe artery and vein are made.

5 The encircled middle lobar artery is triply ligated and divided. The middle lobar vein or occasionally veins are also ligated and divided.

6 The middle lobar bronchus is located within the fissure posterior to the pulmonary arterial stump. The origin of the bronchus is dissected free, stapled closed, and divided. Any parenchymal tissue bridging the major fissure is divided with the cautery. Occasionally, a linear cutting stapler is used to divide the parenchyma to complete the major fissure.

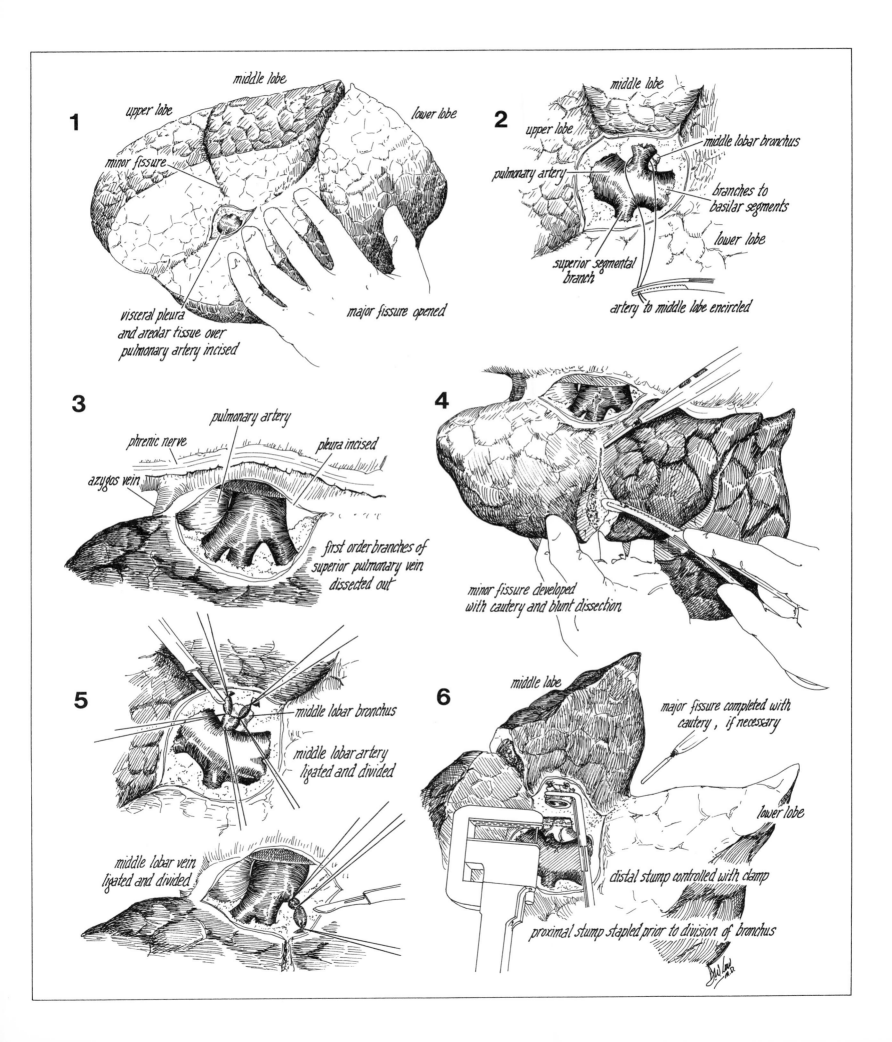

1

upper lobe

middle lobe

lower lobe

minor fissure

visceral pleura
and areolar tissue over
pulmonary artery incised

major fissure opened

2

middle lobe

upper lobe

pulmonary artery

middle lobar bronchus

branches to
basilar segments

lower lobe

superior segmental
branch

artery to middle lobe encircled

3

phrenic nerve

pulmonary artery

pleura incised

azygos vein

first order branches of
superior pulmonary vein
dissected out

4

minor fissure developed
with cautery and blunt dissection

5

middle lobar bronchus

middle lobar artery
ligated and divided

middle lobar vein
ligated and divided

6

middle lobe

major fissure completed with
cautery , if necessary

lower lobe

distal stump controlled with clamp

proximal stump stapled prior to division of bronchus

(7) With traction on the middle lobar bronchus, the minor fissure is further developed. The two lobes can be completely separated by a combination of finger compression and blunt dissection with gauze-tipped clamps as is done in a segmental resection. Partial inflation of the surrounding right lung facilitates this dissection. Bleeding interlobar veins are cauterized.

Alternatively, the minor fissure can be developed by bronchial traction and blunt dissection until a 1 to 2 cm thick bridge of undivided parenchyma remains. This bridge of tissue is sealed and divided using the linear cutting stapler.

The pulmonary ligament is not divided after middle lobectomy.

RIGHT UPPER AND MIDDLE LOBECTOMY

When resection is performed for carcinoma of either the right upper or middle lobes, usually both lobes are resected en bloc. The minor fissure is not divided.

(8) The lung is retracted posteriorly and the mediastinal pleura over the hilum of the right lung is incised. The right superior pulmonary vein and the right main pulmonary artery, which is anterior to the right main and upper lobar bronchi, are dissected out. The anterior and apical segmental arteries are dissected out, triply ligated, and divided.

(9) The major fissure is entered and the posterior segmental and middle lobar arteries are dissected out, positively identified, ligated, and divided.

(10) The superior pulmonary vein is dissected out past first order branches. The entire vein is ligated with a 0 nonabsorbable ligature. Individual first-order veins are separately ligated proximally and either ligated or clipped distally. The individual veins are divided.

(11) The upper lobe bronchus is easily located posterior to the pulmonary artery near the stumps of the anterior and apical segments. This is stapled closed with an RC-30 stapler and divided. The middle lobe bronchus is located posterior to the right pulmonary artery anteriorly. It is also stapled and divided. Both bronchi are transected about 1 cm from the right main bronchus so that the staple line closes the airway flush with the main bronchus and does not reduce the diameter of the main bronchus.

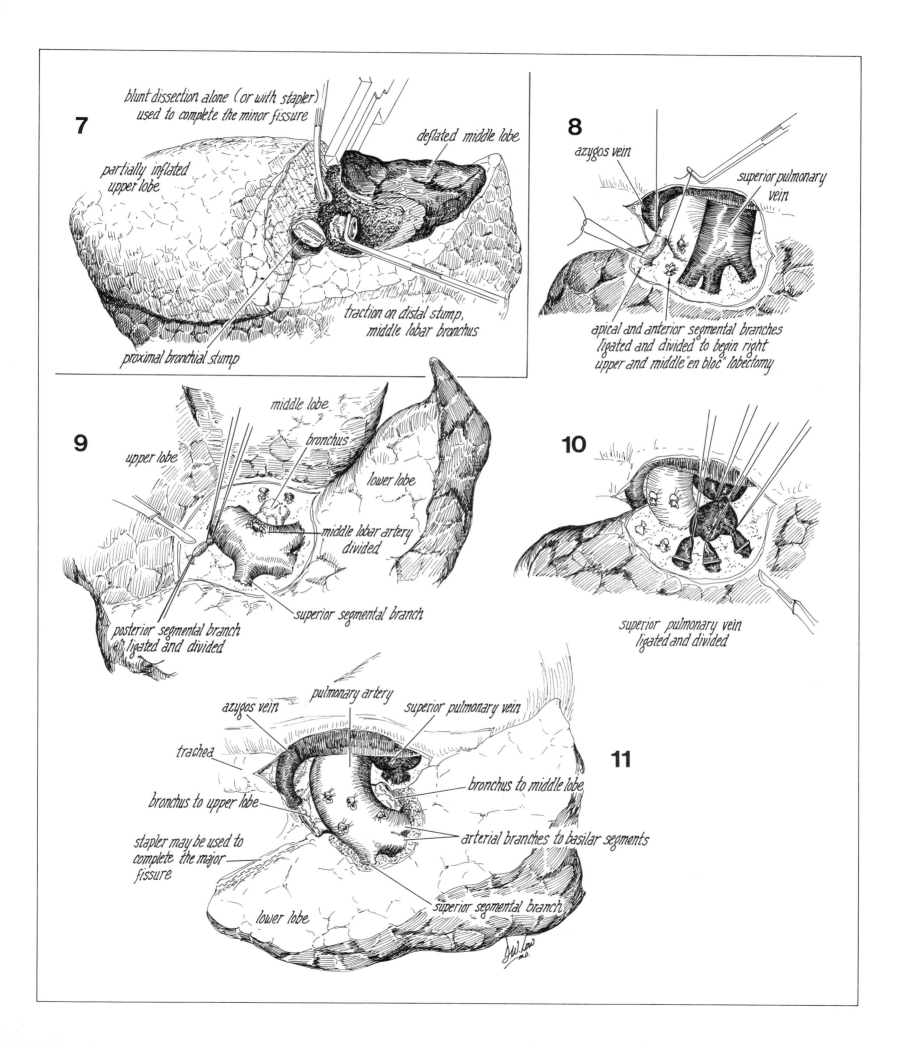

7 blunt dissection alone (or with stapler) used to complete the minor fissure

deflated middle lobe

partially inflated upper lobe

traction on distal stump, middle lobar bronchus

proximal bronchial stump

8 azygos vein

superior pulmonary vein

apical and anterior segmental branches ligated and divided to begin right upper and middle "en bloc" lobectomy

9 middle lobe

bronchus

upper lobe

lower lobe

middle lobar artery divided

superior segmental branch

posterior segmental branch ligated and divided

10 superior pulmonary vein ligated and divided

11 azygos vein

pulmonary artery

superior pulmonary vein

trachea

bronchus to middle lobe

bronchus to upper lobe

arterial branches to basilar segments

stapler may be used to complete the major fissure

superior segmental branch

lower lobe

Right Lower Lobectomy

The chest is entered through a right lateral thoracotomy; a segment of either the fifth or sixth rib is resected. The chest is explored.

1 The major fissure is incised to dissect out the interlobar segment of the pulmonary artery. The arteries to the middle lobe and superior segment of the lower lobe are identified. The superior segmental artery is divided and ligated. The pulmonary artery (arteries) to the basilar segments are then ligated and divided also, just beyond the origin of the middle lobe vessel(s).

2 The lung is retracted posteriorly and superiorly to divide the pulmonary ligament with the cautery. The inferior pulmonary vein is dissected out, including 1.5 cm of the first-order branches. The vein is ligated and divided.

3 The mediastinal pleura posterior to the hilum is incised superiorly from the divided inferior pulmonary vein. The bronchus is palpated to identify the origin of the middle lobe bronchus anteriorly. Peribronchial tissue containing lymph nodes is dissected toward the specimen and bronchial vessels are clipped or cauterized.

4 Parenchymal bridging across the major fissure is now divided. Often, the fissure between the superior segment of the lower lobe and posterior segment of the upper lobe is incomplete. This is divided and sealed using the linear cutting stapler.

5 The closing stapler is placed across the intermediate bronchus approximately 1 cm distal to the origin of the middle lobar bronchus.

6 Occasionally, the intermediate bronchus is short, necessitating closure and division of the superior segmental bronchus and bronchi to the basilar segments separately. After testing for air leaks, the bronchial stump may be covered with a flap of posterior parietal pleura.

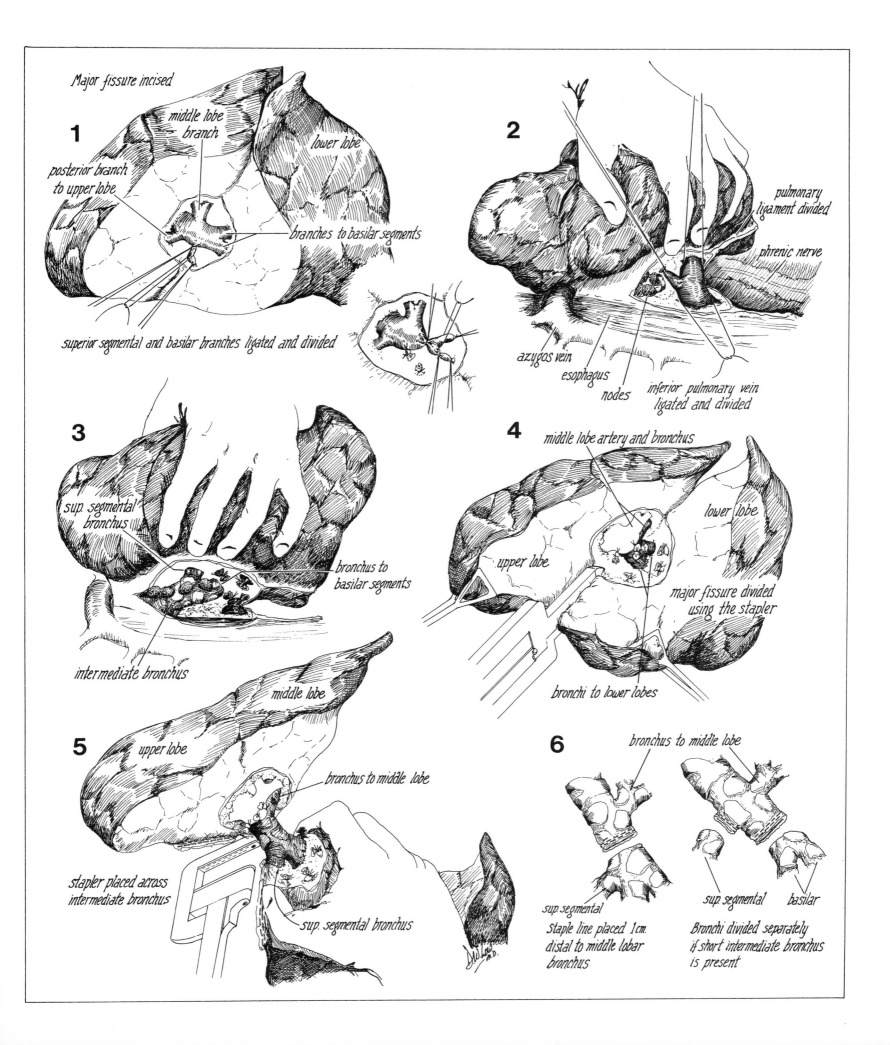

1 Major fissure incised

posterior branch to upper lobe

middle lobe branch

lower lobe

branches to basilar segments

superior segmental and basilar branches ligated and divided

2 pulmonary ligament divided

phrenic nerve

azygos vein

esophagus

nodes

inferior pulmonary vein ligated and divided

3 sup. segmental bronchus

bronchus to basilar segments

intermediate bronchus

4 middle lobe artery and bronchus

upper lobe

lower lobe

major fissure divided using the stapler

bronchi to lower lobes

5 middle lobe

upper lobe

bronchus to middle lobe

stapler placed across intermediate bronchus

sup. segmental bronchus

6 bronchus to middle lobe

sup. segmental

Staple line placed 1 cm distal to middle lobar bronchus

sup. segmental

basilar

Bronchi divided separately if short intermediate bronchus is present

Left Upper Lobectomy

This operation is illustrated for a solitary peripheral nodule. Bronchoscopy, which is usually not prescribed preoperatively for a peripheral nodule, is performed in the operating room to confirm the absence of endobronchial lesions and unusual bronchial anatomy. The patient is positioned right side down for a left lateral thoracotomy.

Because the histologic diagnosis is not known, a small lateral thoracotomy incision is made and a segment of the fifth rib is excised. It is convenient to open the auscultatory triangle just posterior to the tip of the scapula to count ribs and to identify the fifth. The nodule is located with the lung gently ventilated. Careful exploration is carried out to exclude the presence of other nodules and to assess the status of regional and paratracheal nodes. An excisional biopsy of the peripheral lung nodule is performed. Large nodules (2.5 cm) are usually not excised but are removed by lobectomy or, rarely, segmental resection.

(1) Usually the nodule is excised by wedge resection. The nodule is held by fingers and, with a linear cutting stapling device, two incisions are made into the collapsed lung to remove the nodule as a pie-slice or V incision. Staples seal the lung edges. While the histology of the nodule is determined by immediate microscopy of frozen sections, the lung is inflated to see if additional sutures are needed to seal the lung edges.

(2) Dissection of the left upper lobe continues by incision of the mediastinal pleura around the hilum. The pulmonary ligament is incised up to the inferior pulmonary vein. Branches of the vagus nerves to the lung are cut. The apical-posterior or apical and posterior pulmonary arteries are dissected out for approximately 1 cm.

(3) When the lung is retracted posteriorly, the superior pulmonary vein is visible anteriorly. This is dissected out and clearly separated from the inferior pulmonary vein. No vessels are ligated or divided until the pathology report is received. When a decision to do the lobectomy is made, the thoracotomy

incision can be extended anteriorly or posteriorly as needed to improve exposure. With the lung collapsed, it is often not necessary to extend the incision. The apical and posterior pulmonary arteries are triply ligated and divided.

(4) Before ligation of the pulmonary veins, the major fissue is dissected out and the lingular and anterior segmental pulmonary arteries are ligated and divided. The dissection is carried anteriorly a short distance to clearly separate the lingular segments of the upper lobe from the lower lobe. The incompletely divided anterior portion of the major fissure is then divided, using a linear cutting stapler to seal the divided lung edge.

(5) The upper lobe pulmonary veins are triply ligated and divided. Often one ligature is placed around the entire superior vein and individual ties or hemaclips are placed on segmental veins, which are then divided.

(6) Bronchial nodes are swept toward the upper lobe specimen throughout the dissection. The origin of the left upper lobe bronchus is dissected out for approximately 1 cm. The small (RC-30) closing stapler is placed across the bronchus approximately 0.5 to 1 cm from the lower lobe bronchus and applied. The bronchus is cut and the specimen is removed.

Bleeding from small bronchial vessels is controlled by cautery. The left lower lobe is reinflated to 30 to 40 cm H_2O and tested for leaks under warm saline. Usually the bronchial stump is not reinforced or covered, but can be with a flap of mediastinal pleura. Large air leaks in the lower lobe are closed by purse-string sutures.

Intercostal nerves are injected with a long-acting anesthetic. An anterior apical and a posterior basal chest tube are inserted through stab wounds placed so that the patient does not lie on the tubes. A single absorbable suture can be used to fix the inflated lower lobe to the mediastinal pleura to prevent torsion of the lung.

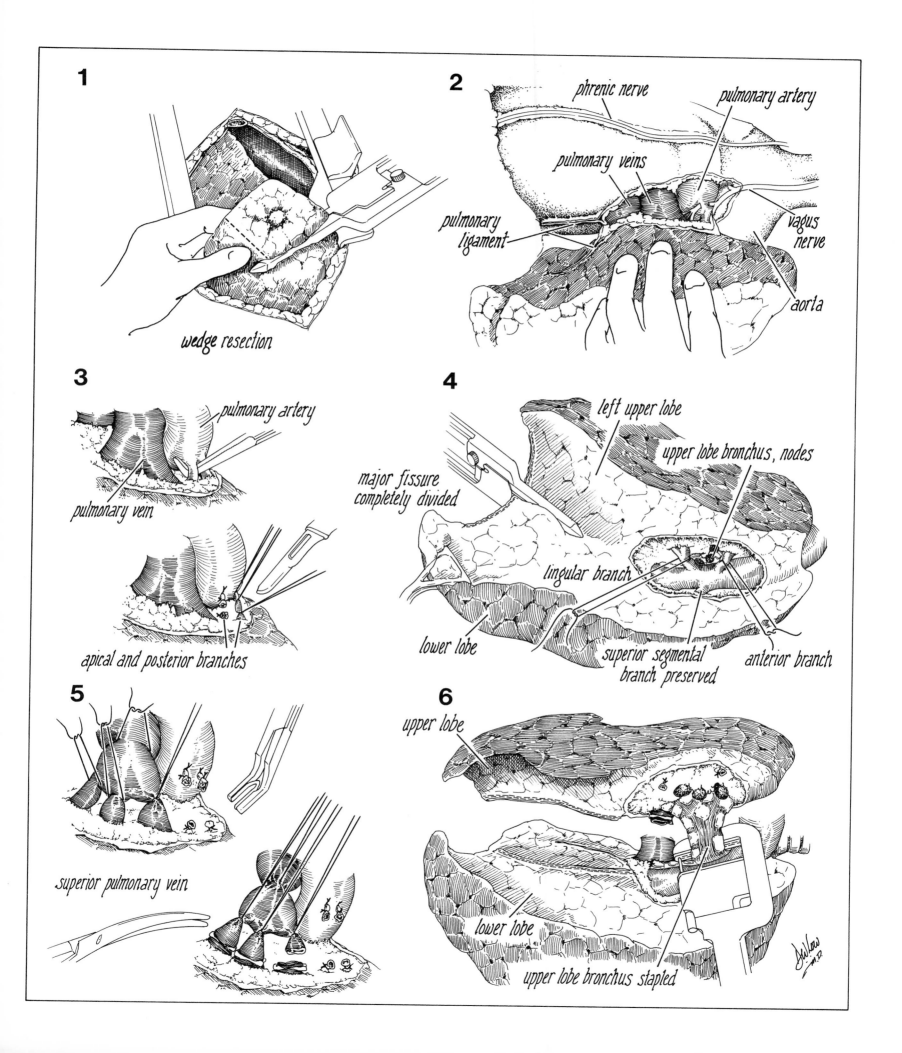

1 wedge resection

2 phrenic nerve · pulmonary artery · pulmonary veins · pulmonary ligament · vagus nerve · aorta

3 pulmonary artery · pulmonary vein · apical and posterior branches

4 major fissure completely divided · left upper lobe · upper lobe bronchus, nodes · lingular branch · lower lobe · superior segmental branch preserved · anterior branch

5 superior pulmonary vein

6 upper lobe · lower lobe · upper lobe bronchus stapled

Left Lower Lobectomy

The chest is entered through the bed of either the fifth or sixth rib. A lateral thoracotomy incision usually suffices if a Robertshaw endotracheal tube is used. The lung, chest cavity, and mediastinum are explored.

(1) The major fissure is opened to expose the interlobar portion of the left pulmonary artery. The lingular and anterior branches to the upper lobe are identified and spared.

(2) The superior segmental branch or branches are dissected out and triply ligated and divided. Sometimes the lower lobar pulmonary artery can be ligated and divided just beyond the origin of the lingular branches. More often, the basilar branches are individually ligated and divided.

(3) The deflated lung is retracted anteriorly and superiorly, and the pulmonary ligament is divided with cautery. The posterior mediastinal pleura is incised, and the inferior pulmonary vein is dissected out and ligated. Individual first-order branches are separately ligated so that at least two ligatures prevent bleeding from the vein stump.

(4) With the lung retracted posteriorly, the anterior mediastinal pleura is incised to the major fissure. The incompletely divided major fissure is now divided using a linear cutting stapler.

(5) The same technique is used to separate the posterior segment of the upper lobe and superior segment of the lower lobe. Completion of the major fissure exposes the lower lobe branches and the surrounding nodes and alveolar tissue.

(6) The bronchus is divided using a closing stapler 1 cm below the origin of the lingular bronchus. Sometimes the superior segmental bronchus arises opposite the lingular bronchus and must be taken separately. Coverage of the bronchial stumps with posterior mediastinal pleura is optional.

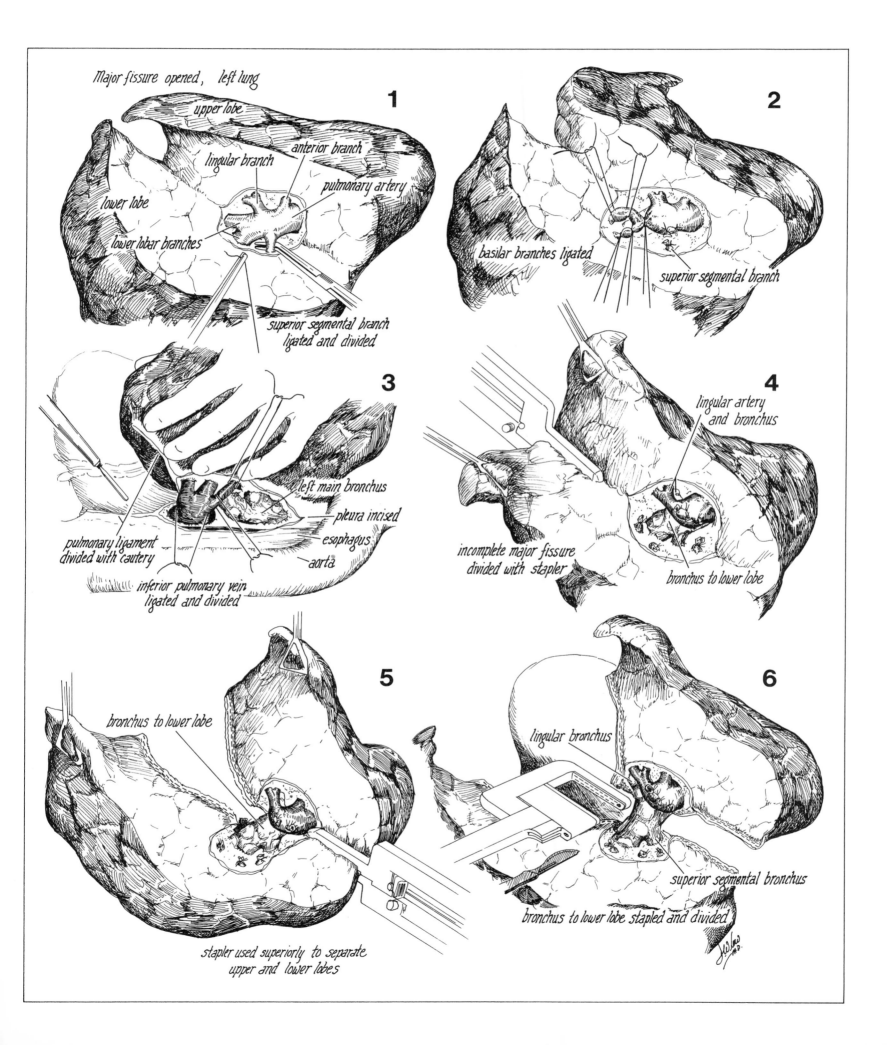

1 Major fissure opened, left lung
- upper lobe
- lingular branch
- anterior branch
- pulmonary artery
- lower lobe
- lower lobar branches
- superior segmental branch ligated and divided

2
- basilar branches ligated
- superior segmental branch

3
- left main bronchus
- pleura incised
- esophagus
- aorta
- pulmonary ligament divided with cautery
- inferior pulmonary vein ligated and divided

4
- lingular artery and bronchus
- incomplete major fissure divided with stapler
- bronchus to lower lobe

5
- bronchus to lower lobe
- stapler used superiorly to separate upper and lower lobes

6
- lingular bronchus
- superior segmental bronchus
- bronchus to lower lobe stapled and divided

Standard Right Pneumonectomy

The patient is placed left side down for a standard right thoracotomy. A Robertshaw divided endotracheal tube is used. A radial arterial catheter, large central venous catheter, and electrocardiographic monitoring leads are in place. The chest is entered through the bed of the excised fifth rib; only a lateral thoracotomy incision is needed.

1 With the right lung collapsed, a circular incision around the hilum of the lung is made in the mediastinal pleura. The incision begins anteriorly, posterior to the phrenic nerve, and overlying the right atrium and lateral superior vena cava, continues superiorly to the azygos vein and swings posteriorly over the esophagus. Inferiorly, the pulmonary ligament is cut up to the inferior pulmonary vein. Often the azygos vein is divided between double ligatures to permit access to right tracheobronchial nodes and paratracheal nodes, if a radical lymph node dissection is desired. As the dissection of the hilum continues, bronchial arteries are clipped or cauterized and lymph nodes are swept toward the specimen.

2 The superior margin of the right superior pulmonary vein is dissected free and gently retracted inferiorly to expose the right main pulmonary artery posteriorly and slightly cephalad. The right pulmonary artery is dissected free of the superior pulmonary vein anteriorly, the superior vena cava medially, and the right main bronchus posteriorly. If necessary, the superior vena cava can be retracted laterally to expose the right pulmonary artery covered by pericardium behind the ascending aorta.

3 Approximately 2 cm of the artery is dissected free of surrounding tissue and doubly ligated with heavy, nonabsorbable ligatures. In some patients, the distal pulmonary artery is ligated downstream to the origin of the apical branch artery. A suture ligature is placed between the two latter ligatures approximately 0.5 cm from the proximal tie. The vessel is divided between the suture and distal ligatures, leaving a 1.0 cm cuff of vessel on the proximal stump. Alternatively, the vessel can be divided between encircling ligatures and the proximal end oversewn with fine nonabsorbable suture. Hemaclips can be used on distal vessels, but for security, sutures and ligatures are preferred for the pulmonary arterial and venous stumps.

4 The lung is retracted posteriorly, and first the superior and then the inferior pulmonary veins are dissected out approximately 1.5 cm beyond the origin of the first-order branches. The veins are triply ligated, usually with one heavy nonabsorbable encircling ligature around the main trunk and two latter ligatures around first-order branches. First-order branches are divided between the two latter ligatures with a cuff between ligature and vein end.

5 If desirable, the pericardium can be opened anterior to the veins and posterior to the right phrenic nerve to ligate and divide the veins within the pericardium. If trunks are divided within the pericardium, a suture ligature is used as the second stump ligature. If a tumor is palpable within the pulmonary veins, a cuff of left atrium may be taken using a Satinsky clamp and a continuous suture closure.

6 The right main bronchus behind the pulmonary arterial stump near the tracheal carina is dissected out, sweeping tracheobronchial lymph nodes toward the specimen. A closing stapling device (with long staples) is placed across the carina. The stapled bronchus is divided and the specimen is removed. Compression of the bronchial walls by the staples 1 cm from the carina minimizes the intraluminal dead space within the bronchial stump.

Alternatively, the bronchus can be closed with interrupted nonabsorbable, monofilament sutures (polypropylene or fine wire). Sutures are placed approximately 0.5 cm from the cut edge approximately 1 mm apart in such a way that the posterior membranous wall of the bronchus is brought forward against the curved, cartilagenous anterior wall. Sutures are tied over the cut end of the bronchus; a bronchial clamp is not used.

7 Usually the bronchial stump is not covered. If coverage is desired, a flap of parietal pleura, mobilized as a pedicle flap from the posterior chest wall, can be tacked over the bronchial stump with fine sutures. Without the pleural flap, the esophagus and mediastinal tissues posteriorly and right pulmonary arterial stump anteriorly cover the bronchial closure.

The chest is closed either without drainage or after insertion of a single chest tube placed near the diaphragm posteriorly. If a chest tube is used, it is connected to balanced drainage. If no chest tube is used, the mediastinum is adjusted after the chest is closed by aspirating air from the right hemithorax by means of a No. 18 needle temporarily placed in the second interspace anteriorly after the chest is closed. Air is aspirated until the syringe barrel can no longer be easily withdrawn. This shifts the mediastinum toward the right hemithorax; however, as fluid accumulates within the right chest, the mediastinum shifts toward the left lung.

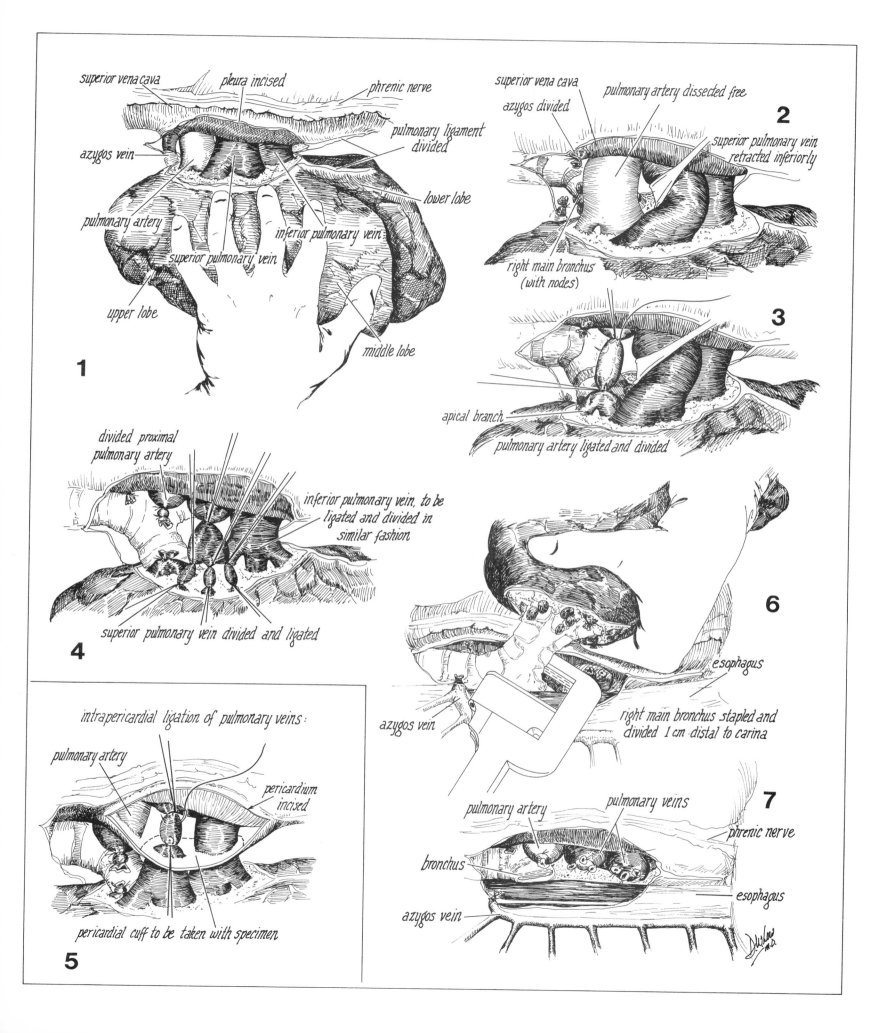

1

superior vena cava — pleura incised — phrenic nerve

azygos vein

pulmonary ligament divided

pulmonary artery

lower lobe

superior pulmonary vein

inferior pulmonary vein

upper lobe

middle lobe

2

superior vena cava — pulmonary artery dissected free

azygos divided

superior pulmonary vein retracted inferiorly

right main bronchus (with nodes)

3

apical branch

pulmonary artery ligated and divided

4

divided proximal pulmonary artery

inferior pulmonary vein, to be ligated and divided in similar fashion

superior pulmonary vein divided and ligated

6

esophagus

azygos vein

right main bronchus stapled and divided 1 cm distal to carina

5

intrapericardial ligation of pulmonary veins:

pulmonary artery

pericardium incised

pericardial cuff to be taken with specimen

7

pulmonary artery — pulmonary veins

phrenic nerve

bronchus

esophagus

azygos vein

Radical Left Pneumonectomy

The operation removes left paratracheal, tracheobronchial, carinal and hilar lymph nodes with the left lung. Because of the recurrent nerve and aortic arch, left radical pneumonectomy is more difficult than right.

(1) After left lateral thoracotomy, the left lung is deflated, and the pathology and lymph nodes are assessed. The mediastinal pleura is incised along the anterior border of the descending thoracic aorta from the pulmonary ligament, over the aortic arch, and parallel and slightly posterior to the left subclavian artery. The highest intercostal vein is ligated and divided. Fat, nodes, and areolar tissue are dissected from the descending thoracic aorta and from the left lateral and anterior esophagus. The pulmonary ligament is incised and the loose tissue and nodes are swept upward to the inferior pulmonary vein.

(2) The left vagus nerve at the aortic arch is identified and dissected free. The recurrent branch passing beneath the ligamentum arteriosum is identified. The left vagus nerve is clipped and divided below the origin of the recurrent nerve. Tissue over the recurrent nerve is carefully dissected inferiorly until it passes beneath the ligamentum arteriosum. The remaining nodes and fat beneath the posterior inferior aortic arch are dissected toward the lung hilum.

(3) The vagus nerve anterior to the left subclavian artery is protected as the left subclavian artery is dissected free from aortic arch to the apex of the left hemithorax. With careful blunt dissection, the recurrent nerve deep to the aortic arch is located and dissected free of surrounding tissue. An umbilical tape is passed around the recurrent nerve and left subclavian artery, and the nerve is dissected free of surrounding tissue from the posteromedial (deep) surface of the aortic arch. When the entire intrathoracic portion of the recurrent nerve is dissected free, an umbilical tape is passed around the aortic arch to facilitate removal of tracheobronchial lymph nodes.

(4) The proximal portion of the esophagus posterior to the left subclavian artery is dissected out, sweeping fat and lymph nodes anteriorly. The lateral and anterior borders of the trachea are palpated anterior to the esophagus. Beginning at the most cephalad segment of the intrathoracic trachea, nodes and fat are dissected caudally from the surface of the trachea and from the anterolateral surface of the esophagus toward the aortic arch. The left subclavian artery and recurrent nerve are retracted anteriorly and laterally to permit complete removal of the left paratracheal nodes.

(5) The aortic arch is retracted laterally to permit removal of tracheobronchial nodes from the trachea just superior to the tracheal bifurcation. Nodes along the posterior surface of the right main bronchus for a distance of 3 to 5 cm are dissected away and toward the tracheal bifurcation. Subcarinal nodes between the superior surface of the left atrium and tracheal bifurcation are dissected free and toward the left main bronchus.

(6) The mediastinal pleura posterior to the left phrenic nerve over the left pulmonary artery is incised to expose the artery inferior to the origin of the left recurrent nerve. The left pulmonary artery between the ligamentum arteriosum and first (apical) segmental branch is dissected out. The artery is ligated and divided, and the proximal stump is oversewn. Fat and nodes lateral to the trachea and left main bronchus are now easily dissected inferiorly to expose the origin of the left main bronchus.

At this point, the left paratracheal nodes, tracheobronchial and subaortic nodes, proximal right bronchial nodes, subcarinal nodes, midparaesophageal nodes, and nodes in the pulmonary ligament have been freed from neighboring structures.

(7) The anterior surfaces of the superior and inferior pulmonary veins are dissected free, the pulmonary ligament is divided, and the dissection is continued outside the pericardium around both veins. The dissection sweeps all tissue from the adjacent pericardium and proximal pulmonary veins toward the specimen. The veins are ligated and divided. Suture closure or a suture ligature is added to reinforce the pulmonary venous stump ligature.

(8) Alternatively, the pericardium may be incised posterior to the phrenic nerve and anterior to the pulmonary veins. A vascular clamp is placed across the junction of the left atrium and left pulmonary veins within the pericardium. A second vascular clamp is applied to the upstream veins. The vein-atrial junction is divided, and the cuff of atrium is sutured closed with a 3-0 vascular suture.

(9) A closing stapler with 4 mm staples is placed across the left main bronchus 1 cm from the carina. Staples are inserted and the bronchus is divided. The lung and all of the dissected lymph nodes are removed.

(10) Because of the extensive paratracheal and right bronchial dissection, coverage of the bronchial stump (after testing for leaks) seems prudent. A flap of pericardium, based on a superior pedicle, is cut to provide a vascular flap to cover the bronchus. This is tacked to the bronchus with fine interrupted sutures.

The left phrenic nerve may be crushed if paralysis of the diaphragm is desired. This step is not essential.

After hemostasis and infiltration of intercostal nerves with a long-acting local anesthesia, the chest is closed without drainage. Air pressure within the left hemithorax is adjusted by needle aspiration at the midclavicular line of the second interspace after the chest is closed.

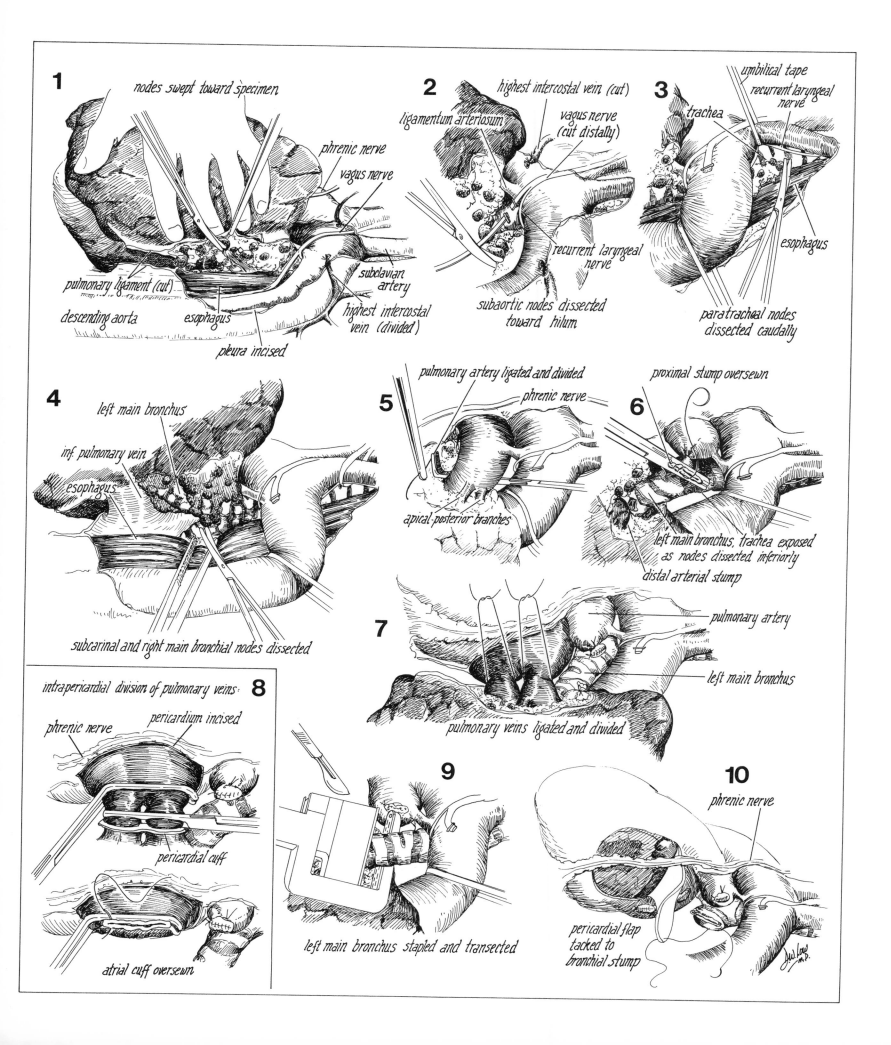

1 nodes swept toward specimen

phrenic nerve

vagus nerve

subclavian artery

highest intercostal vein (divided)

pulmonary ligament (cut)

descending aorta

esophagus

pleura incised

2 highest intercostal vein (cut)

ligamentum arteriosum

vagus nerve (cut distally)

recurrent laryngeal nerve

subaortic nodes dissected toward hilum

3 umbilical tape

recurrent laryngeal nerve

trachea

esophagus

paratracheal nodes dissected caudally

4 left main bronchus

inf. pulmonary vein

esophagus

subcarinal and right main bronchial nodes dissected

5 pulmonary artery ligated and divided

phrenic nerve

apical-posterior branches

6 proximal stump oversewn

left main bronchus, trachea exposed as nodes dissected inferiorly

distal arterial stump

7 pulmonary artery

left main bronchus

pulmonary veins ligated and divided

8 intrapericardial division of pulmonary veins:

phrenic nerve

pericardium incised

pericardial cuff

atrial cuff oversewn

9 left main bronchus stapled and transected

10 phrenic nerve

pericardial flap tacked to bronchial stump

Segmental Resections

Segmental resections remove anatomic units and are preferred to stapled wedge resections when the disease process is limited to one or more segments. The operation conserves functional lung tissue and therefore is particularly useful in patients with reduced pulmonary function. Benign tumors, localized vascular malformations, areas of chronic infection or destroyed lung, apical blebs, metastatic tumors, and occasional small primary tumors are examples of lesions treated by segmental resection. Although lower lobe bronchiectatic segments were frequently resected in the past, now the lingula, apical, and superior segments are most commonly resected. Resection of the lingula and apical segments of the left upper lobe and resection of the superior segment of the right lower lobe are illustrated.

LINGULAR RESECTION

1 The left chest is entered through a lateral thoracotomy incision with resection of a segment of the fifth rib. The left lung may be allowed to collapse to facilitate dissection, but this is not essential. The left pulmonary artery is identified in the major fissure and dissected out so that the artery to the lower lobe and branch to the superior segment are preserved. The branch or branches to the lingula are dissected out and doubly ligated and divided.

2 The upper lobe is retracted posteriorly to reach the left superior pulmonary vein. This vein is dissected out to its major branches and the most inferior or lingular branch is doubly ligated and divided. Only the branch that clearly drains the lingula is divided; if doubt exists, ligation should be deferred until the lingula is dissected from the upper lobe.

3 The upper lobe is now retracted anteriorly to expose the mediastinal pleura over the bronchus below the left pulmonary artery. The pulmonary artery is dissected posteriorly and cephalad from the bronchus. The lingular bronchus is identified coming off anteriorly from the inferior wall of the left upper lobe bronchus. After a 1.5 cm segment of the lingular bronchus is cleared, it is stapled closed and amputated so that the closed stump is 6 to 7 mm. The distal bronchus is grasped with a right-angled or bronchus clamp to apply traction.

4 If the left lung was allowed to collapse, it is now partially inflated to aid in separation of the parenchyma of the lingular and upper lobes. Hyperinflation is avoided to prevent partial inflation of the lingula by means of collateral airways. A line of demarcation between the lingula and upper lobe becomes apparent, and if one looks carefully, sometimes a white line indicating the intersegmental plane is visible on the visceral pleural surface. With a cautery, the visceral pleura is incised 1 to 2 mm to the lingular side of the line of demarcation. With traction on the lingular bronchus and finger-rolling compression along the line of demarcation, the lingula is gradually separated from the inflated upper lobe. Intersegmental veins are preserved, if possible, but branches to the lingula are clipped or cauterized.

5 The thin anterior portion of the lingula is frequently divided from the anterior segment of the upper lobe along the line of demarcation with a linear cutting stapler to avoid tearing part of the upper lobe. As the dissection proceeds anteriorly, the lingular branches of the superior pulmonary vein become apparent and are ligated and divided if not done previously.

The remaining left lung is inflated under warm saline. Any major air leaks are closed with purse-string or figure-of-eight 3-0 absorbable sutures. Two chest tubes are left in the hemithorax for evacuation of air and fluid before the chest is closed.

APICAL SEGMENTAL RESECTION

The apical segment of the left upper lobe is sometimes resected for apical blebs in patients with recurrent pneumothorax. The chest is entered through a lateral thoracotomy incision after removal of a segment of the fourth or fifth rib.

6 The lung is retracted inferiorly and the mediastinal pleura over the anterior and cephalad portion of the hilum is incised. The upper lobe branches of the left main pulmonary artery are dissected out. The most anterior branch of the apical-posterior segmental branch of the left pulmonary artery is doubly ligated and divided. Following this, the most superior branch of the left superior pulmonary vein is identified as the lung is retracted posteriorly. The vein is dissected out, ligated, and divided.

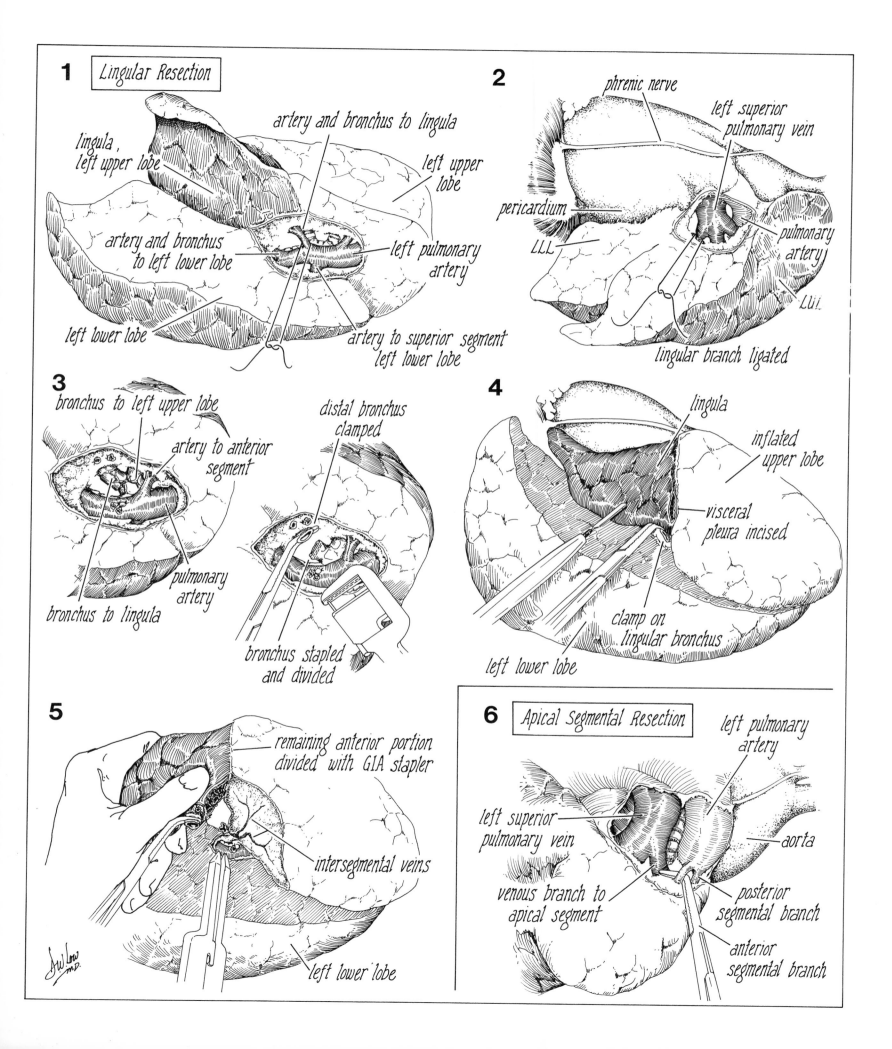

1 Lingular Resection

lingula, left upper lobe

artery and bronchus to lingula

left upper lobe

artery and bronchus to left lower lobe

left pulmonary artery

left lower lobe

artery to superior segment left lower lobe

2

phrenic nerve

left superior pulmonary vein

pericardium

LLL

pulmonary artery

LUL

lingular branch ligated

3

bronchus to left upper lobe

artery to anterior segment

pulmonary artery

bronchus to lingula

distal bronchus clamped

bronchus stapled and divided

4

lingula

inflated upper lobe

visceral pleura incised

clamp on lingular bronchus

left lower lobe

5

remaining anterior portion divided with GIA stapler

intersegmental veins

left lower lobe

6 Apical Segmental Resection

left pulmonary artery

left superior pulmonary vein

aorta

venous branch to apical segment

posterior segmental branch

anterior segmental branch

⑦ The apex of the lung is retracted inferiorly and slightly posteriorly. The lung is allowed to deflate until the apical bronchus is divided. The bronchus to the apical segment is identified adjacent to the inferior surface of the left main pulmonary artery as the most anterior branch of the left upper lobe bronchus. The bronchus is dissected free and either stapled closed or divided and sutured closed with interrupted 3-0 nonabsorbable sutures. The distal bronchus is clamped to apply traction during removal of the segment.

⑧ The lung parenchyma is separated from the anterior and posterior segments using traction and finger compression as described earlier. The cautery is used to incise the visceral pleura along the line of demarcation as established by inflating the left lung after the apical bronchus is divided.

Resection of the apical segment of right or left lung removes a wedge-shaped piece of lung. Small venous bleeders are cauterized. Usually air leaks are small and inconsequential.

SUPERIOR SEGMENTAL RESECTION

The superior segment of the right lower lobe is sometimes destroyed by aspiration pneumonia, tuberculosis, or another chronic inflammatory process. It also may be involved in a malignant or inflammatory process that involves the upper lobe (but spares the middle lobe). The upper lobe and superior segment of the lower lobe are often removed together, but in such circumstances, the middle lobe is not included to avoid space problems when only the basilar segments of the lower lobe remain.

⑨ After right lateral thoracotomy (fifth rib), the major fissure is entered and the pulmonary artery is dissected out.

The posterior branch to the posterior segment of the upper lobe, the branch to the superior segment of the lower lobe, and the branches to the remaining segments of the lower lobe are identified. Sometimes two branches to the superior segment arise from the posterior surface of the pulmonary artery in the major fissure. The superior segmental branch is doubly ligated and divided.

⑩ The lung is retracted anteriorly and the mediastinal pleura over the inferior pulmonary vein and right main bronchus is incised. The vein is dissected out to major branches and the most superior branch is encircled with a ligature, but not tied. The superior segmental bronchus is dissected out and positively identified.

⑪ The major fissure, which is seldom complete posteriorly, is divided with a linear cutting stapler to separate upper and lower lobes. (This is not done, of course, if the superior segment is being resected in continuity with a right upper lobectomy). The superior segmental bronchus is cleared, stapled closed, and divided. If identified correctly, the encircled pulmonary vein to the superior segment is tied and divided.

⑫ Using differential lung inflation as a guide, the visceral pleura along the line of demarcation is incised with a cautery. As traction is applied to the bronchus and with rolling-finger compression along the line of demarcation, the segment is gently separated from the adjacent lower lobe segments from posterior to anterior. Cautery is used for small bleeding vessels and an attempt is made to preserve the intersegmental vein on the surface of the retained segments.

The expanded lung is inspected for air leaks. Two chest tubes for air and fluid are left.

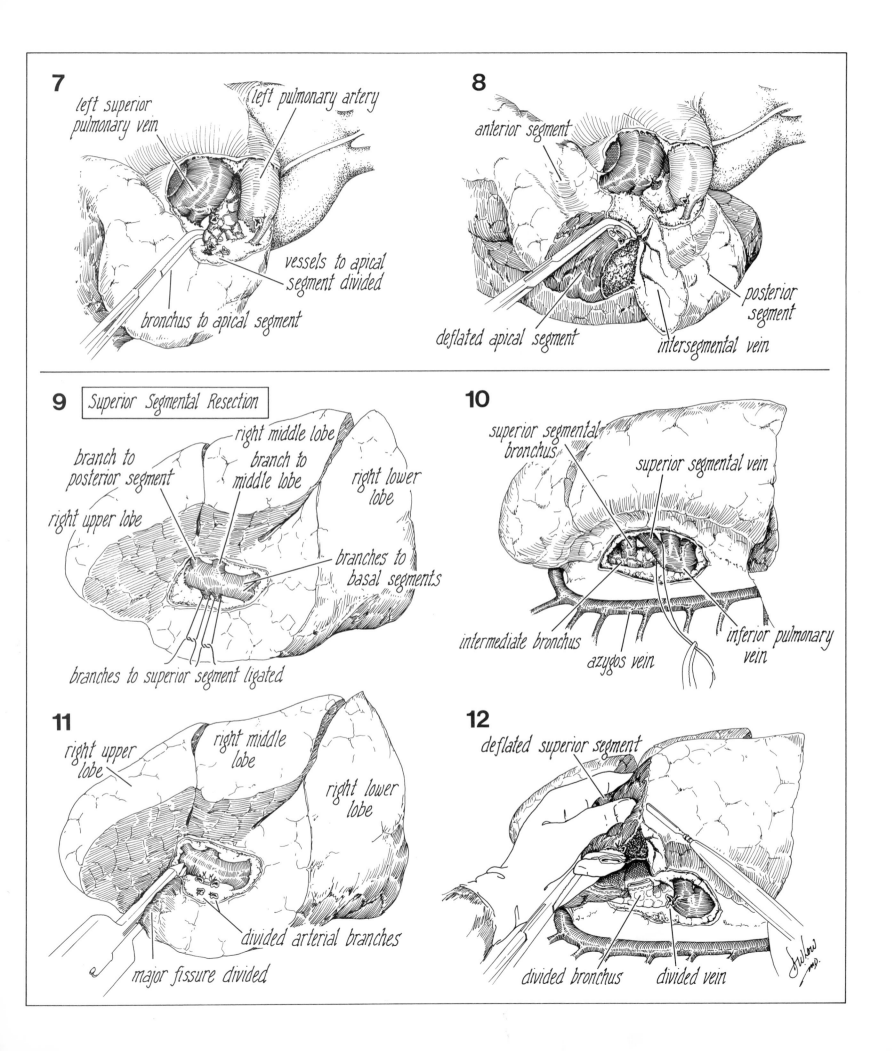

7

left superior pulmonary vein

left pulmonary artery

vessels to apical segment divided

bronchus to apical segment

8

anterior segment

posterior segment

deflated apical segment

intersegmental vein

9 | Superior Segmental Resection |

right middle lobe

branch to posterior segment

branch to middle lobe

right lower lobe

right upper lobe

branches to basal segments

branches to superior segment ligated

10

superior segmental bronchus

superior segmental vein

intermediate bronchus

azygos vein

inferior pulmonary vein

11

right upper lobe

right middle lobe

right lower lobe

divided arterial branches

major fissure divided

12

deflated superior segment

divided bronchus

divided vein

Bronchoplastic Procedures and Sleeve Resections

Bronchoplastic procedures are designed to conserve functioning lungs after traumatic tears or amputation of a bronchus, or after excision of benign or malignant endobronchial tumors. Bronchial anastomoses are required after sleeve resections of lobes or segments. The use of a Robertshaw tube to collapse the ipsilateral lung facilitates these operations.

REPAIR OF LACERATION

1 Lacerations and traumatic amputations are repaired with interrupted monofilament sutures. A minimal amount of parenchyma and soft tissue should be dissected away around the tear to preserve the blood supply to the bronchus. Usually lacerated edges do not require debridement; occasionally ragged edges need to be conservatively trimmed. Sutures are placed 2 to 3 mm from the torn edges and 2 to 3 mm apart. After repair, the lung is reinflated and the suture line checked for air leaks. A flap of pleura may be raised to cover the suture line.

EXCISION OF ENDOBRONCHIAL LESION, LEFT MAIN BRONCHUS

2 The lung is usually retracted anteriorly for excision of endobronchial lesions. Soft tissue, lung parenchyma, and nodes, overlying the bronchial segment to be excised, are dissected away to and only slightly beyond the prospective bronchial incisions. It is important for healing to preserve the blood supply on either side of the bronchial anastomoses.

3 Bronchial incisions are made approximately 270° around the circumference of the bronchus above and below the segment to be removed. The first monofilament suture is placed 2 to 3 mm from the edges of the incisions before the circumferential bronchial incisions are complete. This suture, which is not tied, ensures proper alignment of the divided bronchi.

4 The anastomosis is made with multiple, interrupted 3 or 4-0 monofilament nonabsorbable sutures inserted 2 mm from the cut ends of the bronchi. Simple sutures, 2 to 3 mm apart, are placed in the bronchial walls away from the operator in the cartilagenous bronchi first. Sutures pass from outside in, so that knots lie outside the bronchus. Each suture passes through the full thickness of the bronchial wall, including both the muscular or cartilaginous layer and the bronchial epithelium.

5 After placement of sutures approximately 200 degrees around the bronchial circumference, bronchial ends are approximated, and all sutures are tied. The remaining sutures are placed through all layers of the bronchial wall in the membranous portion to complete the anastomosis.

6 Small discrepancies in diameters of the two bronchi can be adjusted by differential spacing of sutures in the membranous bronchi.

7 Larger discrepancies can be managed by a 2 to 5 mm incision in the membranous portion of the smaller bronchus. It is imperative that minimal tension exist at the anastomotic suture line. Tension must be relieved by lifting adjacent structures off the bronchi without injury to bronchial vessels.

8 After the anastomosis is tested for air leaks under saline, a pleural or pericardial flap is usually placed over the bronchial suture line adjacent to a pulmonary artery to protect against erosion or injury to the artery.

SLEEVE RESECTION, RIGHT UPPER LOBE

9 Sleeve resection of the right upper lobe involves dividing the right main bronchus and intermediate bronchus on either side of the right upper lobe bronchus after the lobe is completely isolated from the remaining lung. Exposure is best obtained by retracting the upper lobe anteriorly and inferiorly. Often the intermediate bronchus must be incised to match the circumference of the right main bronchus.

SLEEVE RESECTION, LEFT UPPER LOBE

10 Sleeve resection of the left upper lobe bronchus is similarly performed. The left upper lobe is retracted anteriorly and inferiorly to expose the upper lobe bronchus anterior to the left pulmonary artery. The left main pulmonary artery must be lifted off the bronchus superiorly and posteriorly after the apical and posterior branches are divided. Traction tapes around the left main and left lower lobe bronchi aid exposure.

SLEEVE RESECTION, LEFT LOWER LOBE

11 Sleeve resection of a lower lobe bronchus is less commonly performed and is usually used to extend the proximal resection margin of a high lower lobar endobronchial tumor. The bronchus is exposed by retracting the entire lung anteriorly and completely dividing the major fissure. Tapes passed around the right or left main bronchus at the origin of the upper lobe aid exposure. The pulmonary artery must be dissected free and lifted anteriorly to obtain proper exposure of the origin of the upper lobe bronchus. Usually the upper lobe bronchus is transected at its origin from the left main bronchus. The left main bronchus is transected above the tumor.

12 An end-to-end bronchial anastomosis is performed, but because of the near right angle between upper lobe and left main bronchus, the left upper lobe bronchus is beveled, and a small wedge is removed from the anterior-superior border of the left main bronchus (the wedge is removed from the cartilagenous portion of the bronchus). With downward displacement of the upper lobe (because of removal of the lower lobe), the resulting bronchial anastomosis is well aligned and without tension.

Sleeve resection of the right lower lobe is seldom necessary because the combination of right lower and middle lobectomy raises the bronchial resection margin to the origin of the upper lobe bronchus.

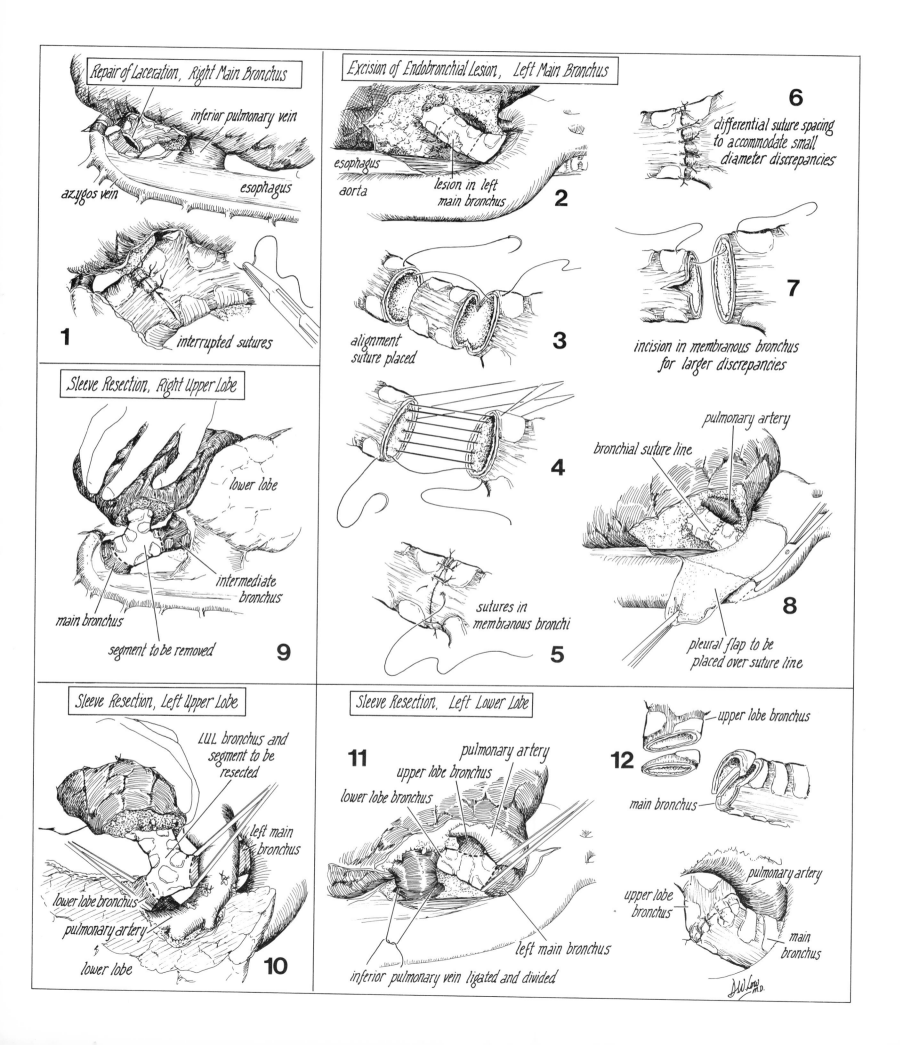

Repair of Laceration, Right Main Bronchus

1 — inferior pulmonary vein; azygos vein; esophagus; interrupted sutures

Excision of Endobronchial Lesion, Left Main Bronchus

2 — esophagus; aorta; lesion in left main bronchus

3 — alignment suture placed

4

5 — sutures in membranous bronchi

6 — differential suture spacing to accommodate small diameter discrepancies

7 — incision in membranous bronchus for larger discrepancies

8 — pulmonary artery; bronchial suture line; pleural flap to be placed over suture line

Sleeve Resection, Right Upper Lobe

9 — lower lobe; intermediate bronchus; main bronchus; segment to be removed

Sleeve Resection, Left Upper Lobe

10 — LUL bronchus and segment to be resected; left main bronchus; lower lobe bronchus; pulmonary artery; lower lobe

Sleeve Resection, Left Lower Lobe

11 — pulmonary artery; upper lobe bronchus; lower lobe bronchus; left main bronchus; inferior pulmonary vein ligated and divided

12 — upper lobe bronchus; main bronchus; upper lobe bronchus; pulmonary artery; main bronchus

D.W. Low M.D.

Pancoast Tumor

The combination of preoperative radiation and subsequent resection of the upper lobe and contiguous chest wall may be prescribed for Pancoast tumors that lack distant metastases, do not invade vertebral bodies or the mediastinum, and do not extensively involve the brachial plexus or subclavian artery. Operation is performed 3 to 4 weeks after completion of radiation therapy and after the extent and location of the tumor are reassessed to determine the wisdom and feasibility of resection.

The patient is anesthetized, intubated, and rebronchoscoped to confirm the absence of endobronchial disease near the proposed resection margin. The endotracheal tube is replaced with a tracheal divider (Robertshaw tube) and the patient placed in the straight lateral position. A right upper lobectomy is illustrated.

The lower neck, entire shoulder, upper arm, chest, and upper abdomen are prepped. The skin is prepped beyond the midline anteriorly and posteriorly.

(1) The incision begins midway between the vertebral spine and medial border of the right scapula at approximately T2 (spine of scapula) and proceeds inferiorly and anteriorly around the tip of the scapula to the anterior axillary line. The trapezius and rhomboid muscles are divided posteriorly, the latissimus laterally, and the serratus anterior anteriorly.

(2) The upper rib insertions of the serratus are divided to permit the entire scapula to be elevated superiorly and anteriorly. This exposes the upper ribs and later permits exposure of the brachial plexus and subclavian vessels. Much of the dissection may be done with electrocautery.

(3) The chest is entered anteriorly, usually in the third intercostal space. Adhesions between lung and chest wall are divided except where the tumor mass adheres and possibly invades the chest wall at the apex of the hemithorax. The presence or absence of tumor involvement of hilar and mediastinal nodes is also determined at this time.

(4) Assuming that the lesion appears resectable, the anterior third and second ribs and intervening intercostal muscles are divided well away from the tumor attachment. The anterior portion of the first rib is exposed by dividing the insertion of the scalenus anterior, anterior to the brachial plexus and scalenus medius and posterior to the plexus.

(5) The subclavian vein and artery and inferior trunk of the brachial plexus are visible in the fat and areolar tissue superior to the first rib. The ligamentous attachment of the first rib and head of the clavicle is divided and the anterior portion of the first rib is disarticulated from the sternum and clavicular head. The subclavian vein and artery are dissected away from the first rib. Before the brachial plexus is transected or dissected free, the posterior attachments of the upper three ribs are divided.

(6) The sacrospinalis muscle is divided in the direction of its fibers to expose the junction of the vertebral spinous process and the transverse process of the first three ribs.

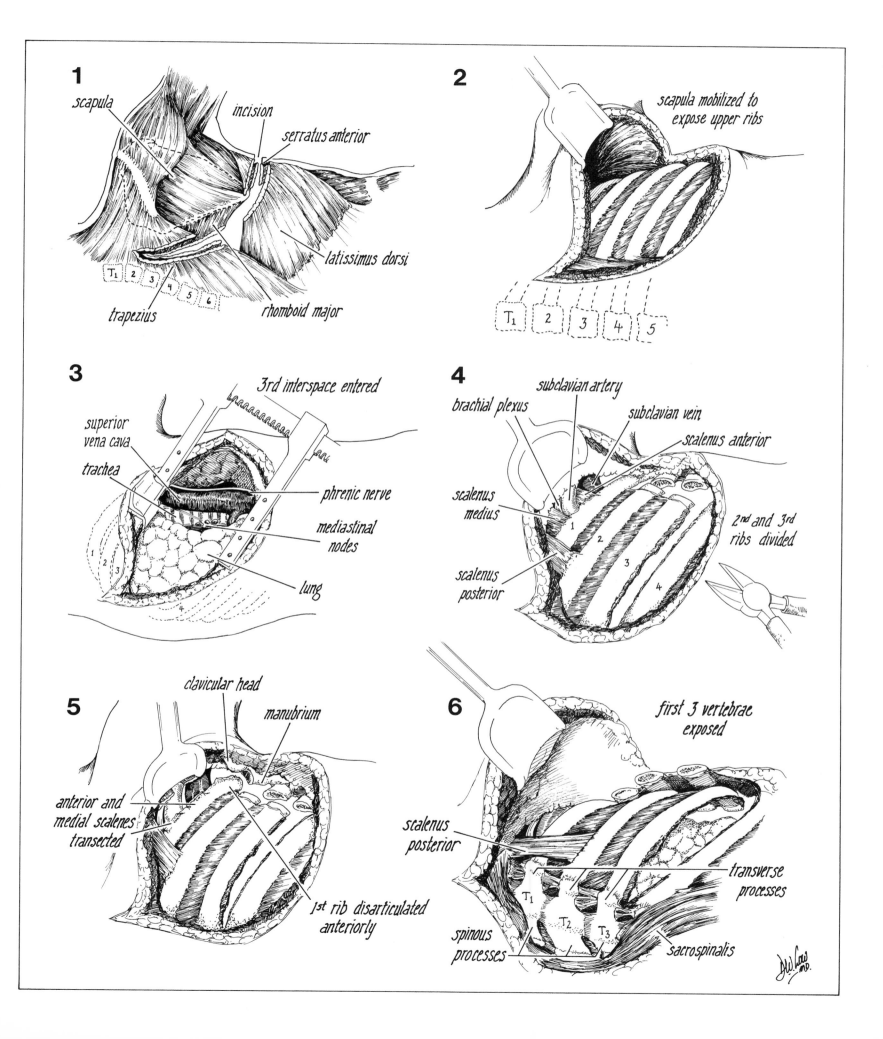

1
scapula
incision
serratus anterior
latissimus dorsi
trapezius
rhomboid major
T₁ 2 3 4 5 6

2
scapula mobilized to expose upper ribs
T₁ 2 3 4 5

3
3rd interspace entered
superior vena cava
trachea
phrenic nerve
mediastinal nodes
lung

4
subclavian artery
brachial plexus
subclavian vein
scalenus anterior
scalenus medius
scalenus posterior
2nd and 3rd ribs divided

5
clavicular head
manubrium
anterior and medial scalenes transected
1st rib disarticulated anteriorly

6
first 3 vertebrae exposed
scalenus posterior
transverse processes
spinous processes
sacrospinalis
T₁ T₂ T₃

7 If the tumor mass involves the junction between vertebral bodies and transverse processes, as it often does, the transverse process of the third thoracic vertebra is chiseled through at its junction with the vertebral body. A portion of the lateral vertebral body may also be removed to obtain a border around the tumor mass. If a portion of the vertebral body is not taken, the articulation with the rib is divided to completely separate rib and transverse body from the vertebrae.

8 Intercostal vessels and nerves are clipped and divided as exposed. The sympathetic chain and superior tributary of the azygos vein are also clipped and divided as the dissection moves superiorly along the lateral portion of the upper three thoracic vertebral bodies. Any margins suspected of tumor are examined by frozen section and recut, if possible, if tumor is encountered.

9 The first thoracic nerve, which contributes to the medial cord of the brachial plexus, is usually divided in this dissection. The eighth cervical nerve, which contributes to both the median and posterior cords of the plexus, can often be spared. The surgeon can now decide whether or not all tumor can be removed before deciding to preserve or divide the median cord of the brachial plexus.

10 The median cord of the brachial plexus is either cut or dissected away from the adherent fibrous tissue and first rib. The attachment of the scalenus posterior muscle to the rib is divided. This frees the right upper lobe and contiguous chest wall from all surrounding structures.

11 A right upper lobectomy is then performed in standard fashion. Usually it is not necessary to remove the middle lobe, but the paratracheal, subcarinal, hilar, and regional lymph nodes should be removed with the specimen (radical lobectomy). The pulmonary ligament is divided to permit movement of the right lower lobe upward.

12 After placement of two chest tubes, the incision is closed by suturing the scapula to the edges of the chest wall defect with interrupted absorbable sutures. Posteriorly, the divided rhomboid muscles are sutured together and to the sacrospinalis. Anteriorly, the serratus anterior is sutured to the anterior portions of the divided second and third ribs and to intercostal muscles at points where the insertions of the serratus were divided inferiorly. The serratus attached to the scapula is sutured to the fourth intercostal muscles to effect airtight closure of the chest. The remaining muscle layers, subcutaneous tissues, and skin are closed with running sutures.

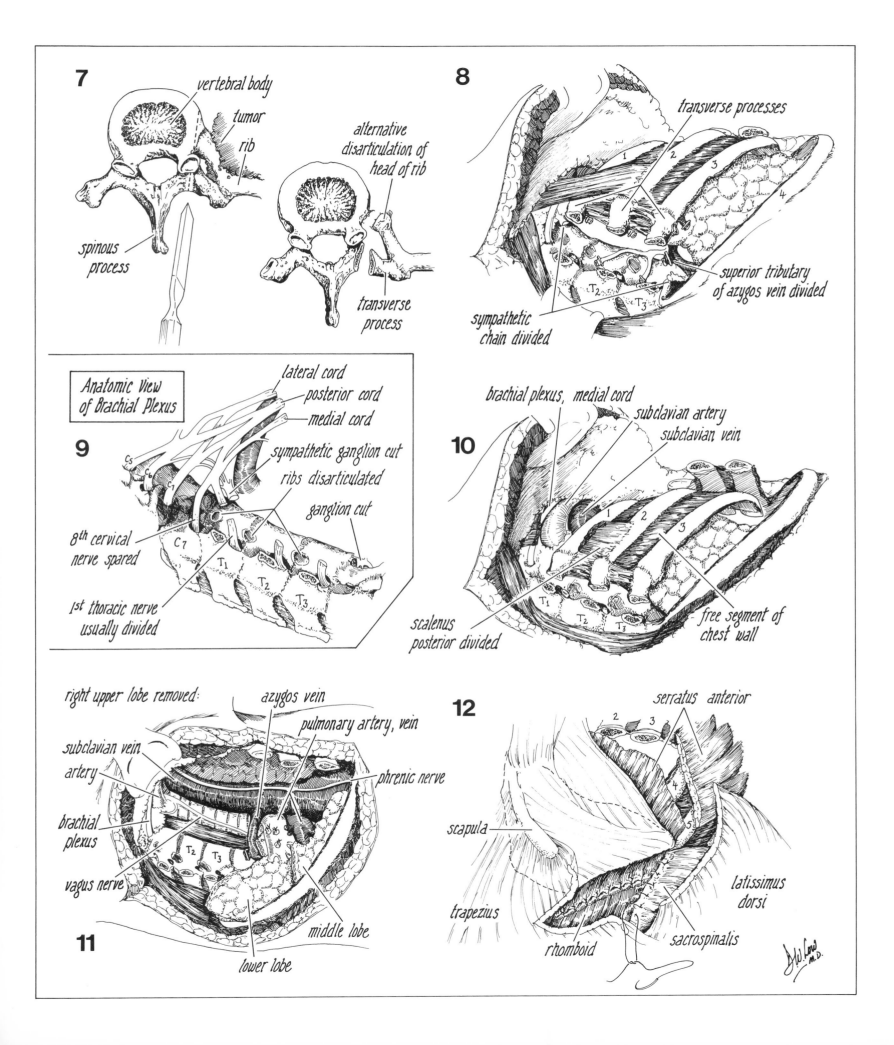

7

vertebral body

tumor

rib

spinous process

alternative disarticulation of head of rib

transverse process

8

transverse processes

superior tributary of azygos vein divided

sympathetic chain divided

T₂

T₃

Anatomic View of Brachial Plexus

9

lateral cord

posterior cord

medial cord

sympathetic ganglion cut

ribs disarticulated

ganglion cut

C₅

C₆

C₇

8th cervical nerve spared

1st thoracic nerve usually divided

C₇

T₁

T₂

T₃

10

brachial plexus, medial cord

subclavian artery

subclavian vein

scalenus posterior divided

free segment of chest wall

T₁

T₂

T₃

11

right upper lobe removed:

azygos vein

pulmonary artery, vein

subclavian vein artery

phrenic nerve

brachial plexus

vagus nerve

T₂

T₃

middle lobe

lower lobe

12

serratus anterior

scapula

trapezius

rhomboid

sacrospinalis

latissimus dorsi

Apical Blebs and Bullae

Spontaneous pneumothorax is often caused by rupture of blebs in the apical segments of either lung. Although recurrent spontaneous pneumothorax is usually treated by tube thoracostomy and tetracycline pleurodesis, an unusual patient may require thoracotomy and plication or resection of ruptured apical blebs.

APICAL BLEBS

1 With the patient in position for a lateral thoracotomy, the chest is entered by resecting a segment of the fourth rib between the pectoralis major anteriorly and latissimus posteriorly. These muscles are retracted and not cut, or if necessary, only the edges of the muscles are incised.

2 After the chest is entered, the lung apex is brought into the wound.

3 The emphysematous blebs in the apical segment are incised if necessary and oversewn with a single purse-string suture started deep to the surface of the lung in the emphysematous alveoli. The suture passes through relatively normal adjacent lung, and when drawn up, plicates the emphysematous tissue and obliterates the blebs both within and on the surface of the lung.

4 The operation is completed by firmly rubbing the parietal pleura of the apical portion of the hemithorax with a dry sponge or by painting this area with a solution of 500 grams of tetracycline in 50 ml of saline. The chest is closed with a single No. 28 Fr chest tube placed up to the apex of the chest to ensure apposition of the lung and apical parietal pleura.

GIANT BULLAE

Occasionally, in carefully selected patients, removal of one or more giant bullae may be indicated to allow expansion of adjacent compressed lung. Usually these patients have a deficiency of alpha-1-antitrypsin, and the disease may be bilateral. The operation is designed to preserve as much functional lung as possible and to create more space for compressed lung. The operation may be done through a midline sternotomy incision to resect bilateral bullae.

5 The hemithorax is entered by means of a full lateral thoracotomy with resection of the fifth rib. If a tracheal divider is used, the ipsilateral lung is allowed to collapse. Bullae collapse slowly, if at all, and the largest ones are easily identified.

6 The visceral pleura over the bullae is incised to enter the honeycombed interior of the bulla.

7 The edges of the visceral pleura are preserved and retracted to permit plication of the interior.

8 The honeycombed interior walls are approximated, using one or two continuous 3-0 absorbable sutures (large, thin curved needle). A purse-string suture is started in the depths of the bulla and continued in concentric fashion toward the visceral pleura. Suture bites are deep enough to hold in the honeycombed wall, but are not so deep as to occlude adjacent vessels and airways.

9 After tying the plication suture(s), the edges of the redundant visceral pleura are twisted together and then ligated to prevent escape of air.

Other large bullae are treated similarly. Thereafter, the lung is gently re-expanded and any major air leaks are controlled by ligation or suture. At least two large bore chest tubes are placed and intercostal nerves are injected with a long-acting local anesthetic before the chest is closed.

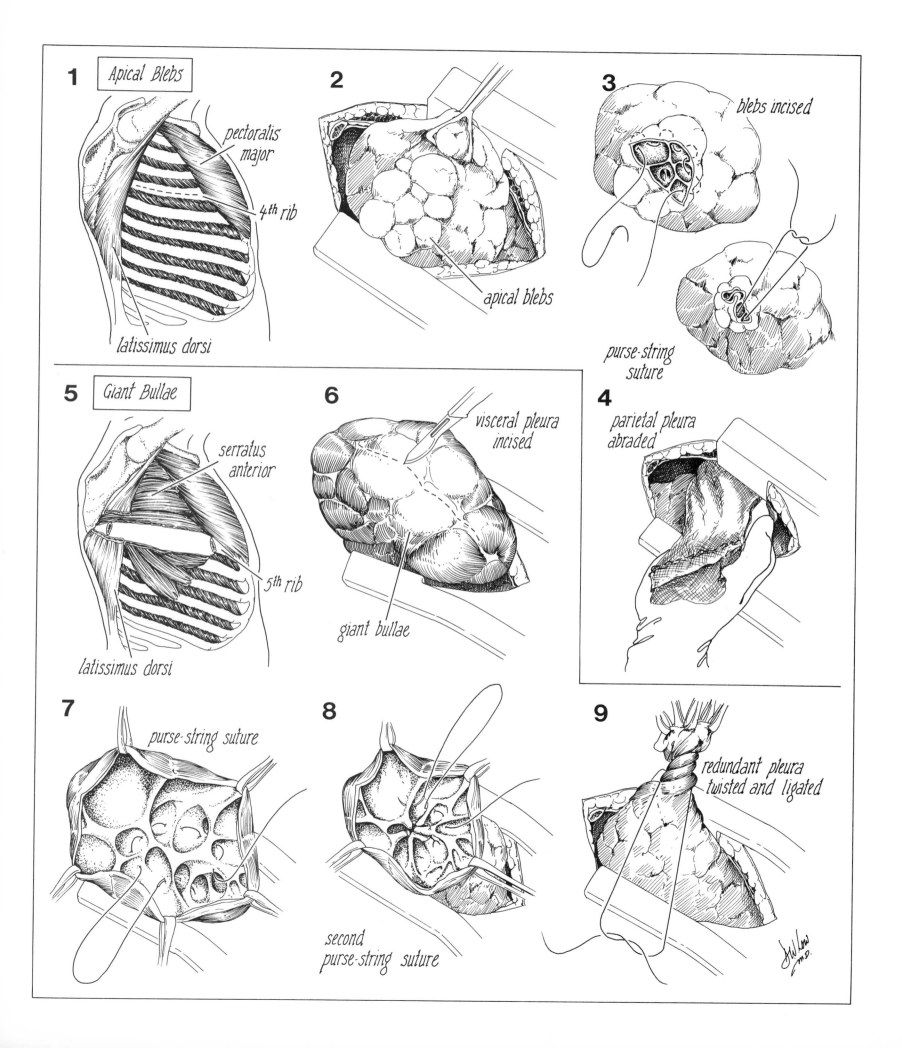

1 Apical Blebs

pectoralis major

4th rib

latissimus dorsi

2 apical blebs

3 blebs incised

purse-string suture

4 parietal pleura abraded

5 Giant Bullae

serratus anterior

5th rib

latissimus dorsi

6 visceral pleura incised

giant bullae

7 purse-string suture

8 second purse-string suture

9 redundant pleura twisted and ligated

Intralobar Sequestration

Intralobar sequestration describes a congenital abnormality wherein systemic arteries supply a portion of the lung. This uncommon condition usually involves a lower lobe on either the right or left side. Airways and pulmonary veins are normal; pulmonary arteries are absent to the portion of the lobe supplied by one or more systemic arteries. Preoperative angiography identifies the number and location of the anomalous systemic vessels that generally arise from the aorta, are large, and may penetrate the diaphragm.

Intralobar sequestration is more common than extralobar sequestration. Extralobar sequestrations are invested with pleura, have both systemic arterial and venous blood supply, and do not have a connection to the bronchial tree. Excision of a left intralobar sequestration is illustrated and described.

(1) The lung is exposed through a lateral or posterolateral thoracotomy incision. The involved lobe is generally inflamed and edematous with enlarged edematous regional lymph nodes. Although the sequestration usually involves the more medial segments of the lower lobe, because of inflammation and difficulty in identifying details of the segmental anatomy, a lobectomy is performed.

(2) On the left, the collapsed lung is retracted anteriorly. The thickened mediastinal pleura over the descending thoracic aorta is incised so that the anomalous systemic vessels can be dissected out and identified. The dissection is extended cautiously to the adjacent diaphragm if one or more of the anomalous vessels penetrate the diaphragm. Anomalous arteries are doubly ligated and divided and oversewn if necessary.

(3) When all of the systemic vessels to the intralobar sequestration are located and divided, the major fissure is entered to locate and divide the branches of the pulmonary artery that supply the nonsequestrated portions of the lobe. When these are ligated and divided, the operation proceeds as for a standard lobectomy because the pulmonary veins and bronchi are normal.

(4) For a right intralobar sequestration, the mediastinal pleura behind the heart lateral to the inferior cava and right atrium is incised and dissected to expose the anomalous arteries anterior to the esophagus. As on the left, one or more anomalous vessels may penetrate the diaphragm. The anomalous vessels are ligated and divided and the sequestrated lobe is excised.

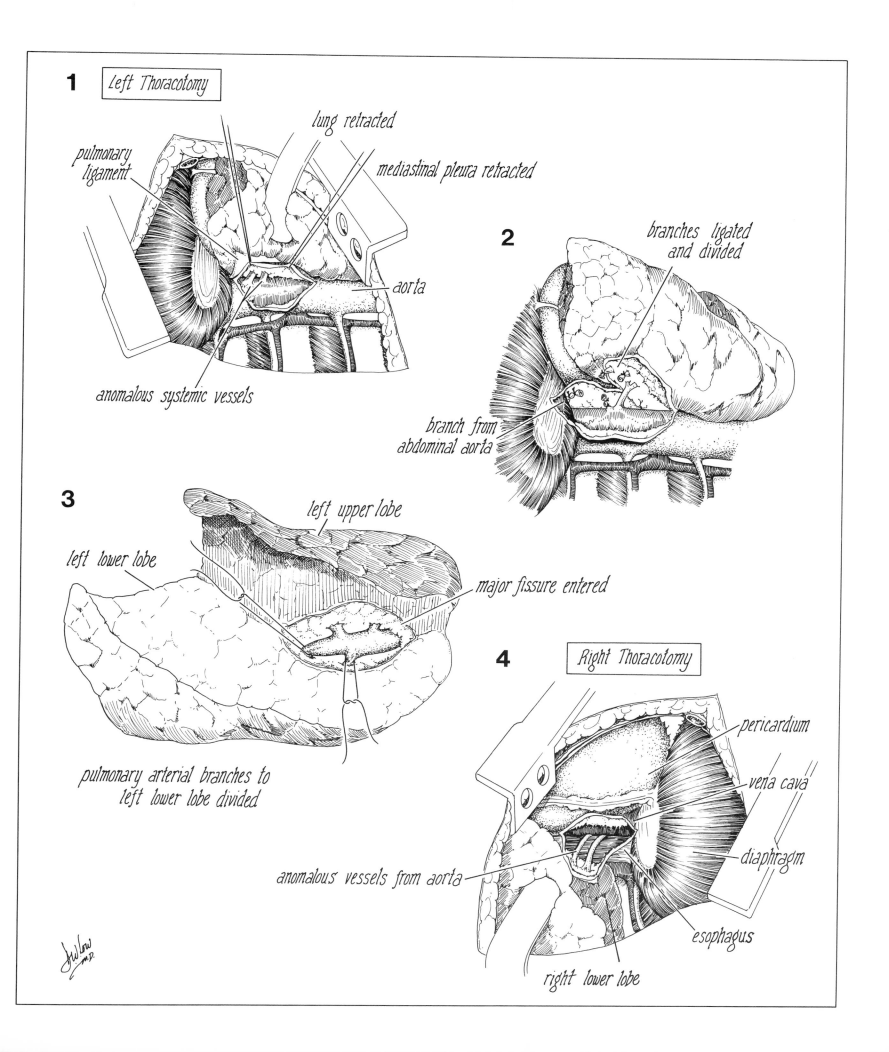

1 Left Thoracotomy

pulmonary ligament

lung retracted

mediastinal pleura retracted

aorta

anomalous systemic vessels

2

branches ligated and divided

branch from abdominal aorta

3

left upper lobe

left lower lobe

major fissure entered

pulmonary arterial branches to left lower lobe divided

4 Right Thoracotomy

pericardium

vena cava

diaphragm

anomalous vessels from aorta

esophagus

right lower lobe

Resection of the Trachea and Carina

Although the adult trachea is only 11 cm long, nearly half of it can be resected by techniques developed over the past two decades. Resection is required primarily for strictures secondary to prolonged endotracheal intubation or tracheostomy and for primary tumors. Lesions of the upper half of the trachea are approached through the neck; those in the lower half or carina are exposed through a posterolateral thoracotomy with resection of the fourth rib. Occasionally a partial sternal splitting incision is used to gain additional exposure of the upper trachea in the region of the innominate artery. A combination of cervical, sternal splitting and right anterolateral incisions exposes the entire trachea, but is seldom needed.

Resection of a benign stricture of the upper trachea and resection of an adenoid cystic carcinoma of the lower trachea are illustrated.

(1) The patient is placed supine on the table with a thin roll under the shoulders. Inhalation anesthesia is carefully induced; then a fiberoptic bronchoscope is passed through the nose to inspect the upper airway proximal to the stricture. If the stricture is less than 5 mm in diameter, a pediatric bronchoscope is used to gently dilate the stricture. The endotracheal tube is inserted down to but not against or through the narrowed area.

The entire neck, chin, and upper chest are prepped and draped into the field. A cervical collar incision is made midway between the laryngeal prominence and sternal notch. The platysma is elevated with skin flaps. The sternohyoid and sternothyroid muscles are retracted laterally, the anterior jugular vein is ligated and divided, and the isthmus of the thyroid is divided.

(2) If exposure is limited, a vertical incision is made in the midline from the collar incision to the midsternum. The sternum is partially transected with a saw, enough to allow placement of a Child retractor. This exposes the thoracic inlet, innominate artery and vein, and midtrachea.

(3) The strictured segment of trachea is dissected out with great care to stay on the surface of the tracheal wall. If the dissection is against the tracheal wall, recurrent laryngeal nerves are protected without being identified. The dissection isolates the strictured segment and no more than 1.5 cm of trachea above and below the planned lines of resection. The trachea is separated from the esophagus posteriorly for a much greater distance, but because blood vessels enter laterally, the circumferential dissection is limited to 1.5 cm from the cut ends of the airway. A sterile endotracheal tube is made available for insertion into the distal trachea after the trachea is incised.

(4) The lower incision is made first at the lowest part of the stricture. Before this incision is made, two 0 gauge nonabsorbable traction sutures are placed firmly into the trachea below the line of incision for traction. The trachea is transected. The lower segment is inspected from inside and an additional segment is resected to reach healthy, unscarred airway. The sterile endotracheal tube is inserted into the lower trachea to resume ventilation. The distal trachea is separated from the esophagus posteriorly but is not dissected from lateral attachments.

(5) A similar incision is made into the trachea at the upper border of the strictured segment. Again additional trachea is resected until healthy, unscarred tissue is reached. Traction sutures are also placed in the upper tracheal segment.

The amount of trachea that can be resected without additional procedures varies with age. In young adults, cervical flexion alone may allow closure of a 4 to 4.5 cm gap without undue (<1000 grams) tension on the suture line. In older individuals with limited cervical flexion and a less elastic airway, only 2 to 2.5 cm may be resected. The neck is now propped in a flexed position and the traction sutures are used to approximate the two ends of the trachea.

SUPRAHYOID RELEASE

(6) If one to two additional centimeters are needed, Grillo recommends the suprahyoid laryngeal release procedure devised by Montgomery. This operation is less likely to injure the superior laryngeal nerve and cause temporary swallowing dysfunction than the infrahyoid release operation devised by Ogura and described by Dedo and Fishman.

The cervical incision must be extended laterally upward to reflect the skin and platysma upward beyond the laryngeal prominence and hyoid bone. This exposes the mylohyoid muscle, the anterior belly of the digastric muscles, and the ligamentous sling that attaches the digastric muscle to the lateral hyoid bone.

(7) The midline muscles attached to the hyoid bone between the two digastric slings are incised carefully using magnification loops. First the mylohyoid, which is thin, then the geniohyoid muscle, which is thick, are separated from the hyoid bone. The deepest muscle attachment is the geniohyoid, which has only a thin attachment to the hyoid bone. This incision exposes the preepiglottic space and genioglossus.

(8) The body of the hyoid bone is cut just medial to the digastric sling and the insertion of the tiny chondroglossus muscle and medial to the lesser and greater cornu of the hyoid bone. Division of the bone causes the unopposed pull of the sternohyoid, thyrohyoid, and omohyoid muscles to pull the body of the hyoid bone downward. The larynx and upper trachea also descend.

INFRAHYOID RELEASE

(9) Infrahyoid release requires division of attachments between the hyoid bone and thyroid cartilage and division of the superior cornua of the thyroid cartilage. The cervical collar incision is extended superiorly on each side, enough to expose the hyoid bone when the platysma and skin flap are retracted upward. The attachments of the sternohyoid and omohyoid muscles to the inferior border of the hyoid bone are cut in the midline to expose the thyrohyoid muscle and superior cornu of the thyroid cartilage. With magnification, the attachment of the thyrohyoid muscle to the upper border of the body of the thyroid cartilage is incised at the superior border of the cartilage. Careful search is made for the internal (superior) laryngeal nerve, artery, and vein, which penetrate the thyrohyoid membrane laterally.

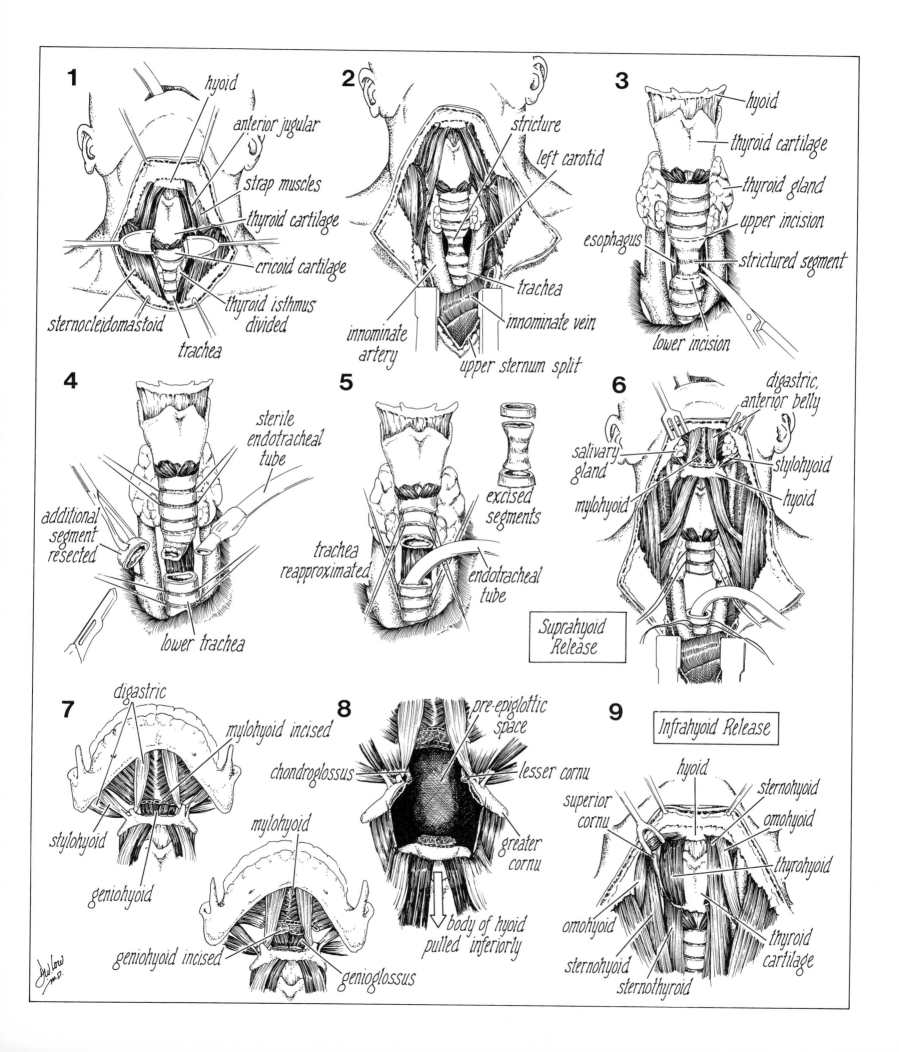

10 The superior cornu, which is close to the internal laryngeal nerve and beneath the incised thyrohyoid muscle, is divided with a scalpel or small powerful "nail" scissors. The thyrohyoid membrane is incised along the superior border of the body of the thyroid cartilage to expose the anterior attachments of the epiglottis to the hyoid bone and to release the body of the thyroid cartilage downward 2 to 2.5 cm.

11 Once the two ends of the divided trachea can be approximated without tension, absorbable (4-0) interrupted sutures are used. All of the posterior sutures are placed (outside in) approximately 3 mm from the cut edges of the trachea. These are divided and brought laterally. The field endotracheal tube is now replaced with one passed by the anesthesiologist from the larynx across the tracheal gap into the lower trachea. With the neck extended to facilitate exposure, the lateral and anterior interrupted sutures are placed. The head is now flexed to approximate the tracheal ends. The head is propped securely in the flexed position. The tracheal sutures are tied (knots outside) and cut. The anastomosis is tested under saline and a small Hemovac drain is left in the wound. The cervical strap muscles are tacked together over the anastomosis and trachea and the platysma muscle is reapproximated. The skin is closed with a subcuticular stitch.

12 A heavy (No. 1) monofilament, nonabsorbable stitch is then passed through the skin just under the mandible and through the skin just below the sternal notch to maintain the head in flexion for the first 7 postoperative days.

More recently developed techniques permit excision of the cricoid and inferior portion of the thyroid cartilage with direct anastomosis of the trachea tailored to fit the residual laryngeal cartilage.

RESECTION OF THE CARINA

13 Lesions of the lower trachea and carina are exposed through a right posterolateral thoracotomy. The chest is entered by excising the fourth rib. The trachea is mobilized by dissecting the lower trachea free from surrounding lymph nodes and the superior cava and aortic arch anteriorly, and from the esophagus posteriorly. Care is taken to preserve bronchial vessels in the region of the carina and main bronchi. The right hilum of the lung is dissected from the investing mediastinal pleura. The right pulmonary ligament is incised. If necessary, the pericardium is opened and the dissection is carried around the right pulmonary vein. This extensive mobilization of lower trachea and right lung generally permits a gap of 4 cm to be closed. With the patient in the lateral thoracotomy position with cervical flexion, an additional 2 to 3 cm of trachea can be removed (total approximately 6 cm).

14 The tumor arises from the trachea just above the carina. After mobilization, heavy traction sutures are placed in the walls of both the right and left main bronchi below the line

of resection. With a sterile long cuff endotracheal tube on the table, the right main bronchus below the tumor is transected. Immediately, the left main bronchus is also transected. The endotracheal tube is placed within the right main bronchus and ventilation is resumed. No attempt is made to clamp the left pulmonary artery because collapse of the left lung will reduce the right-to-left shunt and maintain an adequate paO_2.

15 After placing two traction sutures, the trachea is transected above the tumor and the tumor-bearing segment is removed. The specimen is inspected by frozen section microscopy to be sure that resection margins are free.

16 It is not always possible to reconstruct the carina by suturing the medial walls of the two major bronchi together. More often, the end of the trachea and the end of the left main bronchus are anastomosed with interrupted 4-0 nonabsorbable sutures. The discrepancy in diameter is managed by plicating the membranous trachea and slightly stretching the membranous portion of the left main bronchus. Occasionally the anterior surface of the first bronchial cartilaginous ring is cut to widen the bronchus slightly and improve the fit. Once the tracheal–left bronchus anastomosis is completed, the endotracheal tube is advanced into the left main bronchus from above and the left lung is re-expanded. The endotracheal tube is removed from the right lung.

17 With traction sutures, the right main bronchus is brought to the side of the trachea. Usually the bronchus is not beveled but is sutured directly end-to-side to the trachea 1 cm or more above the tracheal–left bronchial anastomosis.

At the selected site, a small vertical incision is made into the right side of the trachea. With sharp-pointed scissors, a round hole is made in the tracheal cartilage. The diameter of the hole should be approximately 90% of the diameter of the right main bronchus. The anastomosis is then made with interrupted 4-0 absorbable sutures. When it is completed, both suture lines should be tested under saline for air leaks and neither suture line should be under tension. Cervical neck flexion should be maintained throughout the remainder of the operation and for the first week postoperatively.

18 The anastomoses should be covered with a flap of pleura. This is raised laterally with the axis approximately 45 degrees from that of the trachea. The pleura is wrapped around the underside (posterior) surface of the anastomosis and tucked to itself and the trachea and bronchus. The chest is closed with two drainage tubes.

Grillo has developed a variety of individualized carinal lower tracheal reconstructions to accommodate specific situations. These include implantation of the left main bronchus into the bronchus intermedius of the right main bronchus or into the trachea above an end-to-end tracheal–right main bronchial anastomosis. The right main bronchus has also been implanted into the side of the left main bronchus.

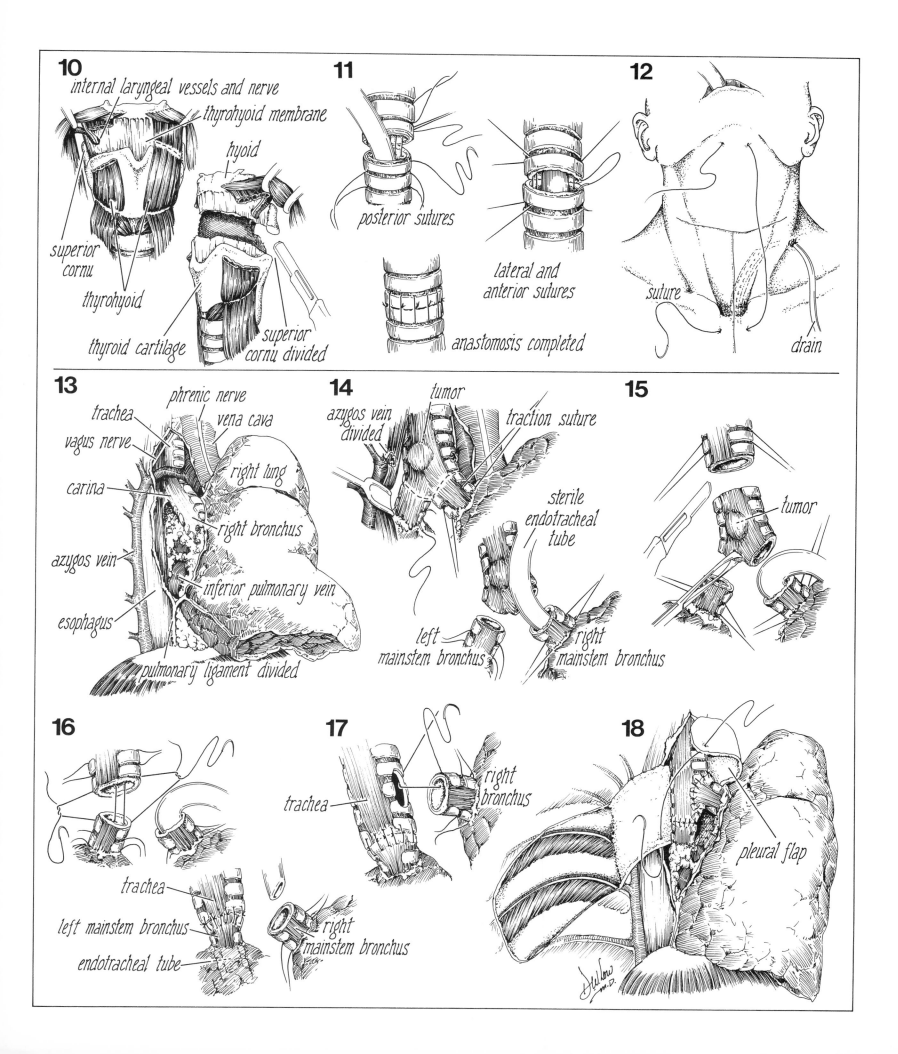

Decortication of the Lung

Decortication is prescribed for patients with unresolved hemothorax or empyema wherein the inflammatory process causes fibrous tissue to grow over the visceral pleura of the atelectatic or partially inflated lung. Usually a blood clot or infection occupies considerable space within the hemithorax. The underlying trapped lung must be able to re-expand to fill this space once the fibrous peel overlying the visceral pleura is removed. Whenever possible, early operation is recommended as soon as any pneumonia or consolidation of the trapped lung is resolved and before the fibrous peel organizes and becomes more difficult to remove.

1 The sagittal diagram illustrates the concept of the operation. The organizing blood clot or abscess develops a fibrous peel or envelope between the visceral pleura of the partially collapsed lung and parietal pleura overlying the chest wall diaphragm and mediastinum. The operation removes the envelope of blood or pus and allows the trapped lung to expand into the space created.

2 The patient is positioned for a lateral thoracotomy (right is illustrated); a divided endotracheal tube is recommended so that ventilation of the trapped lung can be separately managed. If a subacute or chronic empyema cavity is to be removed, several units of blood should be available. The thoracotomy incision is placed over the fourth through seventh ribs and anteriorly or posteriorly to center it over the pleural space mass. Usually a segment of rib is removed. The intercostal muscles are incised carefully in an effort to identify the plane between the parietal pleura and the adjacent fibrous peel.

3 If this plane is found, it may be developed in all directions and an attempt may be made to excise the fibrous envelope containing pus (empyema) in toto. Usually this is difficult, particularly over the diaphragm; thus the cavity is generally entered, cultured, and evacuated completely.

4 The parietal peel is usually separated from the chest wall first by blunt and sharp dissection. Bleeding and dissection are minimized if the exact plane between peel and pleura can be identified and separated. Small patches of peel in inaccessible areas need not be removed because they do not appreciably reduce chest wall respiratory motion.

5 Separation of the peel from the diaphragm is usually more difficult. The plane between fibrous peel and diaphragmatic muscle and central tendon is often indistinct and the recesses created by the diaphragmatic attachments to the chest wall are difficult to reach.

6 Separation of the peel from the visceral pleura and underlying lung must be done patiently. If the fibrin exudate is not organized or is only partially organized, the peel can be lifted off primarily by blunt dissection. Again the exact plane between visceral pleura, which is still shiny, and the peel must be found to prevent dissection into the underlying lung, which produces air leaks and bleeding. If the peel is more organized, a scalpel incision is made to find the plane of the visceral pleura. Several incisions may be required before a dissection in the proper plane can be started. Once the proper plane is found, the peel is painstakingly dissected off the underlying, somewhat shiny visceral pleura with knife and scissors, with careful attention to cauterization of small bleeding vessels.

7 The underlying lung expands progressively as the peel is dissected off. Control of the expansion and ventilation made possible by the tracheal divider is helpful. The peel is removed from the entire lateral surface of the lung, diaphragmatic surface, over the apex and down into the fissures. When the job is completed, the inflated lung should fill the entire hemithorax to prevent recurrence.

8 Major air leaks and incisions and tears of the lung parenchyma are oversewn with 3-0 absorbable figure-of-eight, purse-string or continuous sutures. Two or more chest tubes are placed so that the released lung can be kept fully expanded against the chest wall. The tubes must prevent reaccumulation of blood and serum and also removal of air, which invariably leaks from the released lung. Hemostasis must be thorough. If infection was present, the chest may be irrigated with saline or dilute povidone-iodine solution to reduce contamination. Recurrent infection is prevented by appropriate and specific systemic antibiotics and complete obliteration of the space between re-expanded lung and chest wall.

The chest (including the skin) is closed completely in the usual manner.

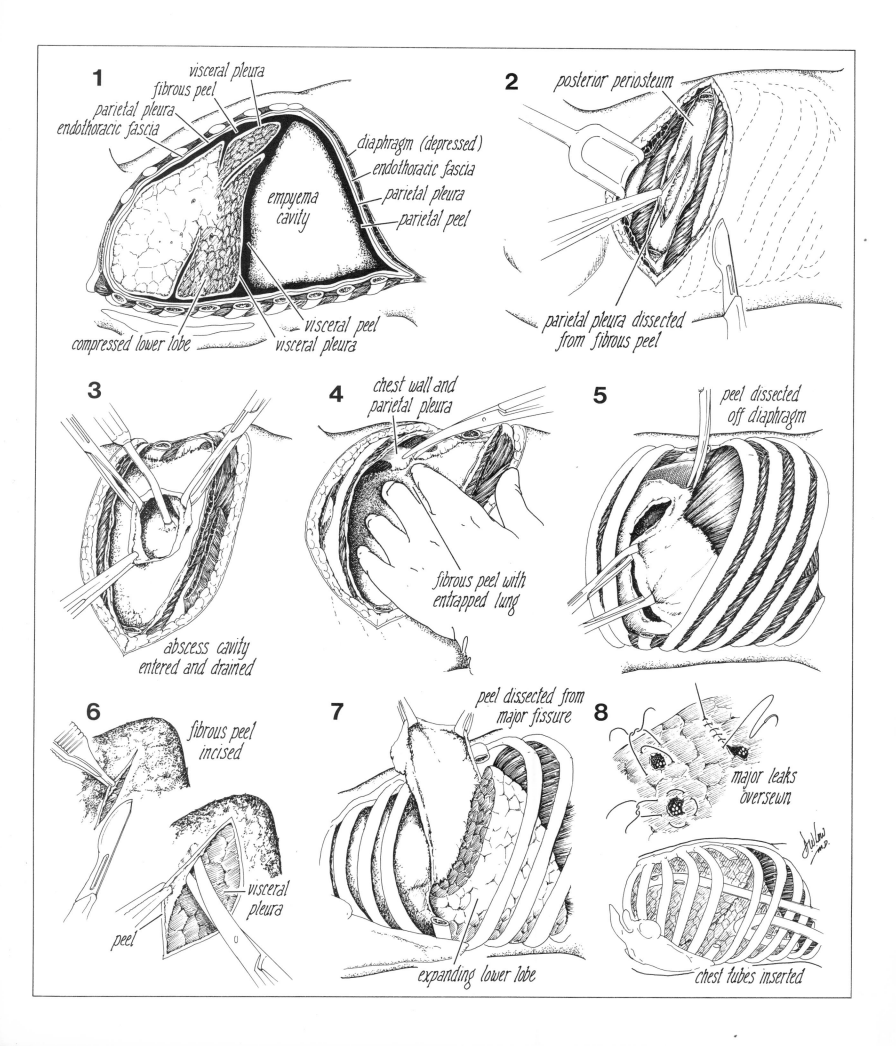

1 parietal pleura · endothoracic fascia · fibrous peel · visceral pleura — diaphragm (depressed) · endothoracic fascia · parietal pleura · parietal peel — empyema cavity — visceral peel · visceral pleura — compressed lower lobe

2 posterior periosteum — parietal pleura dissected from fibrous peel

3 abscess cavity entered and drained

4 chest wall and parietal pleura — fibrous peel with entrapped lung

5 peel dissected off diaphragm

6 fibrous peel incised — visceral pleura — peel

7 peel dissected from major fissure — expanding lower lobe

8 major leaks oversewn — chest tubes inserted

Drainage of Empyema, Eloesser Flap, and Schede Thoracoplasty

Empyema and bronchopleural fistula are preferably treated by tube thoracostomy, with or without simultaneous excision of the empyema cavity, decortication, or lung resection; however, in a few patients these preferred operations are not applicable, and operations developed largely in the preantibiotic era are prescribed.

DRAINAGE OF EMPYEMA

When tube thoracostomy drainage is inadequate and decortication is impossible or inappropriate, open drainage of chronic empyema may be necessary. This operation may be done under local anesthesia, but general anesthesia is strongly preferred. The lung surrounding the empyema cavity must be stuck to the chest wall so that collapse does not occur when the opening in the chest wall is made and maintained.

The patient is usually positioned for a lateral thoracotomy, although occasionally other positions, including an upright position, may be better. The lowermost border of the cavity should be determined from study of axial tomograms before operation, but may be confirmed by needle aspiration with the patient in the upright position just before induction of anesthesia.

(1) A 5 to 6 cm incision parallel to and over the selected site is made and the underlying segment of rib is resected. The ends are rongeured smooth. An ellipse of posterior periosteum and thickened parietal pleura is excised with cautery. The contents of the cavity are evacuated with suction and debridement. One or two large bore silicone or polyvinyl tubes (40 Fr or larger) are inserted into the cavity to provide dependent drainage. Each tube is sutured to the skin edge with one or two heavy monofilament sutures to prevent dislodgement. The soft tissues around the tube or tubes may be approximated with a few absorbable sutures or left open. The outside ends of the tubes are amputated 2 to 3 cm from the skin edge, and the entire wound and tube ends are covered with a fluffed gauze dressing which is changed often to maintain local hygiene. If the cavity is expected to granulate over several months, the tubes are gradually shortened and finally removed as the cavity disappears.

ELOESSER FLAP

An Eloesser flap is designed to produce permanent open drainage of a chronic empyema cavity by suturing a pedicle of skin from either the upper or lower border of the drainage tract to the edge of the empyema cavity. The flap can be made at the time of initial drainage or later and the pedicle can be located either anteriorly or posteriorly.

(2) A rectangular flap 2 to 4 cm in width of skin and subcutaneous tissue is raised either above or below the incision or drainage tract. The length of the flap is dictated by the thickness of the chest wall.

(3) After the flap is raised, the tip is sutured to the parietal edge of the empyema cavity with heavy (0) absorbable sutures. This maneuver produces an epithelial lining of one side of the tract and prevents closure even when the chest tubes are removed. Usually it is possible to slide some adjoining soft skin over the flap bed to reduce the size of the raw area.

SCHEDE THORACOPLASTY

A Schede thoracoplasty unroofs a chronic empyema cavity by excising the overlying ribs and intercostal muscles to allow the soft tissues of the chest wall to collapse inward and adhere to the base of the cavity. The operation is usually bloody and leaves the patient with a large raw area, which must be kept clean with frequent dressing changes. The wound granulates over several months; however, once the deep infection and pockets of infection have been obliterated, the granulating base can be covered with skin flaps or skin grafts.

(4) The patient is usually in the lateral thoracotomy position. A long curved skin incision, roughly parallel to the ribs and through the center of the drainage site, is made. The incision is deepened through the muscles and soft tissues to the ribs and intercostal muscles. The soft tissues over the ribs and intercostal muscles, which overlie the empyema cavity, are elevated from the chest wall. The edges of the empyema cavity are located by palpation.

(5) Using rib shears, cautery, and heavy ligatures of absorbable material to ligate intercostal vessels, overlying *ribs and intercostal muscles* are cut along the edges of the cavity. The overlying plate of ribs and muscle is removed and bleeding points are ligated or cauterized to achieve hemostasis. Bone edges are rongeured smooth and back to the edges of the cavity. Any hardened scar around the drainage tract in the soft tissues and skin is excised.

(6) The soft tissues of the chest wall are allowed to fall inward against the edges of the cavity and visceral pleura. Petrolatum gauze may be placed over the skin edges; the cavity is covered with a large fluffy gauze dressing which is changed two to three times daily.

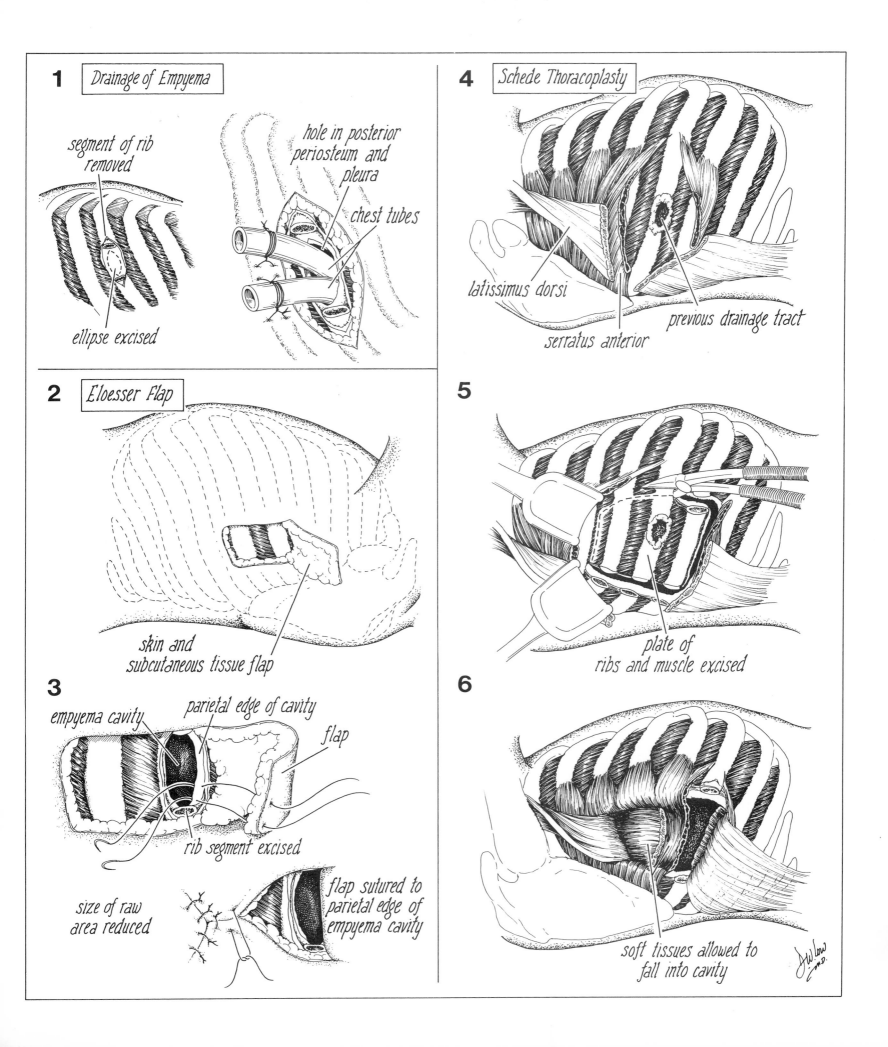

1 — Drainage of Empyema

segment of rib removed

ellipse excised

hole in posterior periosteum and pleura

chest tubes

2 — Eloesser Flap

skin and subcutaneous tissue flap

3

empyema cavity

parietal edge of cavity

flap

rib segment excised

size of raw area reduced

flap sutured to parietal edge of empyema cavity

4 — Schede Thoracoplasty

latissimus dorsi

serratus anterior

previous drainage tract

5

plate of ribs and muscle excised

6

soft tissues allowed to fall into cavity

Standard Thoracoplasty

A standard thoracoplasty differs from a Schede thoracoplasty in that only ribs are removed and not intercostal muscles and periosteum. This operation is more appropriate for patients with high empyema cavities and those with chronic bronchopleural fistulas that cannot be managed by resection and closure of the bronchial stump. If the empyema cavity is large, the operation is usually staged with a 10-day to 2-week interval. The purpose of the operation is to remove the bony support of the chest wall over the cavity to allow the soft tissues to collapse inward to abut the visceral surface (floor) of the cavity.

(1) The uppermost ribs are removed first, and complete removal of the entire rib and ipsilateral transverse processes is important to completely obliterate the cavity. To remove the first four or five ribs, the patient is positioned for a lateral thoracotomy. A posterolateral thoracotomy incision is made; however, the incision should start midway between the vertebral column and medial edge of the scapula beginning at about T2, and curve around the tip of the scapula over the sixth rib. The trapezius and rhomboid muscles are divided and the sacrospinalis muscle fibers are split to expose the posterior ribs and ipsilateral transverse processes.

(2) The posterior segment of the first through fourth or fifth ribs and adjacent transverse processes are cleared of muscle fibers. The periosteum over the posterior ribs is stripped away. The junctions of the transverse processes and ribs are divided with rib shears. The transverse processes are also divided with rib shears, dissected free of muscle and ligamental attachments, and removed.

(3) Division of rhomboids and trapezius muscles posteriorly and the latissimus dorsi and serratus anterior muscles allows the scapula to be elevated superiorly and moved anteriorly. This exposes the lateral and anterior segments of the second through fifth ribs. The second rib is removed first and is either disarticulated from the sternum or transected anterior to the edge of the cavity. Removal of the second rib exposes the first, which is also stripped of periosteum and removed.

(4) The first rib must be removed carefully to avoid injury to the brachial plexus and the subclavian and axillary vessels. The attachment of the anterior scalene muscle is divided, remembering that the subclavian artery is behind this muscle and the subclavian vein and phrenic nerve are anterior to the muscle. When the rib is free of attachments, it is transected posteriorly and then anteriorly and removed. It is not necessary to trim the transverse process, but it is important to push the parietal wall of the cavity inward to obliterate the space. If the cavity does not collapse, the extrapleural plane outside the parietal pleura can be opened over the cupola of the lung. This is easily freed up by a combination of blunt and sharp dissection. Some of this thickened pleura can be resected and removed to allow the overlying intercostal muscles and chest wall to collapse against the visceral pleura.

(5) Ribs 3 through 5 are similarly removed. This should allow the intercostal muscles and adjacent tissues to collapse inward to obliterate the upper portion of the empyema cavity.

(6) If a bronchopleural fistula is present, the empyema cavity is entered in the line of the skin incision. The edges of the bronchus are dissected out, freshened, and closed with 2-0 absorbable sutures. The collapsing parietal wall is sutured over the fistulous opening. Sometimes the thick fibrous peel of the parietal wall of the empyema cavity must be removed from inside the cavity to obtain enough mobility to bring the chest wall over the fistula. Even when a fistula is not present, it may be necessary to remove part of the fibrous parietal wall of the cavity to collapse the chest wall inwards.

The divided rhomboid and trapezius muscles are resutured with interrupted or continuous 0 gauge absorbable sutures. The last two inches of the tip of the scapula are amputated to prevent the scapula from impinging on the sixth rib and adjacent soft tissues. The other muscles are reapproximated and the wound is closed in layers with one or more drains left in the residual empyema cavity.

At the second stage, ribs 5, 6 through 9, or 10 are removed if necessary. The same posterolateral incision is opened at least partially to expose the target ribs. These ribs are removed without periosteum, serratus, and pectoralis muscle attachments and the ipsilateral transverse processes are trimmed as described above. If it is necessary to remove the remaining ribs, this operation is done at the third sitting and through a limited posterior incision that ends in the midaxillary line over the tenth rib.

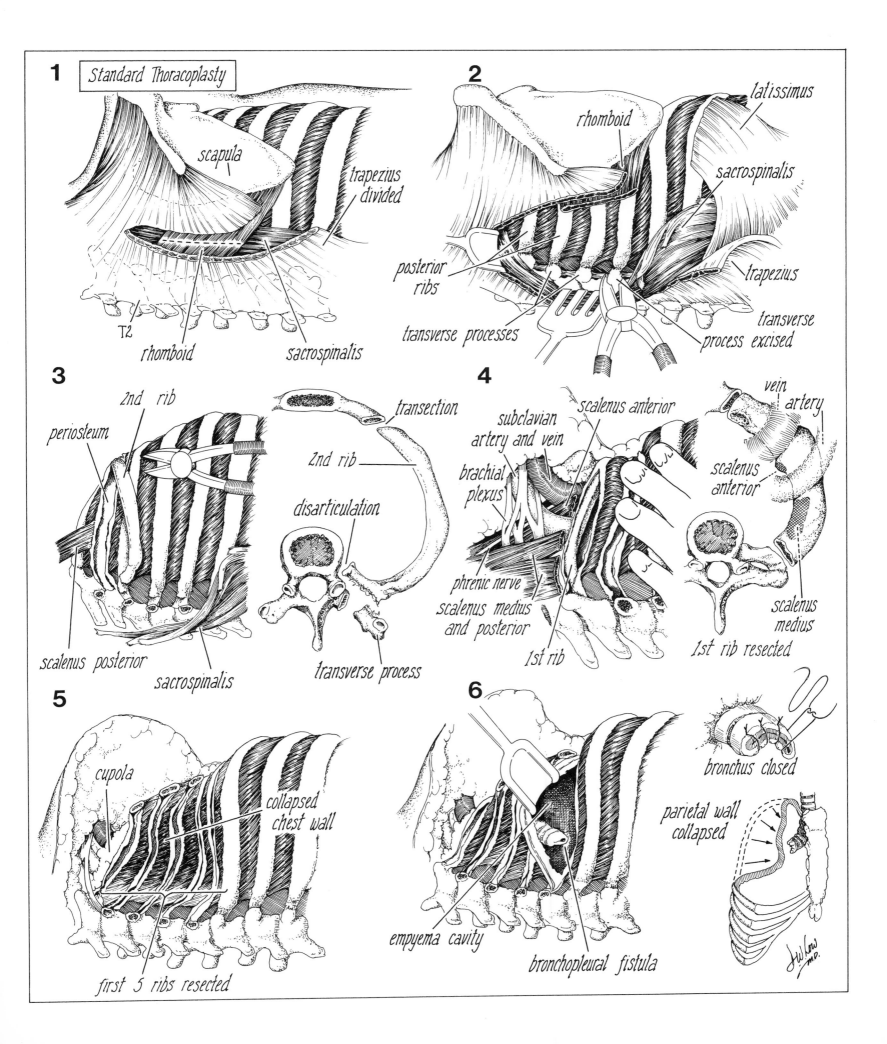

1 Standard Thoracoplasty

scapula

trapezius divided

T2

rhomboid

sacrospinalis

2 rhomboid

latissimus

sacrospinalis

trapezius

transverse process excised

posterior ribs

transverse processes

3 periosteum

2nd rib

transection

2nd rib

disarticulation

scalenus posterior

sacrospinalis

transverse process

4 subclavian artery and vein

scalenus anterior

vein

artery

brachial plexus

scalenus anterior

phrenic nerve

scalenus medius and posterior

scalenus medius

1st rib

1st rib resected

5 cupola

collapsed chest wall

first 5 ribs resected

6 bronchus closed

parietal wall collapsed

empyema cavity

bronchopleural fistula

J.W. Low M.D.

Pectus Excavatum and Carinatum

Pectus excavatum, which is more common by far than pectus carinatum, is usually repaired before or at school age. Many adolescents and adults with unrepaired pectus deformities request repair for primarily cosmetic reasons. The operation is performed under general anesthesia with the patient supine and consists of subperichondral resection of deformed anterior ribs and relocation and stabilization of the sternum.

PECTUS EXCAVATUM

1 In women, a bilateral submammary incision is used whenever possible; we prefer a vertical incision in men. The insertions of the pectoralis major, rectus abdominis, and serratus anterior muscles are elevated from the deformed ribs from the xiphoid to the manubrium.

2 Beginning at the highest and usually least deformed of the ribs, a longitudinal incision is made in the perichondrium. The perichondrium is elevated and stripped from around the deformed cartilagenous rib using a periosteal elevator. The rib is transected laterally at the point where the abnormal direction of the rib begins. Rib shears are often required laterally to transect either bone or cartilage; the cartilage is easily disarticulated from the sternum or cut with the scalpel.

3 In succession, all of the deformed ribs (4 to 6 pairs) are removed without injuring the underlying internal mammary vessels or entering either pleural cavity. Narrow extensions of the seventh, eighth, and even ninth ribs may require resection if the cartilages are involved in the deformity. The xiphoid is mobilized by cutting the rectus and diaphragmatic attachments.

4 A transverse osteotomy is made with osteotomes across the anterior table of the sternum near the junction of the manubrium and body. A thin wedge of bone is excised to permit elevation of the sternal body. In patients with an asymmetric pectus excavatum, the transverse osteotomy may be made full thickness on each side to facilitate rotation of the sternal body. A central slab of posterior sternal table is left intact to maintain continuity and blood supply from the manubrium.

5 The sternum is elevated and, if necessary, rotated into the desired position. This usually improves the position of the xiphoid process; however, in some patients, the xiphoid is amputated and removed or detached, realigned, and reattached with simple sutures.

6 A stainless steel strut, approximately 1 cm in width, is used to maintain the new position of the sternum until costal cartilages regenerate. The length of the strut is determined by distance between the amputated rib ends. The strut should overlap the lateral ribs by 2 to 3 cm and should be bent with sterile vise-grip pliers to follow the curvature of the chest wall. The strut passes beneath the sternum (anterior to the internal mammary vessels and thoracus muscle) and rests on the unresected ribs on both sides. After the strut is finally shaped so that the rounded ends do not protrude beneath the skin over the lateral ribs and the sternum is lifted and held in the desired position, a single wire suture is passed through the rib and through one hole of one strut end. A No. 1 absorbable suture is used for the same purpose at the opposite end. These stitches fix the strut in position during the healing period.

If necessary, interrupted sutures are used to anchor the superior rectus attachments to perichondrium and intercostal muscles. Overlying soft tissues are reapproximated with interrupted or continuous sutures. The skin is closed with a subcuticular stitch.

If one or both pleural cavities are entered, a small chest tube is placed and brought out through a stab wound to remove accumulated fluid. Occasionally, a small Hemovac chain is used between the sternum and intercostal muscles and the overlying soft tissues to evacuate blood and fluid.

The strut may be left in place indefinitely. In some patients, the bar causes real or imagined discomfort. It can be easily removed by making an incision over the end with the wire suture, grasping the strut, and sliding it out through the small incision. This procedure, although quick, should be done in the operating room, preferably with brief general anesthesia or local anesthesia and sedation.

PECTUS CARINATUM

7 The operation for pectus carinatum is similar to that for pectus excavatum. In patients with prominence of the manubrium, the incision and resection of deformed ribs begin at the second pair. Two or more sternal osteotomies may be required to realign and flatten the angulated sternum. A metal strut may be necessary to securely elevate the lower portion of the sternum to correct the depression that patients with high pectus carinatum deformities usually have.

8 When pectus carinatum primarily involves the lower anterior ribs, lower sternum and xiphoid, the deformed cartilages are resected. The xiphoid process is completely detached from the sternum and some of the muscle attachments that are holding the bone in a protruding position. The anterior table of the sternum is transected with osteotomes and the posterior table is fractured by forcibly bending the lower body of the sternum backward. Sometimes full-thickness cuts from each side are necessary to realign the lower body of the sternum.

9 With the sternum realigned, the xiphoid is reattached with two or three simple sutures. Any residual bony prominences are shaved off with the osteotome. To maintain position, the overlying skin and muscle flaps are dissected laterally to obtain mobility and then sutured together over the realigned sternum. The completed repair is carefully inspected to ensure a satisfactory appearance after the flaps have been approximated. A metal strut is not necessary for repair of pectus carinatum that involves only the lower body of the sternum and xiphoid.

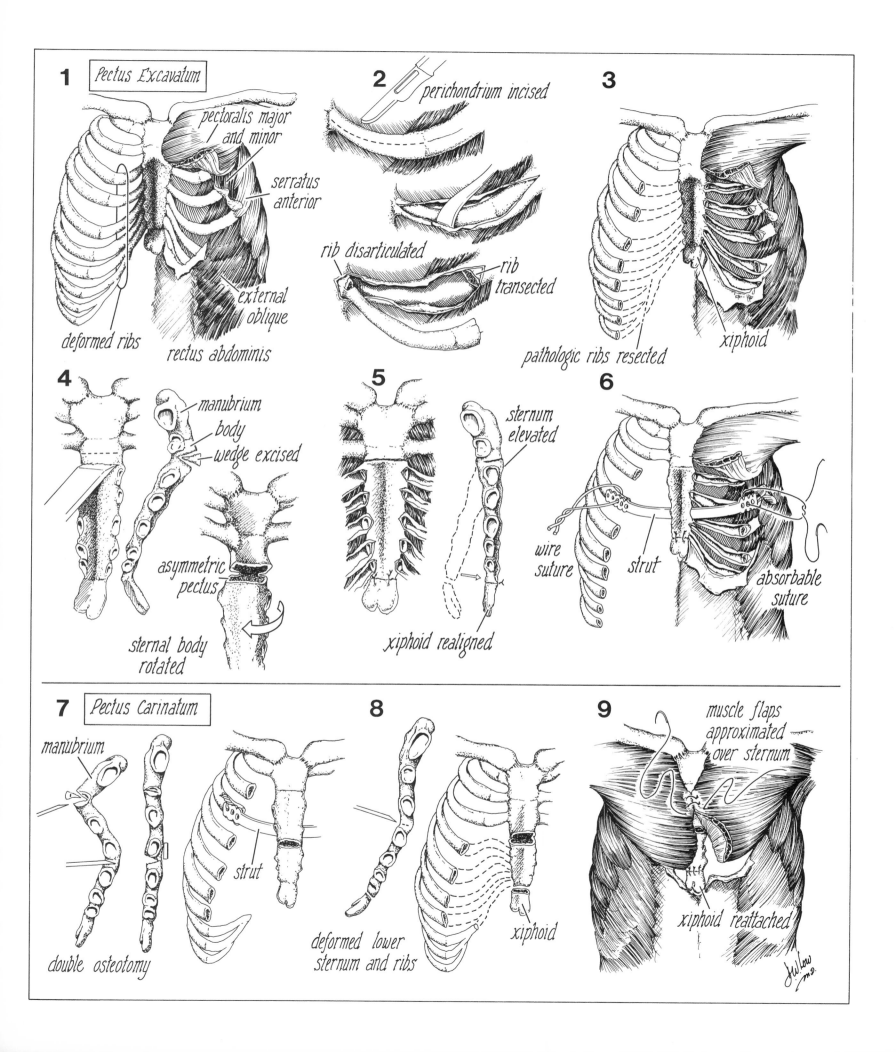

1 Pectus Excavatum

pectoralis major and minor

serratus anterior

deformed ribs

external oblique

rectus abdominis

2 perichondrium incised

rib disarticulated

rib transected

3 pathologic ribs resected

xiphoid

4 manubrium

body

wedge excised

asymmetric pectus

sternal body rotated

5 sternum elevated

xiphoid realigned

6 wire suture

strut

absorbable suture

7 Pectus Carinatum

manubrium

double osteotomy

strut

8 deformed lower sternum and ribs

xiphoid

9 muscle flaps approximated over sternum

xiphoid reattached

J.W.Low M.D.

Excision of Sternal Tumor

Approximately 90% of primary sternal tumors are malignant; therefore, incisional biopsy for diagnosis is not recommended. Radical en bloc excision of the sternal tumor and overlying muscle and fascia with reconstruction is recommended as the initial procedure.

1 The chest, neck, and upper abdomen are prepped and draped widely. If the skin and subcutaneous tissues are freely movable over the tumor, a midline incision through these tissues is made. The skin and subcutaneous tissue are dissected away from the underlying muscle fascia to both midclavicular lines.

2 A line of incision in the muscles and ribs is established laterally at least 3 cm from the edge of the sternum using electrocautery. The anterior ribs are transected, and the intercostal muscles are divided to establish the lateral border of the en bloc dissection. The muscle and rib transection is repeated on the opposite side. If the entire sternum must be removed to achieve adequate resection margins, ribs 1 through 6 are transected bilaterally.

The xiphoid cartilage is dissected free, and the rectus muscle attachments to the medial portions of the sixth and seventh ribs are divided to establish the inferior margin of the en bloc dissection. The anterior attachments of the diaphragm to the chest wall are divided. This permits a hand to be passed under the sternum to palpate the underside of the tumor.

3 The superior border of the en bloc dissection is developed by separating the ligamentous attachments of the medial portions of the first ribs and clavicles. Both clavicular heads are detached from the manubrium. Sternocleidomastoid and strap muscle attachments to the superior border of the sternum are severed, but attachments to the clavicular heads are not divided. The proximal internal mammary arteries and veins are ligated and divided after first locating the arteries by palpation beneath the sternal-chondral junctions. By tipping the specimen cephalad, the remaining ligamentous, pleural, and muscular attachments are easily divided. Any attachments of the thymic capsule to the underside of the sternum are divided.

4 After the specimen is removed, careful hemostasis is achieved, and chest tubes are placed in both pleural cavities and brought out through stab wounds. The thymus gland, pericardium, and anterior portion of the lungs comprise the floor of the wound.

A piece of Marlex mesh of medium weave is cut to equal the size of the defect plus a 4 cm border. Separation of the clavicular heads is maintained by traction on two towel clips. The Marlex mesh is sutured to the edges of the defect with heavy interrupted sutures. Cut edges of sternocleidomastoid, strap, diaphragm, and rectus abdominis muscles are sutured to the edge of the mesh. Tension on the mesh is maintained so that it does not rest on the pericardium, but rather creates a shallow dish approximately the thickness of the chest wall.

5 Sufficient methyl methacrylate to fill in the defect in the anterior chest wall is dissolved and stirred to a pasty consistency according to the manufacturer's specifications in a disposable container provided by the manufacturer. With lungs expanded by 10 to 15 cm positive end-expiratory pressure (PEEP) and with lateral traction on the clavicular heads and lateral chest walls, the plastic is placed into the Marlex mesh dish and pushed into the corners and smoothed over with wooden tongue blades. A second piece of Marlex mesh is placed on the anterior surface of the nearly hardened plastic so that it becomes adherent to the material. After the methyl methacrylate hardens completely (a few minutes), PEEP and lateral traction on the clavicles and chest wall are released. The edges of the anterior sheet of Marlex mesh are sutured to the intercostal muscles and the anterior rectus abdominis and sternocleidomastoid muscles.

6 The skin flaps are permitted to fall over the reconstructed chest wall. Small Hemovac drains are placed between the skin flaps and anterior mesh. The subcutaneous tissue and skin are closed without tension using two layers of running absorbable sutures. With suction on the Hemovac drains, the skin flaps fall against the plastic reconstruction. Because skin has not been removed, the entire reconstruction is easily covered by healthy skin flaps without tension.

If an incisional biopsy has been performed (and indicates a malignant tumor), the operation must be modified to remove the biopsy incision with 4 to 5 cm borders. Mobilization of lateral skin and muscle flaps is required to cover the chest wall reconstruction with healthy tissue. Skin grafts are often required to cover the donor beds of the pectoralis or latissimus muscle-skin flaps.

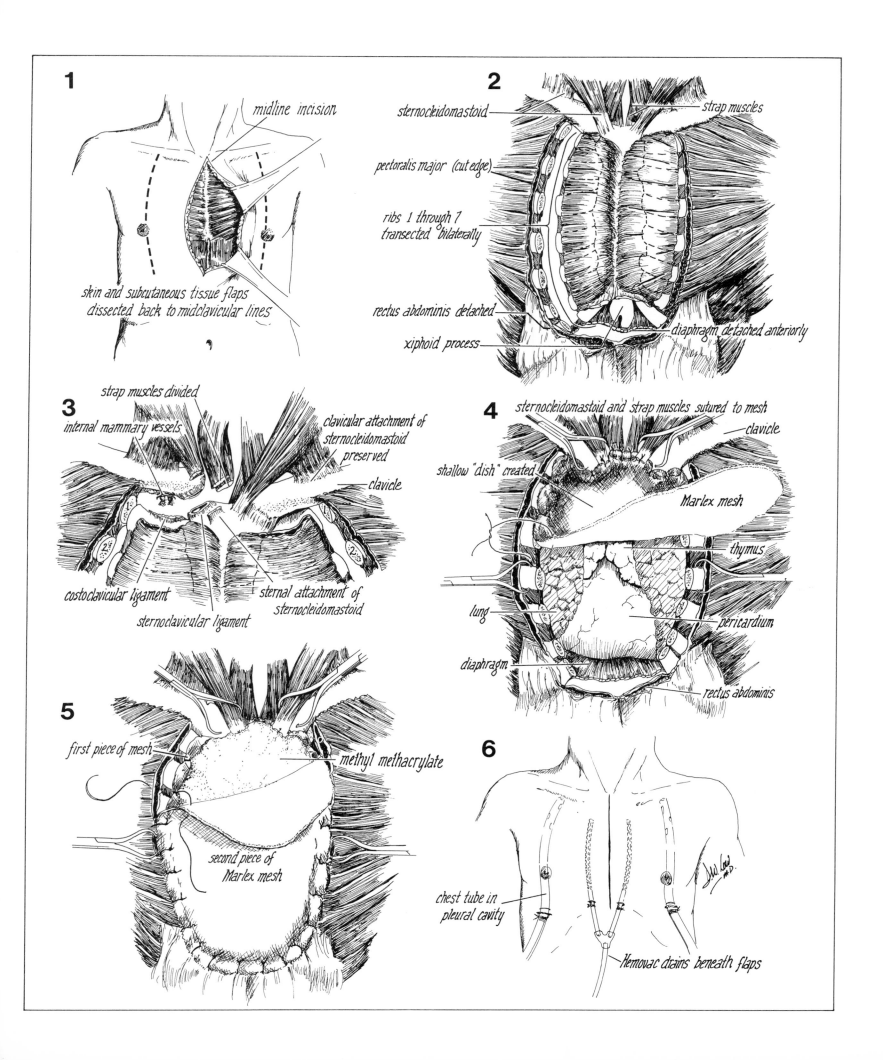

1   midline incision

skin and subcutaneous tissue flaps
dissected back to midclavicular lines

2

sternocleidomastoid   strap muscles

pectoralis major (cut edge)

ribs 1 through 7
transected bilaterally

rectus abdominis detached

xiphoid process

diaphragm detached anteriorly

3

strap muscles divided

internal mammary vessels

clavicular attachment of
sternocleidomastoid
preserved

clavicle

costoclavicular ligament

sternoclavicular ligament

sternal attachment of
sternocleidomastoid

4

sternocleidomastoid and strap muscles sutured to mesh

clavicle

shallow "dish" created

Marlex mesh

thymus

lung

pericardium

diaphragm

rectus abdominis

5

first piece of mesh

methyl methacrylate

second piece of
Marlex mesh

6

chest tube in
pleural cavity

Hemovac drains beneath flaps

Excision of Cervical and First Ribs

The axillary approach is used to excise cervical and first ribs in selected patients with the thoracic outlet syndrome. The operation is performed with the patient in the lateral thoracotomy position, with the ipsilateral arm draped into the operative field and the anesthesiologist placed above and in front of the patient so that the arm can be retracted above the head.

(1) The transverse incision just at the lower border of the axillary hair line and parallel to skin lines is made in the axilla between the pectoralis major and latissimus dorsi muscles.

(2) The incision is deepened to the chest wall, which is covered by the serratus anterior muscle. The dissection continues upward in areolar tissue on the surface of the serratus beneath the axillary contents. Intercostal sensory nerves that penetrate the serratus are protected as much as possible; the supreme thoracic artery, which originates from the axillary artery at the first rib, is ligated or clipped and divided. The thin fascia attached to the first rib is ruptured by finger dissection to expose the axillary vessels and brachial plexus.

The arm is now pulled upward and over the patient's head. This pulls the subclavian-axillary vessels and brachial plexus upward and medial to the first rib.

(3) The insertion of the scalenus anterior muscle is identified between the subclavian vein anteriorly and the axillary artery posteriorly. With gentle blunt dissection, the pleura, which is immediately beneath the scalenus anterior, is pushed medially to allow a right-angled clamp to be passed around the insertion of the muscle into the first rib. The insertion is cut with a No. 15 scalpel blade on a long handle. The anterior portion of the first rib is cleared. Part of the origin of the subclavius

muscle at the costochondral junction of the first rib with the sternum is incised with scissors.

(4) A raspatory is used to clear the exposed first rib of pericostal attachments and to push the scalenus medius muscle posteriorly. The attachments of the intercostal muscles below are cleared from the inferior border of the rib. With care not to perforate the pleura, a right-angle clamp is used to clear the inner medial border of the rib.

(5) The first rib is cut posteriorly as close to the vertebral transverse process as possible with a right angle rib cutter. A clean cut is made and any bone spicules that develop are immediately smoothed away. Anteriorly, the rib is avulsed from the costochondral junction by lateral traction and twisting after cutting some more of the ligamentous attachments of the subclavius muscle. Occasionally a rib cutter must be used.

(6) A cervical rib is removed after excision of the first rib, or occasionally at the same time if the ribs are attached anteriorly. Often a short cervical rib ends with a strong abnormal ligament that attaches to the scalenus anterior tubercle on the first rib. If the rib is short, only the ligament is excised.

(7) After excision of the first rib, the scalenus medius is pushed posteriorly and the cupola of the pleura is pushed downward. The posterior attachment of the cervical rib is felt and with a right angled rib cutter is transected. This is done by palpation only because it is difficult to expose beneath the scalenus medius muscle. The cervical rib or ligament, which is now attached only to the scalenus anterior tubercle, is removed when the first rib is avulsed.

The wound is closed by closing the subcutaneous tissue and placing a subcuticular stitch of 4-0 absorbable suture in the skin. No drainage is needed.

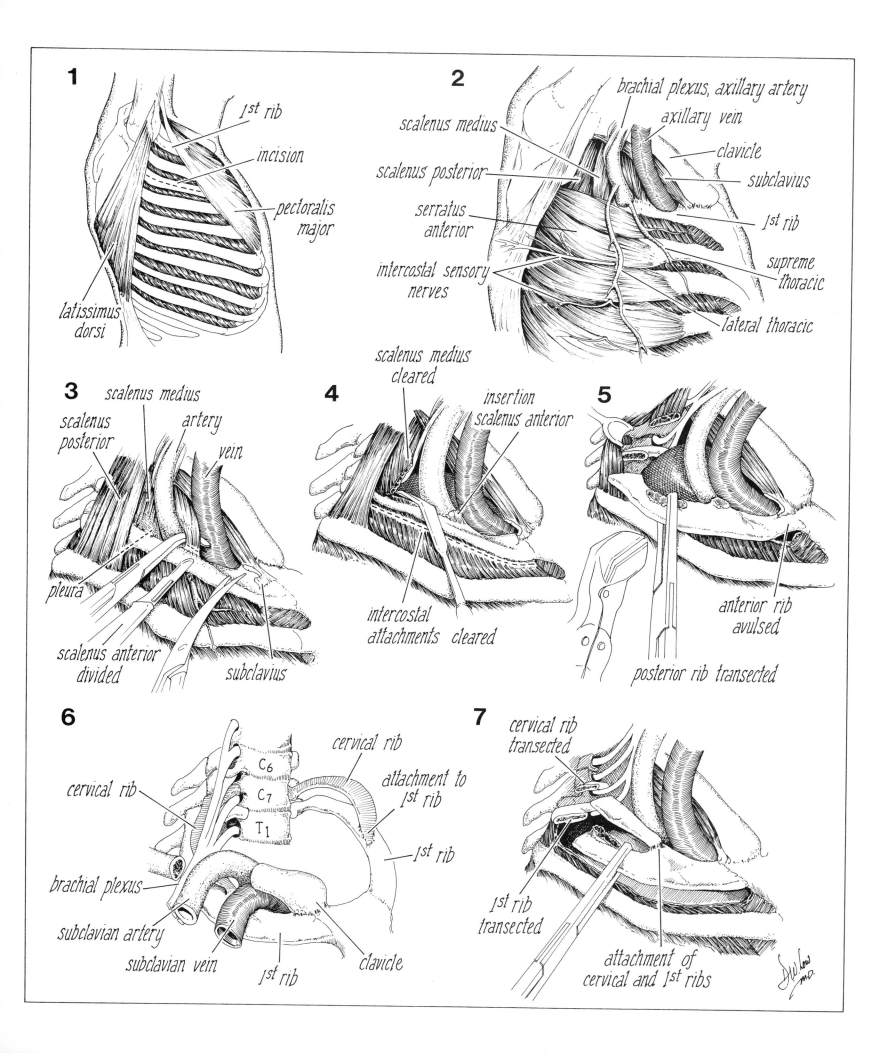

Excision and Reconstruction of the Chest Wall

Many benign and malignant chest wall tumors are amenable to local resection. Because over 50% of chest wall tumors are malignant, we recommend excisional biopsy, not needle or incisional biopsy. Large tumors, prior excisional attempts, or damage from radiation therapy may necessitate extensive resection for complete removal. Development of prosthetic materials and omental and myocutaneous flaps permits reconstruction of large chest wall defects.

CHEST WALL TUMOR

1 If skin and subcutaneous tissue move freely over a tumor that has not been previously biopsied, a long skin incision is made over the tumor in the axis of the rib. Skin and superficial tissues are dissected back to expose the localized tumor on rib, cartilage, or soft tissue. The affected rib is transected 5 to 7 cm away from the tumor edge. Adjacent intercostal muscles are incised and uninvolved ribs immediately above and below the tumor are transected to permit en bloc removal of the specimen and underlying pleura. If the tumor has been previously biopsied, a generous ellipse of skin, fat, and underlying muscle is taken with the specimen to prevent local recurrence.

2 For defects 10 × 15 cm or less with mobile, healthy skin flaps, simple reconstruction with Marlex mesh is adequate. A piece of Marlex mesh is cut to cover the defect. After insertion of chest tubes, the Marlex is sutured to the edges of the defect with a few interrupted 2-0 polyester sutures and a running monofilament suture.

3 For larger defects, methyl methacrylate is placed over the Marlex mesh and allowed to harden into a thin shell in the defect. This prevents paradoxical expansion of overlying soft tissues when the patient later develops positive pressure within the chest. A second piece of Marlex can be placed over the still-soft methyl methacrylate for defects of this size. The overlying superficial muscles are reapproximated and the skin and subcutaneous tissues are closed primarily.

OMENTAL GRAFT

Excision of large tumors, malignant ulcers, or large areas of irradiated skin requires more extensive reconstruction. Two methods, not mutually exclusive, are available and have largely replaced rotated skin flaps and split-thickness skin grafts. A pedicled graft of omentum, covered with split-thickness skin grafts, can be used to cover huge chest wall defects that have been closed with methyl methacrylate and Marlex mesh. Myocutaneous flaps of latissimus dorsi, pectoralis major, serratus anterior, or rectus abdominis can also be used.

For large tumors and extensive lesions, both the excision and reconstruction must be carefully planned. Blood loss can be substantial because operations are necessarily long. The patient's circulation must be carefully monitored and maintained. The lesion is excised en bloc. Usually resections do not include important structures such as the wall of the aorta or large veins, but may include the lobe of a lung, part of the diaphragm, and the abdominal wall. Once the lesion is excised, careful hemostasis is obtained, and remote chest tubes are placed. After the omental pedicle is prepared, the defect is covered by one or more pieces of Marlex mesh sutured to the edges of the defect and, if necessary, to the abdominal wall and diaphragm.

4 The omentum is freed through either the abdominal portion of the thoracoabdominal incision or a separate midline abdominal incision. The greater omentum is reflected off the transverse colon and mesocolon and the left and right gastroepiploic vessels are identified. The gastroepiploic arcade is inspected and the right or left gastroepiploic vessel chosen as the pedicle base. The omentum is separated from the greater curve of the stomach and the unselected gastroepiploic vessel is temporarily clamped before it is ligated and divided.

5 Methyl methacrylate is prepared and contoured to form a smooth shell between the inner and outer layers of marlex mesh. Because this material sets rapidly, surgeon and assistants must work quickly to smooth the paste over the inner mesh and apply the outer mesh before the plastic hardens. The outer mesh is also sutured to the edges of the defect.

6 The omentum is brought up and sutured to the soft tissues surrounding the prosthesis with simple nonabsorbable sutures. The abdominal wound is closed. The exit port of the omentum through the diaphragm or abdominal wall is closed to allow two fingers to fit easily alongside the pedicle. The circumference of the skin, subcutaneous tissues, and superficial muscles that surround the defect is reduced by tucks. This reduces the area of omentum that must be covered by split-thickness skin grafts and buries the edges of the Marlex prosthesis beneath full-thickness soft tissues.

Split-thickness grafts are harvested from the exposed upper thigh or abdomen, meshed if desired, and placed on the entire surface of the uncovered omentum. Petrolatum dressings are applied over the grafts and donor site; absorptive dressings are placed over the remaining areas of the reconstruction.

PECTORALIS MAJOR FLAP

Myocutaneous flaps are reliable and increasingly popular for reconstruction of large chest wall defects. Flaps are constructed from pectoralis major, latissimus dorsi, serratus anterior, and rectus abdominis. Although each muscle can be transposed without a skin island, most retain a central island to place in the center of the chest wall defect. Perforating vessels nourish the overlying skin so that slough is uncommon. The pectoralis major muscle easily reaches the ipsilateral anterior chest wall and even crosses the midline. The latissimus reaches all of the back and lateral chest wall and part of the anterior chest wall and sternum. The serratus anterior, which is attached to the tip and undersurface of the scapula and supplied by the lateral thoracic branch of the thoracoacromial artery, can reach large defects on the anterior or posterior chest wall. The rectus flap based on the superior epigastric artery will reach the sternum and part of the anterior chest wall. Free musculocutaneous flaps are also possible with microvascular techniques, but we have not used them.

7 The pectoralis major muscle is supplied by the thoracoacromial artery. This vessel arises from the axillary artery medial to the pectoralis minor and passes on the undersurface of the pectoralis major in the direction of its fibers along with a vein and the lateral pectoralis nerve. Many perforating vessels pass between muscle and skin; therefore large areas of skin and muscle can be transposed as a unit.

8 A right pectoralis major myocutaneous flap to reconstruct the defect produced by excision of osteomyelitis involving the upper half of the sternum and right costochondral cartilages is illustrated. Part of the overlying indurated infected skin and the upper half of the sternum, costochondral cartilages of the first three ribs, and part of the medial head of the right clavicle have been excised to healthy bleeding bone. Granulation tissue covers exposed mediastinal structures. A chest tube is inserted.

9 An incision is made below the right clavicle between the medial right clavicular head and deltopectoral groove. The clavicular attachment of the pectoralis major is incised to enter the infraclavicular space containing the pectoralis minor and thoracoacromial vessels on the medial border of the pectoralis minor. The vessels are carefully preserved.

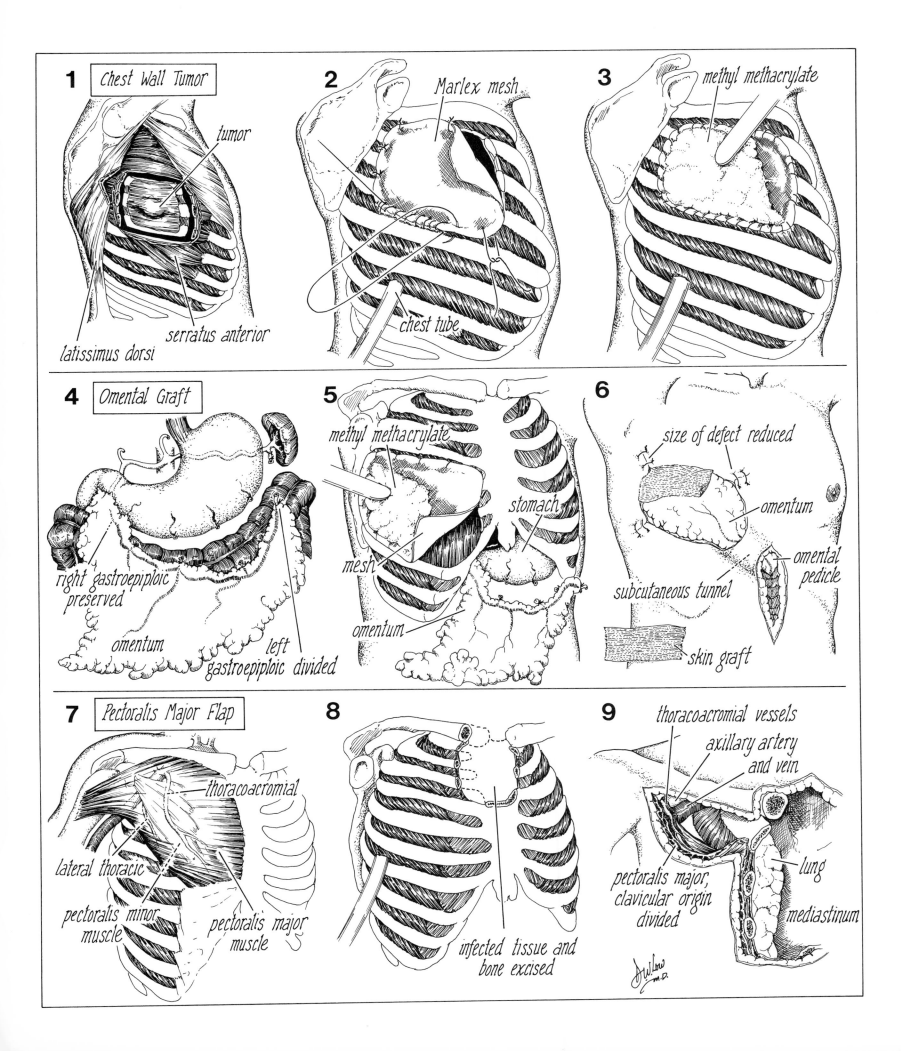

1 Chest Wall Tumor

tumor

serratus anterior

latissimus dorsi

2 Marlex mesh

chest tube

3 methyl methacrylate

4 Omental Graft

right gastroepiploic preserved

omentum

left gastroepiploic divided

5 methyl methacrylate

mesh

omentum

stomach

6 size of defect reduced

omentum

omental pedicle

subcutaneous tunnel

skin graft

7 Pectoralis Major Flap

thoracoacromial

lateral thoracic

pectoralis minor muscle

pectoralis major muscle

8 infected tissue and bone excised

9 thoracoacromial vessels

axillary artery and vein

pectoralis major, clavicular origin divided

lung

mediastinum

(10) An incision is now made in the deltopectoral groove over the humeral attachment of the pectoralis major. The humeral attachments of the pectoralis are incised to release the muscle from the arm. A third incision is made from a point just lateral to the nipple to the lower edge of the defect parallel to the clavicle.

(11) The pectoralis major muscle is elevated by incising its attachments to the anterior first four ribs. Care is exercised to preserve the muscle blood supply, which enters the superior border of the muscle and courses in the muscle near the posterior surface. After elevation and careful hemostasis, the myocutaneous flap easily extends over the defect. The muscle edges are sutured to the edge of the defect with interrupted absorbable sutures; the skin is approximated with interrupted nylon. No drains are used if the debrided area is dry; otherwise a small Hemovac drain is brought out through stab wounds in the left chest. The nipple is slightly distorted and moved medially by this flap; this can be revised later if necessary.

Pectoralis major muscle flaps can also be used to reinforce precarious closures of mediastinal airways and great vessels, to cover infected vascular prostheses that cannot be removed, and to fill empyema cavities in lieu of thoracoplasty. When used inside the chest, the mobilized muscle is passed through the chest wall by resecting a segment of the second rib near the neurovascular bundle of the muscle. The serratus anterior muscle and latissimus dorsi muscles can also be used within the chest as pedicled flaps.

LATISSIMUS DORSI MYOCUTANEOUS FLAP

A left myocutaneous flap of latissimus dorsi used to close a large anterolateral defect is illustrated. A previously excised chondrosarcoma of the left fifth rib recurred locally.

The patient is positioned for a left thoracotomy and draped widely so that the tumor bed can be widely excised, the latissimus can be mobilized, the left arm can be moved freely, and the left thigh is available to harvest split-thickness skin grafts.

(12) The tumor area is widely excised. The excision includes ribs 3 through 7 with the overlying skin and muscle and entire previous scar. It is helpful to outline the area of excision before starting with a marking pencil. A full thickness of chest wall is removed at least 5 cm away from known tumor beginning medially and superiorly. Part of the left costal margin is excised, as well as part of the uninvolved left edge of the sternum. The excision extends to the midaxillary line posteriorly. The specimen is inspected by a pathologist to determine if margins are free of microscopic disease.

(13) The myocutaneous flap is mobilized by an incision along the anterior border of the latissimus dorsi posteriorly and inferiorly to its aponeurosis near the left iliac crest. From this point, the incision turns superiorly to curve upward, roughly parallel to the spine along the insertion of the muscle into the aponeurosis. The incisions are carried deep to the undersurface of the muscle, which is carefully reflected with the overlying skin from the external oblique and serratus anterior. As the flap is mobilized, the posterior incision is continued superiorly, curving toward the axilla as the superior border of the muscle is reached in line with the tip of the scapula.

(14) After freeing the entire latissimus from the underlying chest wall muscles, the flap can be rotated to cover the chest wall defect. The skin and subcutaneous tissues over the superior edge of the muscle and anterior to the anterior edge of the scapula may not have to be incised to allow the bulk of the flap to rotate anteriorly to close the defect. After careful hemostasis, the flap and donor bed are covered with wet lap pads while a Marlex mesh-methyl methacrylate prosthesis is made for the chest wall defect.

(15) The mesh is cut to size and sutured to the edges of the defect with nonabsorbable interrupted and continuous sutures. Before closure of the defect, a chest tube is inserted from the upper abdomen near the midline beneath the sternum and into the left hemithorax for drainage.

(16) The methyl methacrylate shell is made and smoothed, and a second piece of Marlex mesh is placed on top of the soft paste to form the outer surface of the prosthesis. The edges of this mesh are trimmed and sutured to the edges of the defect.

(17) As the prosthesis cools, split-thickness skin grafts are harvested from the exposed left thigh with a dermatome. The myocutaneous flap is now rotated into place over the prosthesis. Both muscle and skin are separately sutured to the edges of the wound with nonabsorbable sutures. The flap is long enough that there is no tension, and preservation of the thoracodorsal artery and thoracodorsal nerve ensure an adequate blood supply and minimal atrophy of the muscle. The inferior border of the rotated flap is tacked to the chest wall with absorbable sutures.

(18) Split-thickness skin grafts are now laid on the donor bed overlying the external oblique and serratus anterior muscles. Petrolatum dressings are applied to the split-thickness grafts. The myocutaneous flap and entire wound are covered with an absorptive dressing.

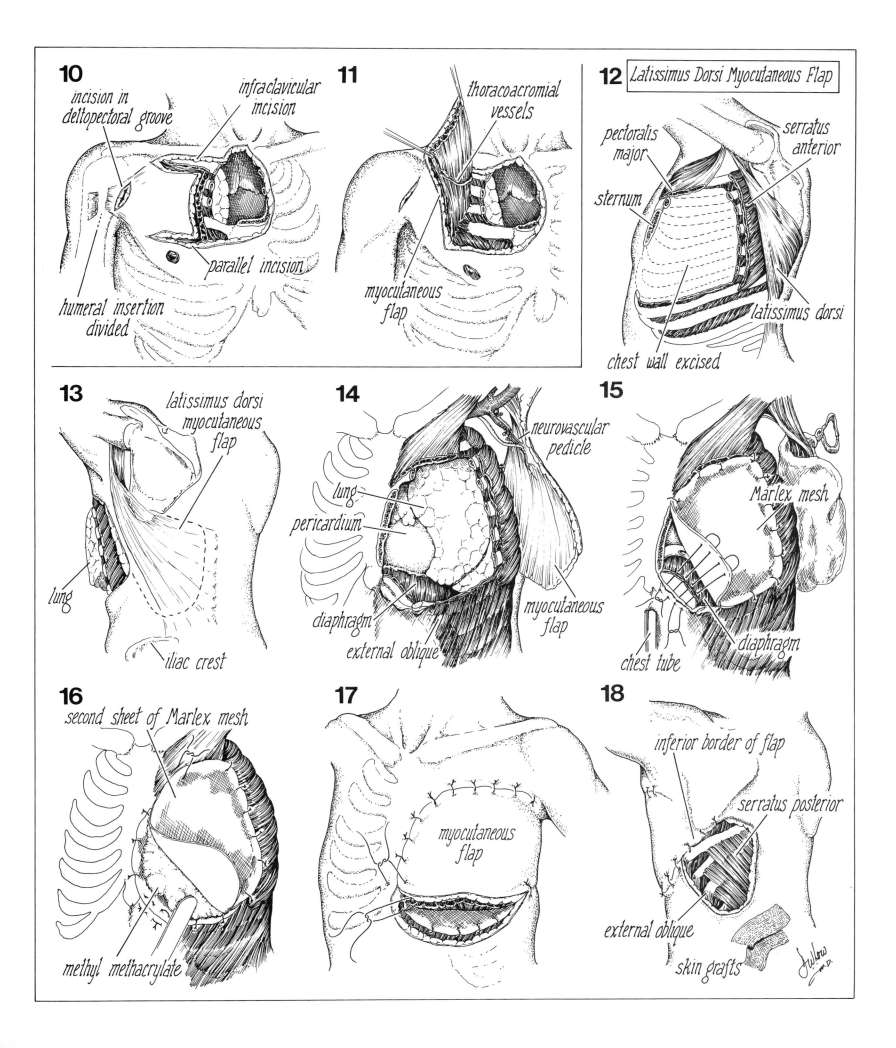

10

incision in deltopectoral groove

infraclavicular incision

parallel incision

humeral insertion divided

11

thoracoacromial vessels

myocutaneous flap

12 Latissimus Dorsi Myocutaneous Flap

pectoralis major

serratus anterior

sternum

latissimus dorsi

chest wall excised

13

latissimus dorsi myocutaneous flap

lung

iliac crest

14

neurovascular pedicle

lung

pericardium

diaphragm

external oblique

myocutaneous flap

15

Marlex mesh

chest tube

diaphragm

16

second sheet of Marlex mesh

methyl methacrylate

17

myocutaneous flap

18

inferior border of flap

serratus posterior

external oblique

skin grafts

Repair of Ruptured Diaphragm

1 Blunt trauma to the chest or abdomen may cause a radial tear in the diaphragm and herniation of abdominal contents into the chest. The tear nearly always involves the left diaphragm and is usually associated with other injuries, particularly abdominal injuries.

2 These tears are best closed during laparotomy, at which time associated abdominal injuries can be discovered and treated. Interrupted mattress sutures of nonabsorbable 0 gauge suture are used after the hernia is reduced and the left colon, spleen, and stomach are retracted to provide exposure.

Occasionally a ruptured diaphragm is overlooked at the time of acute trauma. The patient may develop dyspnea or the herniated bowel may become obstructed. Old diaphragmatic ruptures are best treated by thoracotomy so that adhesions to the lung and chest wall can be lysed.

3 The patient is positioned for a left lateral thoracotomy. The incision is made over the left sixth or seventh rib and a segment is excised. The pleural space is entered cautiously to avoid injury to the viscera.

4 Adhesions between the chest wall and the lung and intestines are taken down. Usually the colon and small bowel are in the chest; occasionally the spleen and part of the stomach are found.

5 When the abdominal viscera are mobilized and returned to the abdomen, the edges of the torn diaphragm are brought together with a single layer of interrupted mattress sutures of 0 gauge nonabsorbable suture. The chest is then closed with drainage.

6 Illustration shows the repaired laceration and its relationships to other intrathoracic structures.

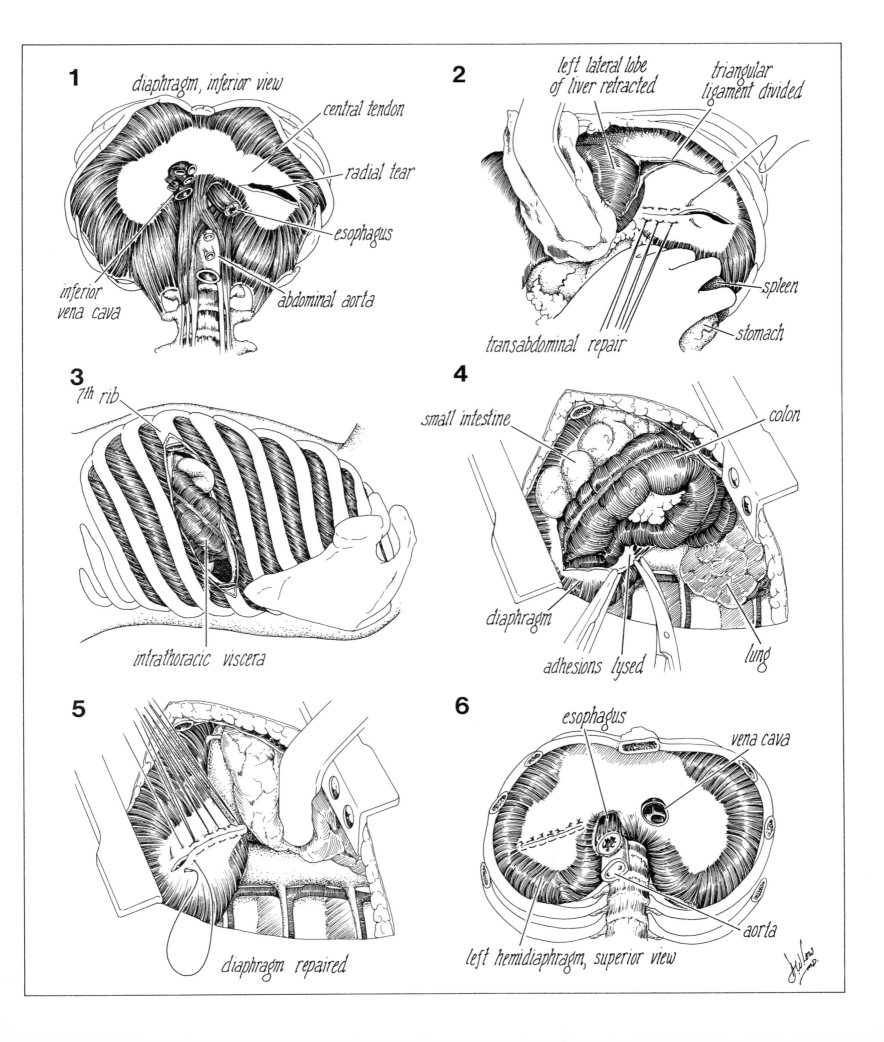

1 diaphragm, inferior view

central tendon

radial tear

esophagus

inferior vena cava

abdominal aorta

2 left lateral lobe of liver retracted

triangular ligament divided

spleen

stomach

transabdominal repair

3 7th rib

intrathoracic viscera

4 small intestine

colon

diaphragm

adhesions lysed

lung

5 diaphragm repaired

6 esophagus

vena cava

aorta

left hemidiaphragm, superior view

Pulmonary Thromboendarterectomy

This operation is designed to remove organized adherent thrombus, which obstructs pulmonary blood flow and causes pulmonary hypertension, cor pulmonale, and right heart failure. The presence of organized thrombus is determined by pulmonary arterial angiography.

The operation is performed during intermittent periods of total circulatory arrest after cooling the patient to nasopharyngeal temperatures of 15° C. The ECG, systemic arterial pressure, and nasopharyngeal and rectal temperatures are monitored. A Swan–Ganz catheter to monitor central venous pressure and pulmonary arterial pressure is placed before operation, withdrawn partially during the thrombectomy, and replaced during rewarming after thrombectomy. Arterial blood gases and thermodilution cardiac outputs are measured periodically.

(1) A median sternotomy is made. Bleeding from dilated veins is meticulously controlled. The lower poles of the thymus gland are dissected from the pericardium. The right pleura is opened widely. The right phrenic nerve is dissected from the superior vena cava and pericardium carefully for approximately 10 cm and retracted with an elastic tape. The pericardium is incised vertically. With the aid of a tongue blade, an incision is made over the aorta to the attachment of the pericardium to the right pulmonary artery. Pericardial edges are tacked to the wound. All bleeding points are cauterized or clipped.

(2) The left pleura is opened. The left phrenic nerve is carefully dissected off the pericardium and hilum of the lung and retracted with an elastic tape. The pericardium is incised over the left main pulmonary artery and tacked to the wound. After heparin administration, the ascending aorta is cannulated. Both cavae are cannulated by means of separate purse-string sutures in the right atrium. Because of high right atrial pressure, each loop of the purse-string suture is passed through Teflon felt pledgets to control bleeding from needle holes.

(3) Bypass is started and the patient is cooled. Slings are passed around both cannulated cavae to direct all flow into the caval catheters. When the heart fibrillates, the aorta is clamped and cold cardioplegic solution is administered. The main pulmonary artery just downstream to the pulmonary valve is opened and a venting No. 18 Ferguson catheter is inserted. Myocardial septal temperature is monitored. When the heart is arrested and decompressed, the pericardial attachments to the left pulmonary artery are dissected away. The left pulmonary artery is dissected out beyond the upper lobe branch to and beyond the origin of the lingular and lower lobe branches beneath the superior left pulmonary vein.

(4) The right pulmonary artery is dissected free from the overlying aorta and superior vena cava. Some of this is done before bypass and is aided by retracting loops of umbilical tape, which lift the great vessels away from the right main pulmonary artery. The entire right main pulmonary artery is exposed beyond the upper lobe branch to the origin of the middle and lower lobe branches.

(5) After at least 30 minutes of cooling and with the nasopharyngeal temperature at 15° C or less, bypass is stopped. Venous catheters are drained to partially exsanguinate the patient. The airway is opened to atmospheric air. The left main pulmonary artery is opened longitudinally from its origin from the main pulmonary artery beyond the upper lobe branches to a point near the origin of the lingular and lower lobe branches. Retraction of the ascending aorta to the patient's right facilitates exposure. When the circulation is stopped and the patient is exsanguinated, only small amounts of blood should be present in the pulmonary arteries.

The thrombectomy dissection is aided by 2.5 power magnification loupes. Sometimes fine traction sutures to hold the edges of the pulmonary artery open are helpful. A pediatric Yankauer suction catheter tip is valuable for aspirating blood away from the intra-arterial dissection.

Initially, the inside of the pulmonary artery may appear normal. Occasionally, an obvious thrombus occludes a branch artery. Often the "intima" appears slightly yellowish and uneven. Close observation reveals a slight elevation or ridge in the proximal left main or distal main pulmonary artery. With a blunt periosteal elevator, the edge of the organized thrombus is elevated and the plane between thrombus and true intima is developed. The plane is gently expanded around the circumference of the artery and then distally to and into the various branches. The organized thrombus forms a cast of varying thickness of the proximal pulmonary arteries. Once the proper plane of dissection is found, this cast can be lifted from the true intima as far out as the third order pulmonary arterial branches. The cast is removed as far out distally in each branch as possible by the combination of gentle dissection with the elevator and retraction of the cast. Totally obstructed branches are revealed and opened as the organized thrombus is removed. Care must be taken not to strip off intima or to perforate the wall of the artery.

The first period of circulatory arrest is limited to 15 minutes. Subsequent periods are extended to 20 minutes. After 15 minutes, bypass is restarted and continued for 10 minutes. Cooling is continued to maintain the nasopharyngeal temperature at 15° C or less. Cardioplegic solution is reinfused into the aortic root to maintain cardiac arrest and myocardial temperature below 12° C.

One or two periods of circulatory arrest are generally needed to remove all thrombus from the left pulmonary artery. When all branches are free of obstructing or constricting thrombus, the arteriotomy is partially closed with a running horizontal mattress suture of 4.0 monofilament suture followed by a continuous over-and-over stitch.

(6) The right main pulmonary artery is opened longitudinally posterior to the ascending aorta and superior vena cava. Retraction of the aorta leftward and the cava first rightward and then leftward permits an incision to the middle lobe branches of the pulmonary artery.

The plane between organized thrombus and intima is found and developed with the periosteal elevator. The dissection usually starts in the distal main pulmonary artery left of the aorta. If thrombus is present, it is dissected from the proximal right pulmonary arterial wall to the proximal site of the arteriotomy, which is on the right side of the retracted aorta. The superior cava is retracted to permit the dissection to progress to the origin of the apical and anterior branches of the artery to the right upper lobe. These branches are dissected free of thrombus and then the middle lobe and lower lobe vessels are cleared. Every effort should be made to tease the organized fibrous thrombus from second- and third-order branches to open the vessels as completely as possible. Again, one or two periods of circulatory arrest for up to 20 minutes are generally needed to completely open all possible vessels. The right pulmonary arteriotomy is closed and reperfusion and rewarming are begun.

The aortic clamp is removed during rewarming, but the heart is kept decompressed with the pulmonary artery venting catheter and by manual compression until coarse ventricular fibrillation occurs. At about 23 to 25° C, the heart is defibrillated and paced by means of temporary ventricular pacing wires. Suture lines are carefully inspected and leaks are stopped during the long period of rewarming. The lungs are inflated before the pulmonary arterial venting catheter is clamped or removed. The Swan–Ganz catheter is repositioned in the main pulmonary artery before bypass is stopped.

Successful thromboendarterectomy causes an immediate decrease in pulmonary arterial and right heart pressures.

After cannulas are removed and protamine is given, both pleural cavities and the mediastinum are drained. When bleeding is controlled, the chest is closed in routine fashion.

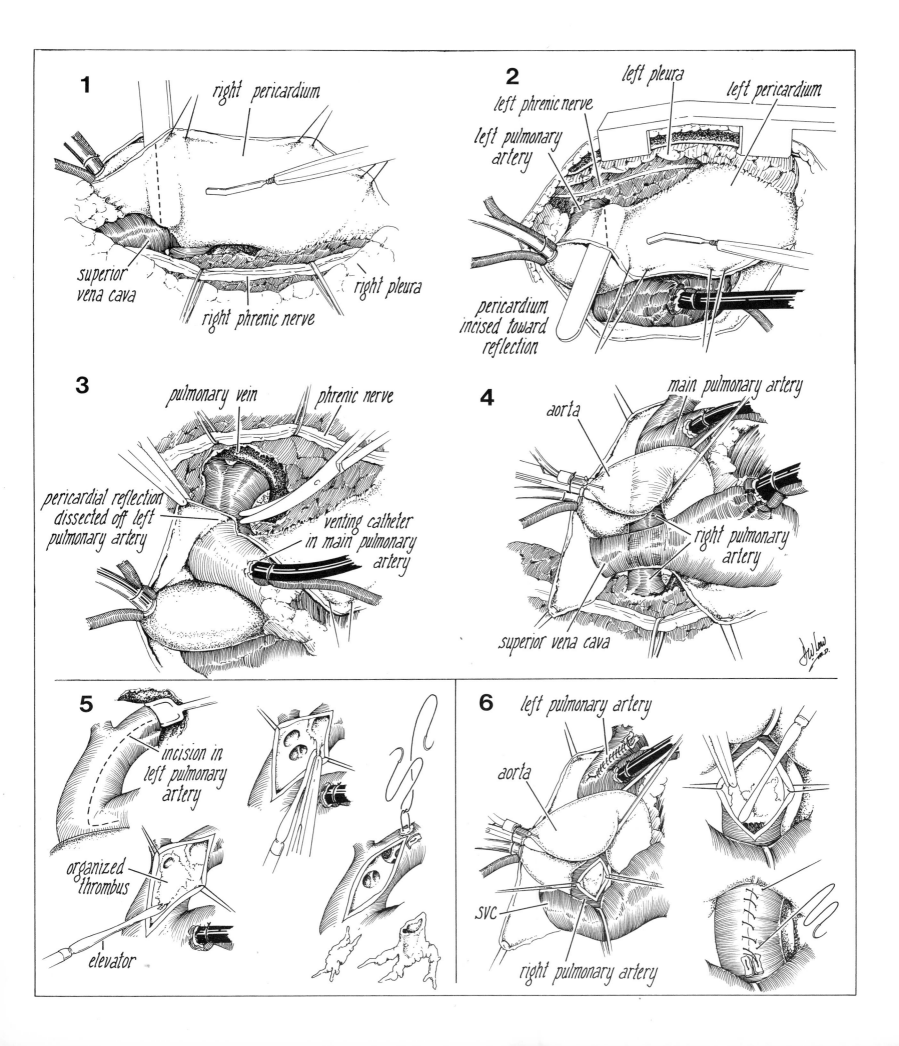

Thymectomy

This operation is identical for patients without thymoma and those with either a thymic cyst or an encapsulated benign thymoma. Because of the presence or possibility of future myasthenia gravis, the entire thymus gland is removed. Very low placement of the midline sternotomy skin incision in women spares the skin of the upper chest and neck and produces a very satisfactory cosmetic result. The incision provides adequate exposure for removal of the entire gland and for that reason is preferred over the cervical approach.

(1) The skin incision is midline and begins at the level of the *third* intercostal space, approximately 7 to 10 cm below the sternal notch. The incision extends to the tip of the xiphoid.

(2) The skin and subcutaneous tissue between the top of the incision and sternal notch are lifted from the chest wall to allow placement of the Stryker saw in the sternal notch. The skin is stretched during this maneuver. The sternum is transected from notch to xiphoid and separated by a small Finochetto retractor.

(3) A 4 cm thymoma in the right lower lobe of the gland is illustrated. This encapsulated tumor touches but does not invade the right pleura and pericardium and is removed along with the entire thymus gland.

(4) The right lateral border of the thymus and thymoma is identified abutting the pleura. With scissors, the filmy covering over this junction is incised from lower pole cephalad to the lateral edge of the upper pole in the neck. The lateral edge of tumor and gland are then easily separated from the pleura by blunt and sharp dissection.

(5) The tumor and lower right pole are elevated and, with scissors, the plane between gland and pericardium is separated to the inferior border of the innominate vein. Often it is difficult to distinguish fatty tissue at the lower poles of the gland from thymic tissue; fat is slightly more yellow, is less co-hesive, shreds easily, and is less meaty than thymus. After the tumor and right lower pole are dissected free, the left is addressed similarly. The phrenic nerves are well lateral to the gland and need not be exposed.

(6) Small or medium-sized veins draining from the thymus directly into the innominate vein are clipped and cut. One or more arteries entering the lateral borders of the thymic lobes at the level of the innominate vein are dissected out, clipped, and divided. The gland is now free of the innominate vein posteriorly, and only the upper poles must be dissected out and removed.

(7) Because of the low sternal incision, a small Deaver retractor is inserted to elevate the sternal flap and cervical strap muscles, which are dissected from the anterior surfaces of both upper lobes. The lateral borders of each upper lobe are then rapidly and easily dissected toward the midline. Finally, the posterior dissection of each lobe is completed separately as the gland and tumor are retracted anteriorly by the Deaver retractor.

(8) The Deaver is repositioned to expose the top of the right upper lobe. This is carefully inspected to identify a possible parathyroid gland before the polar artery and vein are clipped and transected. The maneuver is repeated for the left pole and the entire gland is removed.

(9) After removal, the specimen is inspected carefully to ensure that all of the gland has been removed. Bleeding is controlled by hemoclips and cautery. The sternum is closed by interrupted wire sutures. No drainage tubes are left even if one or both pleural cavities are opened. If the pleura is opened, the lungs are fully inflated to 20 cm H_2O as the sternal wires are twisted. Positive end expiratory pressure is maintained until the soft tissues are reapproximated with running 3-0 absorbable sutures. The skin and subcutaneous tissues are closed with running subcutaneous and subcuticular absorbable sutures.

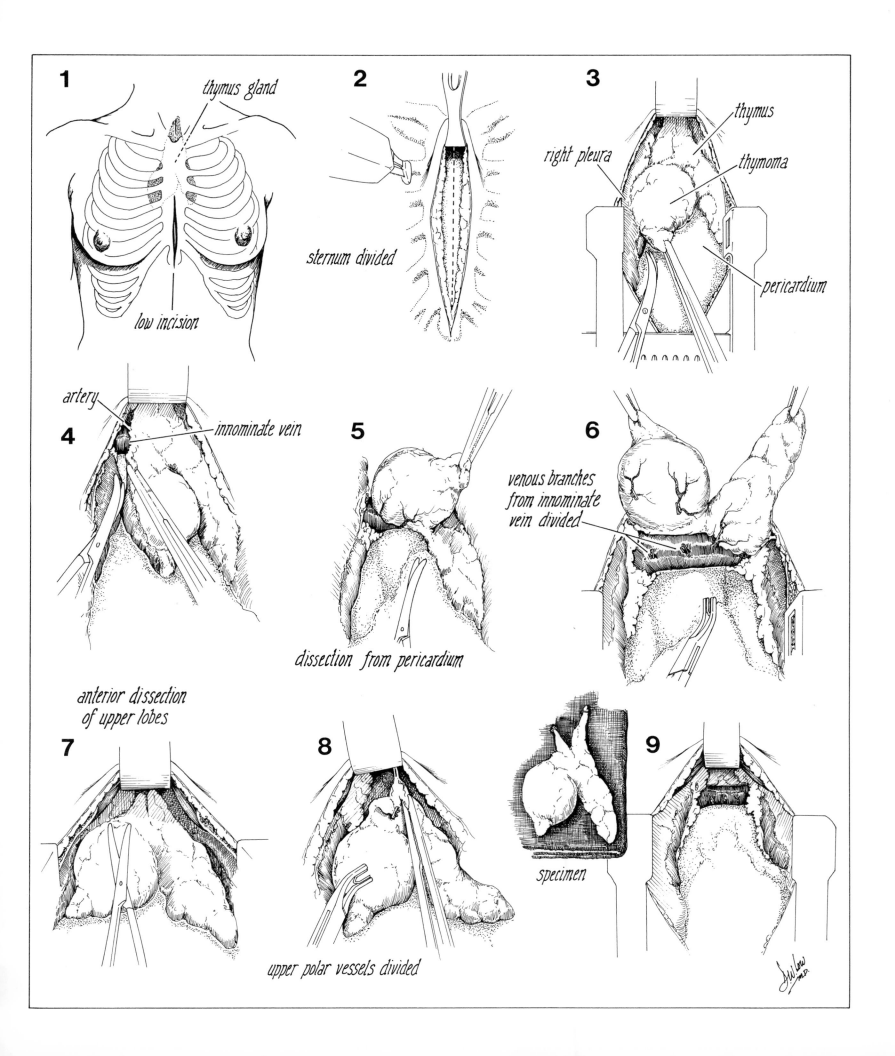

1 thymus gland

low incision

2 sternum divided

3 thymus

right pleura

thymoma

pericardium

4 artery

innominate vein

5 dissection from pericardium

6 venous branches from innominate vein divided

anterior dissection of upper lobes

7

8

specimen

9

upper polar vessels divided

Excision of Anterior-Superior Mediastinal Tumors

The anterior-superior mediastinal compartment occupies the space between the pericardium and great vessels posteriorly and the underside of the sternum and cervical strap muscles anteriorly. Tumors and cysts of the anterior-superior mediastinum arise from the thymus, thyroid, mesenchymal tissues, and lymph nodes and include thymoma, thyroid goiter, germ cell tumors, lymphomas, and a smattering of uncommon lesions.

Because encapsulated thymomas and teratomas are benign and do not recur if completely excised, biopsy of an undiagnosed anterior mediastinal tumor is not recommended. During excision of encapsulated tumors, great care is taken to avoid injury to the capsule. Large tumors (>500 g) are often malignant (locally invasive) thymomas or germ cell tumors or Hodgkin's disease. Biopsy of these tumors may be justified in some instances if benign teratoma can be ruled out.

Preoperative evaluation of anterior-superior mediastinal tumors generally includes computerized axial tomography (CT scan) in addition to PA and lateral chest roentgenograms. If thyroid tumor is suspected, a radioactive iodine scan and blood thyroid and thyroid-stimulating hormone concentrations are measured. Blood tumor markers (beta-human chorionic gonadotropin and alpha-fetoprotein) for possible germ cell tumors are measured in males with anterior mediastinal tumors. Invasive malignant and metastatic tumors may produce the superior vena cava syndrome and preclude attempts at excision.

Anterior-superior mediastinal tumors and cysts are removed through a midline sternotomy incision. This well-tolerated incision provides full access to the anterior-superior mediastinum and permits full assessment of the relationship of the tumor to adjacent structures. Although postoperative morbidity and discomfort are somewhat greater than those produced by mediastinotomy or mediastinoscopy, the advantages of complete exposure and preservation of the option to remove the undiagnosed mass completely outweigh the disadvantages of the larger incision.

Benign teratomas (desmoid tumors), most thymomas, and thymic cysts are easily removed from a midline sternotomy. Small and moderate-sized thyroid goiters that extend into the anterior-superior mediastinum can be completely excised from a cervical collar incision. Large goiters that extend to the aortic arch and cause compression and dislocation of mediastinal structures are best removed through a midline sternotomy. These large goiters often derive part of their blood supply from mediastinal vessels. A low collar cervical incision can be added if all or part of the cervical thyroid is removed.

INTRATHORACIC GOITER

1 The patient is placed supine on a shoulder roll with the neck extended. Neck, anterior chest, and upper abdomen are draped into the surgical field. Because the goiter extends well into the neck, a low transverse cervical (collar) incision is made. This is followed by a connecting midline sternotomy incision.

2 The anterior surface of the tumor mass is inspected and upper and lower borders are determined. Cervical strap muscles are retracted laterally from the surface of the tumor in the neck. The right and left pleurae are reflected from the surface of the tumor by blunt and sharp dissection. The plane between the inferior border of the thyroid mass and pericardium is entered and separated by incising areolar attachments as the mass is lifted.

3 Small vessels that enter the goiter from the mesenchymal tissue overlying the great vessels and innominate vein are clipped or cauterized and divided. The superior extension of the tumor is removed by rolling the tumor medially and dissecting cervical muscles and carotid sheath laterally. Tumor vessels are clipped or cauterized as discovered. Both the inferior and superior thyroid arteries are identified.

4 As the dissection proceeds laterally, the right recurrent laryngeal nerve is identified on the prevertebral fascia between the trachea and esophagus. The nerve is behind but very close to the inferior thyroid artery. After protecting the nerve, the superior pole of the thyroid gland is dissected free by ligation and division of the superior thyroid vessels. The isthmus can be divided between clamps if all or part of the left lobe is not removed.

SEMINOMA (INVASIVE GERM CELL TUMOR)

If an anterior-superior mediastinal tumor is locally invasive in one or two areas, these points of invasion are excised with the tumor. Most often these tumors prove to be thymomas, which are malignant by definition because of local invasion; however, complete excision and postoperative radiation therapy improve the prognosis.

5 If an anterior mediastinal tumor is *extensively* invasive so that complete extirpation is impossible or extensive surgery is required, with patch reconstruction of great vessels and other vital structures, a generous incisional biopsy is made. Frozen section is valuable.

6 If a seminoma or Hodgkin's lymphoma is found, subtotal resection of the tumor may (or may not) be beneficial. Subtotal resection is performed, often with cautery, and with care to avoid great vessels and other vital structures. Subtotal resection of a very large seminoma is illustrated. When the tumor is removed, the field is inspected for bleeding and small chest tubes are placed in the hemithorax (if the pleura is opened) and mediastinum for drainage. The wound is closed in standard fashion.

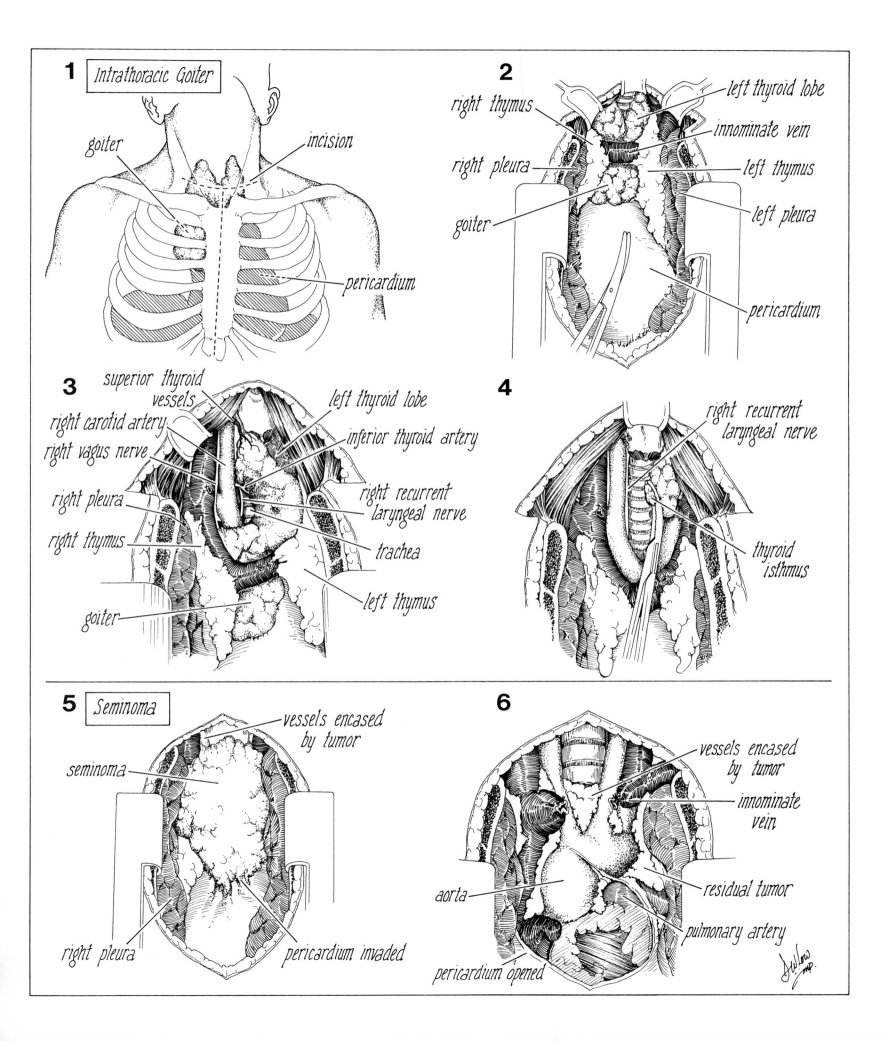

Excision of Posterior and Middle Mediastinal Lesions

Middle and posterior mediastinal lesions are best exposed by lateral thoracotomy. The middle mediastinum contains the heart, pericardium, aorta, trachea, and main bronchi. Carcinoma of the lung is the most common tumor involving the middle mediastinum. Primary lesions include lymphoma and pericardial and bronchogenic cysts. Pericardial cysts, which are usually located in the crease between the diaphragm and the pericardium, are usually asymptomatic, are differentiated from solid tumors by ultrasound and can be aspirated.

BRONCHOGENIC CYST

Bronchogenic cysts arise in the middle mediastinum, often near the tracheal bifurcation. Cysts bulge to either the right or left and may or may not be attached by a small stalk to the bronchi or trachea. Cysts vary in size, but are commonly 5 to 8 cm in diameter. Infection may occur in those cysts with a patent connection to the airway.

(1) The cyst is exposed by means of posterolateral thoracotomy on the side to which the cyst presents on chest x-ray. The encapsulated cyst is easily located by retracting the lung anteriorly. The cyst usually has a thick wall, which is dissected from adjacent lung and mediastinal structures toward the tracheal bifurcation. Sometimes only blunt dissection is required. Often the cyst is attached to the carina, trachea, or major bronchus by a narrow stalk.

(2) If a stalk is present, ligation and division of the stalk near the airway are all that is required to complete the excision. Only one chest tube is required if the adjacent lung does not have an air leak.

GANGLIONEUROMA

The posterior mediastinum contains the esophagus, descending thoracic aorta, sympathetic chains, and intercostal nerves. Lymphoma may involve paraesophageal nodes; thus lymphoma may present in any mediastinal compartment. Esophageal diverticula and duplication cysts are presented with esophageal lesions; aortic lesions are illustrated in that section. Neurogenic tumors, which include pheochromocytoma and a variety of other benign and malignant cell types, are predominant primary tumors of the posterior mediastinum. Most adult neurogenic tumors are benign, but may occasionally recur if incompletely resected. The incidence of malignancy is higher in children.

Posterior mediastinal tumors are usually found by chest roentgenogram and precisely located by computerized axial tomography. Urinary vanillylmandelic acid is measured preoperatively. If spinal cord symptoms are present, a myelogram and neurosurgical consultation are advisable. Excision of a left ganglioneuroma extending from T2 to T5 is illustrated.

(3) With the patient positioned for a left thoracotomy, a hockey-stick posterolateral thoracotomy incision is made. The incision is carried high between the scapula and spine so that a segment of the third rib can be removed. The scapula is pulled anteriorly. Retraction of the lung reveals a lobulated tumor of the left sympathetic chain in the vertebral gutter.

(4) The parietal pleura over the ribs lateral to the tumor and over the vertebrae medial to the tumor is incised. Because the tumor does not invade ribs or vertebrae or extend into the vertebral foramen, a plane is developed between the parietal pleura beneath the tumor and rib. Frequently tumor tissue bulges into the intercostal space, but as the dissection proceeds along the lateral border of the tumor, the entire tumor can be rotated medially. It is usually easier to develop the plane between tumor and vertebrae medially. Every effort is made to avoid cutting into the tumor.

(5) The sympathetic chain from which this tumor arises is identified, clipped, and cut above and below.

(6) Beginning inferiorly, the tumor is lifted from the transverse processes until it can be removed completely.

Dumb-bell-shaped tumors that extend into the spinal cord through a vertebral foramen are best managed by a thoracic surgeon and a neurosurgeon working together. Occasionally the thoracic portion of the tumor must be amputated to facilitate exposure for the neurosurgeon.

Radical excision of malignant tumors of the posterior mediastinum is rarely recommended.

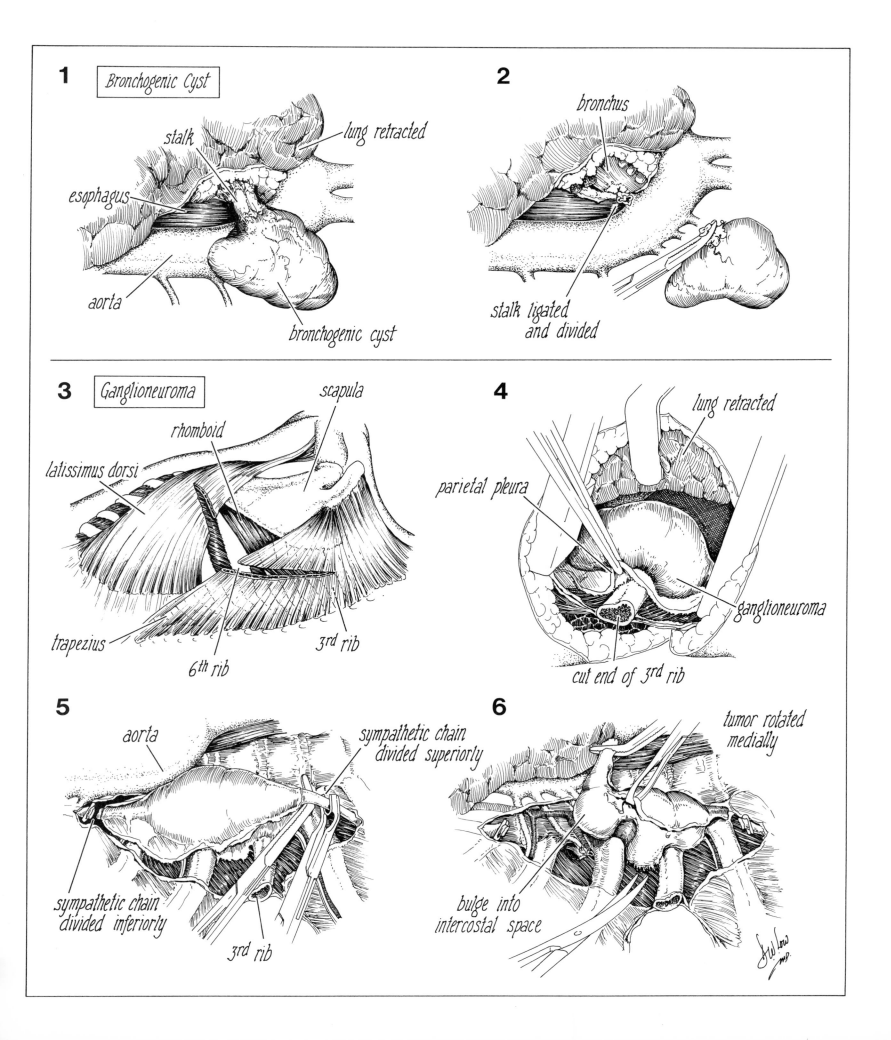

1 Bronchogenic Cyst

stalk

lung retracted

esophagus

aorta

bronchogenic cyst

2

bronchus

stalk ligated
and divided

3 Ganglioneuroma

scapula

rhomboid

latissimus dorsi

trapezius

6th rib

3rd rib

4

lung retracted

parietal pleura

ganglioneuroma

cut end of 3rd rib

5

aorta

sympathetic chain
divided superiorly

sympathetic chain
divided inferiorly

3rd rib

6

tumor rotated
medially

bulge into
intercostal space

Section 6

Esophageal Disease

Esophageal Myotomy

Incision of either the upper or lower esophageal sphincter is recommended for highly selected patients who develop dysphagia with or without secondary changes of the esophagus caused by pharmacologically resistant dysfunction of the sphincter. Spasm of the upper sphincter may lead to Zenker's diverticulum; lower esophageal sphincter spasm is associated with achalasia.

ZENKER'S DIVERTICULECTOMY

(1) A pharyngoesophageal (Zenker's) diverticulum is usually approached from the left with the patient supine, shoulders elevated and face turned toward the right. An incision along the anterior border of the sternocleidomastoid provides the best exposure; a more transverse incision parallel to skin folds can be used and provides a better cosmetic result. The right-sided approach is often used if myotomy of only the upper sphincter is performed.

(2) The dissection is deepened lateral to the left lobe of the thyroid gland and strap muscles and medial to the carotid-jugular sheath. The omohyoid muscle is usually divided, as are the inferior thyroid artery and several thyroid veins. The recurrent laryngeal nerve is carefully avoided, with the thyroid and trachea retracted anteriorly and to the right.

(3) After the prevertebral space is entered, the diverticulum and lower pharynx are readily apparent. The diverticulum is usually easily mobilized and is completely dissected to delineate its moderately broad neck which presents between the thin oblique fibers of the inferior constrictor muscle above and the slightly thicker cricopharyngeus muscle below. Care must be taken to avoid aspiration if the diverticulum is large and filled with fluid. A nasogastric tube is not used.

(4) With minimal traction on the diverticulum, a clamp is placed across the neck to control the contents of the sac. The clamp is placed parallel to the longitudinal axis of the esophagus and care is taken not to pull normal esophagus into the clamp. The neck of the diverticulum, consisting of mucosa and submucosal tissue, is partially incised below the clamp. Interrupted full-thickness 4-0 nonabsorbable sutures are placed, tied, and held until the diverticulum is completely amputated. Alternatively, a stapler can be placed across the neck in lieu of a clamp and the mucosa stapled closed.

(5) The inferior constrictor and cricopharyngeus muscles above and below are approximated with interrupted sutures to secure the closure.

(6) The cricopharyngeus muscle and about 2 to 3 cm of the circular muscle fibers of the upper esophagus are incised down to but not through the mucosa in the posterior midline after amputation of the diverticulum. The muscle fibers are spread apart to allow the mucosa to protrude.

(7) If the diverticulum is small (4 cm or less), it need not be amputated. The diverticulum can be sutured to the inferior constrictor muscle to prevent filling. The myotomy incision in the cricopharyngeus and upper esophagus is sufficient to alleviate the problem.

Because of the possibility of a mucosal nick, a 1/4" Penrose drain is brought out through the incision and left for three days.

HELLER MYOTOMY

(8) Achalasia is well treated by Heller myotomy, which is performed through a left posteriolateral thoracotomy, usually with resection of the sixth rib. The mediastinal pleura is incised and a Penrose drain is placed around the lower esophagus for traction.

(9) A vertical incision in the longitudinal muscle fibers proximal to the lower esophageal sphincter is made with the scalpel and deepened with incision of the circular muscle fibers. Traction sutures in the muscle layers can be used to lift muscle off the mucosa. As the intact mucosa appears, circular muscle fibers are gently but firmly separated to allow the mucosa to pout out between the muscle edges for nearly half the circumference of the esophagus.

(10) The incision is carried downward across the lower esophageal sphincter onto the anterior gastric wall for about 1 cm and upward through all the thick-walled esophagus. The incision stops at the aortic arch or when the esophageal musculature becomes attenuated and dilated.

(11) After separation of the circular muscle bands to allow the mucosa to pout, the mucosa is carefully inspected for leaks. The chest is closed with a single chest tube placed near but not touching the distal esophagus.

A long myotomy is sometimes prescribed for diffuse esophageal spasm. If function of the lower esophageal sphincter is normal, the myotomy is not carried across the sphincter onto the cardia but is extended the full length of the intrathoracic esophagus, behind and above the aortic arch.

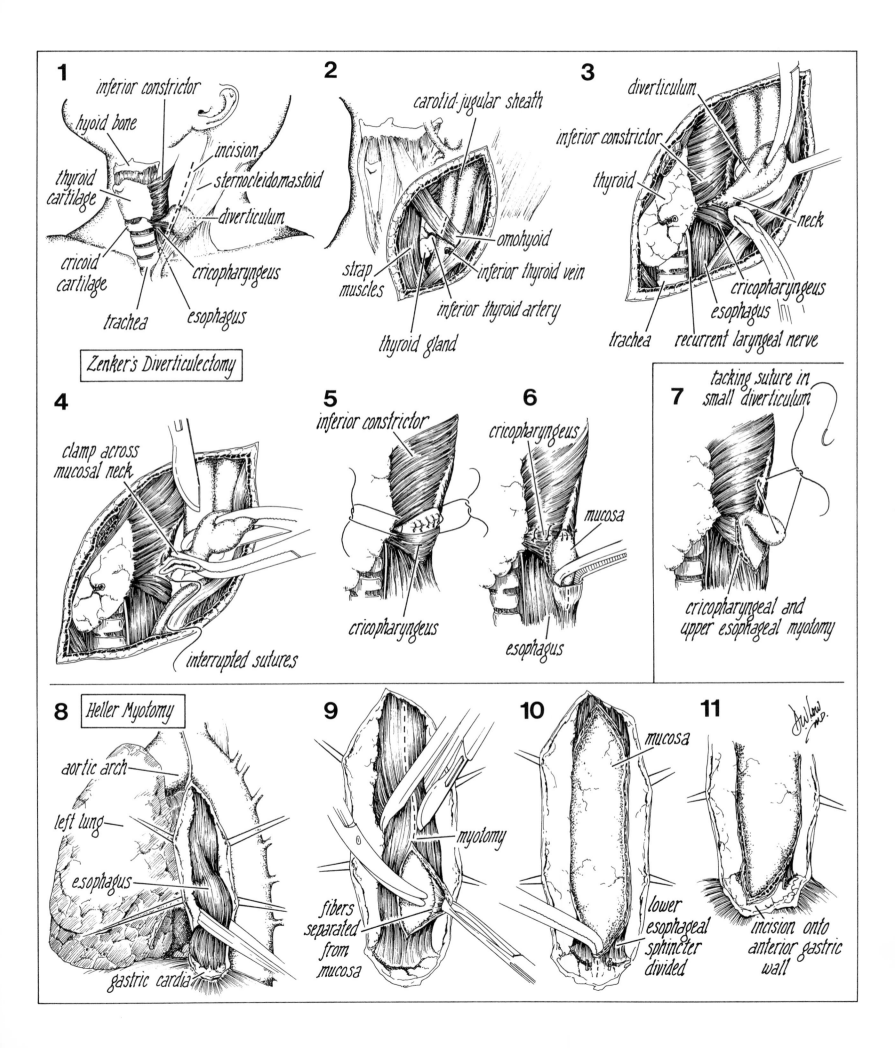

1

inferior constrictor

hyoid bone

thyroid cartilage

cricoid cartilage

trachea

incision

sternocleidomastoid

diverticulum

cricopharyngeus

esophagus

Zenker's Diverticulectomy

2

carotid-jugular sheath

omohyoid

strap muscles

inferior thyroid vein

inferior thyroid artery

thyroid gland

3

diverticulum

inferior constrictor

thyroid

neck

cricopharyngeus

esophagus

trachea

recurrent laryngeal nerve

4

clamp across mucosal neck

interrupted sutures

5

inferior constrictor

cricopharyngeus

6

cricopharyngeus

mucosa

esophagus

7

tacking suture in small diverticulum

cricopharyngeal and upper esophageal myotomy

8 *Heller Myotomy*

aortic arch

left lung

esophagus

gastric cardia

9

myotomy

fibers separated from mucosa

10

mucosa

lower esophageal sphincter divided

11

incision onto anterior gastric wall

Transsthoracic Nissen Fundoplication

Although the transabdominal approach is more commonly used, Nissen fundoplication can be performed through a left posterolateral thoracotomy (with resection of the sixth or seventh rib). The transthoracic approach may be preferable in patients with dilatable stricture and some degree of esophageal shortening.

(1) The pulmonary ligament is divided to permit retraction of the left lung. The lower esophagus and both vagal nerves are mobilized and encircled with a Penrose drain. The nerves are carefully protected.

(2) The diaphragm is incised radially 4 to 5 cm. The short gastric vessels are clipped or ligated and divided to mobilize approximately 8 to 10 cm of the greater curvature of the stomach. On the lesser curvature, branches of the left gastric artery in the gastrohepatic ligament are clipped and divided. This mobilizes the fundus of the stomach for the wrap.

(3) A 40 Fr bougie is passed into the stomach by the anesthesiologist. The gastric fundus is then passed behind the lower esophagus and sutured to the anterior gastric wall with multiple interrupted 2-0 nonabsorbable sutures over a distance of 5 cm.

(4) The sutures do not include bites into the anterior esophagus, as is usually the procedure in the transabdominal approach. When these sutures are tied, it should be possible to pass a finger between the wrap and the anterior esophagus. The wrap is then rotated toward the patient's right so that the plication sutures are aligned with the lesser curve of the stomach in the right anteromedial axis. Multiple 4-0 nonabsorbable sutures are placed between the esophageal wall and the wrapped fundus to secure the location of the wrap.

(5) If the diaphragmatic hiatus is patulous, one or more mattress sutures of 0 polyester can be used to approximate the right and left diaphragmatic crura. These are usually placed before the fundus is wrapped around the esophagus, but are tied after the wrap is completed. The diaphragmatic incision is closed with 0 polyester mattress sutures so that a finger, the esophagus, and the bougie fit snugly in the opening and the fundoplication is below the diaphragm.

(6) If the esophagus is shortened, the fundoplication is left above the diaphragm. The edges of the diaphragm are sutured to the plicated fundus around the entire circumference with 2-0 polyester sutures.

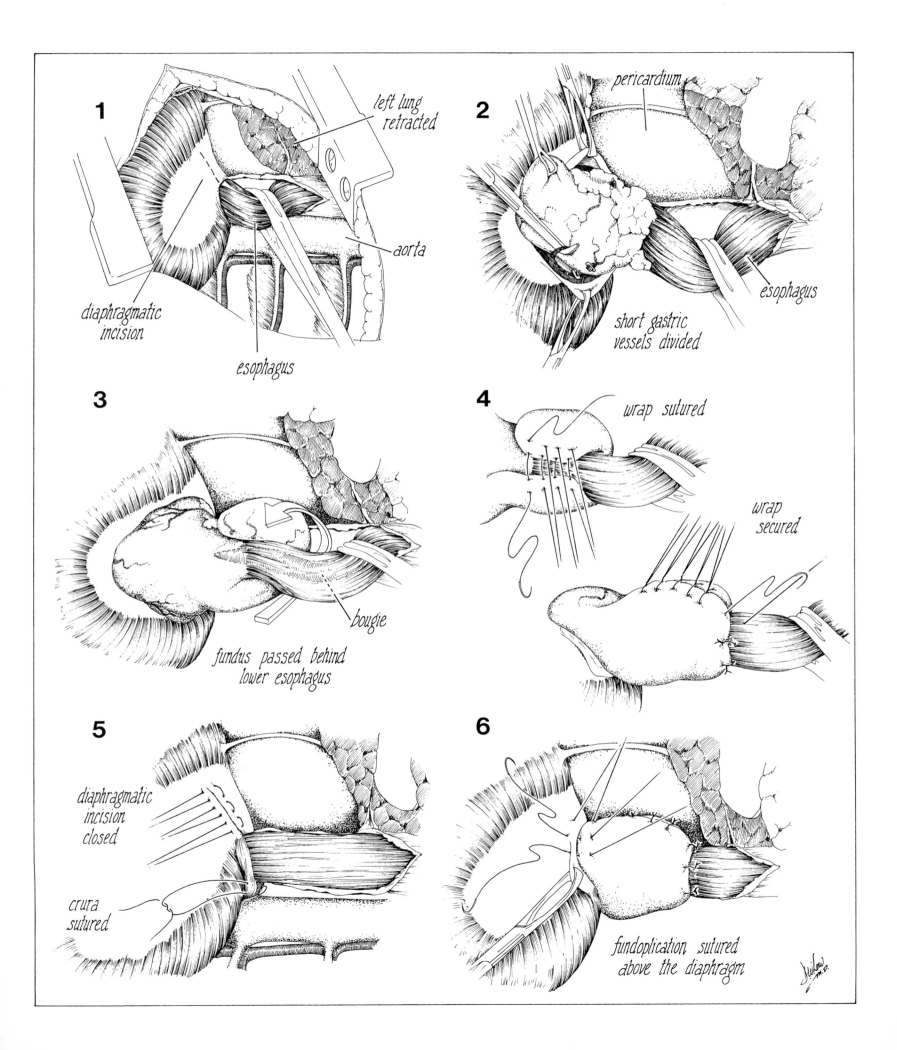

1
left lung
retracted

aorta

diaphragmatic
incision

esophagus

2
pericardium

esophagus

short gastric
vessels divided

3
bougie

fundus passed behind
lower esophagus

4
wrap sutured

wrap
secured

5
diaphragmatic
incision
closed

crura
sutured

6
fundoplication sutured
above the diaphragm

Belsey Repair of Hiatus Hernia

1 The Belsey repair (Mark IV) is also performed through a left posterolateral thoracotomy with resection of the sixth rib. The repair is made without a nasogastric tube in place. The mediastinal pleura is incised over the esophagus from diaphragm to aortic arch. The pulmonary ligament is divided to the inferior pulmonary vein. Esophageal branches of the aorta are ligated and divided. Near the diaphragm, the right pleura is gently dissected away from the esophagus. With upward traction on the esophagus, the pleural reflection is incised around the anterior circumference of the esophagus. The two vagus nerves are mobilized at the lower esophagus and allowed to drop posteriorly.

2 The peritoneal reflection is divided anteriorly around the gastric cardia. This incision is carried laterally and one or two short gastric vessels are ligated and divided. The upper 2 to 3 cm of the gastrohepatic ligament and branches of the left gastric artery are similarly ligated and divided. Fat on the anterior portion of the stomach and esophagus is removed. This dissection completely frees the lower esophagus and upper stomach from all attachments to the diaphragm and surrounding tissues.

3 The esophagus and gastric cardia are retracted anteriorly to expose the two divisions of the right diaphragmatic crus that form the esophageal hiatus. Two to five 2-0 polyester sutures are placed posteriorly in the crura, but are not tied.

When tied later, they approximate the two divisions of the right crus to form a posterior buttress.

4 Three or four interrupted 2-0 polyester mattress sutures are placed through the muscle layers of the esophagus 2 cm above the gastroesophageal junction and then through the muscular layers of the gastric wall 2 cm below the junction at the approximate line of the incised peritoneal reflection. When tied, these sutures in-fold the gastro-esophageal junction over an arc of approximately 240 degrees anteriorly and laterally.

5 A second row of three or four 2-0 polyester mattress sutures is placed in the esophagus 2 cm above the first row. Small Teflon felt pledgets may be used to buttress these sutures on the esophageal wall if the muscle layers are thin. The sutures pass through the muscular layers of the stomach 2 cm below the first suture line and then through the diaphragmatic hiatus and below upward through the diaphragm. When all are placed around a 240 degree arc, the sutures are tied firmly but not so tight as to cause necrosis or tearing. When these sutures are tied, the plicated stomach and gastroesophageal junction are imbricated below the diaphragm into the abdomen.

6 The previously placed crural sutures are now tied so that a finger can be inserted between the crura and posterior gastroesophageal junction. A nasogastric tube is now passed. The chest is closed with one drainage tube.

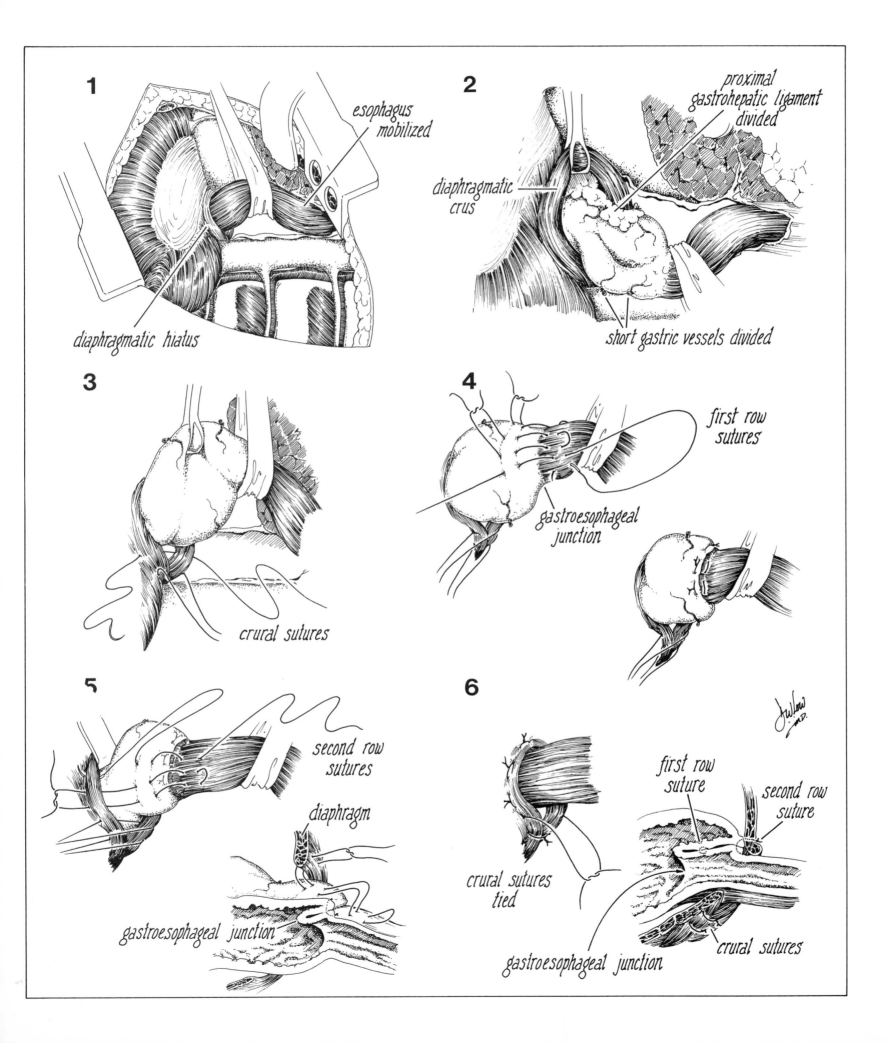

1

esophagus mobilized

diaphragmatic hiatus

2

proximal gastrohepatic ligament divided

diaphragmatic crus

short gastric vessels divided

3

crural sutures

4

first row sutures

gastroesophageal junction

5

second row sutures

diaphragm

gastroesophageal junction

6

first row suture

second row suture

crural sutures tied

gastroesophageal junction

crural sutures

Collis-Belsey Operation for Short Esophagus

This operation is prescribed for patients who have lost esophageal mobility due to local scarring and stricture ("short esophagus"). The stricture must be successfully dilated; if it is not, resection of the diseased esophagus with or without interposition of colon or jejunum is recommended.

1 The gastroesophageal junction is exposed by means of a left posterolateral thoracotomy. A segment of the sixth rib is excised. The esophagus with both vagi is mobilized below the aortic arch, pleural and peritoneal attachments to the diaphragmatic hiatus are divided, and short gastric vessels and upper branches of the left gastric artery in the gastrohepatic ligament are ligated and divided. The esophagus and gastric cardia are mobilized as completely as for a Belsey repair of hiatal hernia. These maneuvers allow the upper stomach and gastroesophageal junction to be brought through the diaphragmatic hiatus into the chest.

2 A 50 Fr Maloney mercury weighted bougie is passed down the esophagus into the stomach. With the bougie pushed against the lesser curvature, a cutting stapler is positioned parallel to the axis of the esophagus across the gastric fundus against the bougie.

3 The stapler is fired to divide the fundus into an anterior gastric extension of the esophagus and a deep fundus. The stapler can be reloaded and fired again to extend the gastric esophagus to a length of between 5 and 8 cm or whatever length of gastric esophagus is necessary to place the new gastroesophageal junction within the abdomen.

4 The gastric "esophageal" staple line is oversewn with 3-0 nonabsorbable suture to approximate serosa to serosa. The bougie should remain in place so that the lumen is not narrowed. The fundic portion of the stapled closure is infolded with a running 3-0 nonabsorbable suture.

5 Interrupted nonabsorbable sutures are placed in the crura, but are not tied. The distal stomach is now enfolded onto the new "gastric esophagus" around a 270° arc with mattress sutures. This produces a new gastroesophageal junction.

6 A second row of enfolding sutures is placed to roll a total of 4 to 5 cm of stomach onto the "gastric esophagus." These sutures are brought through the diaphragm as shown. The crural sutures are now tied. Space for a finger should remain between the anterior stomach and posterior crura. The bougie is now withdrawn.

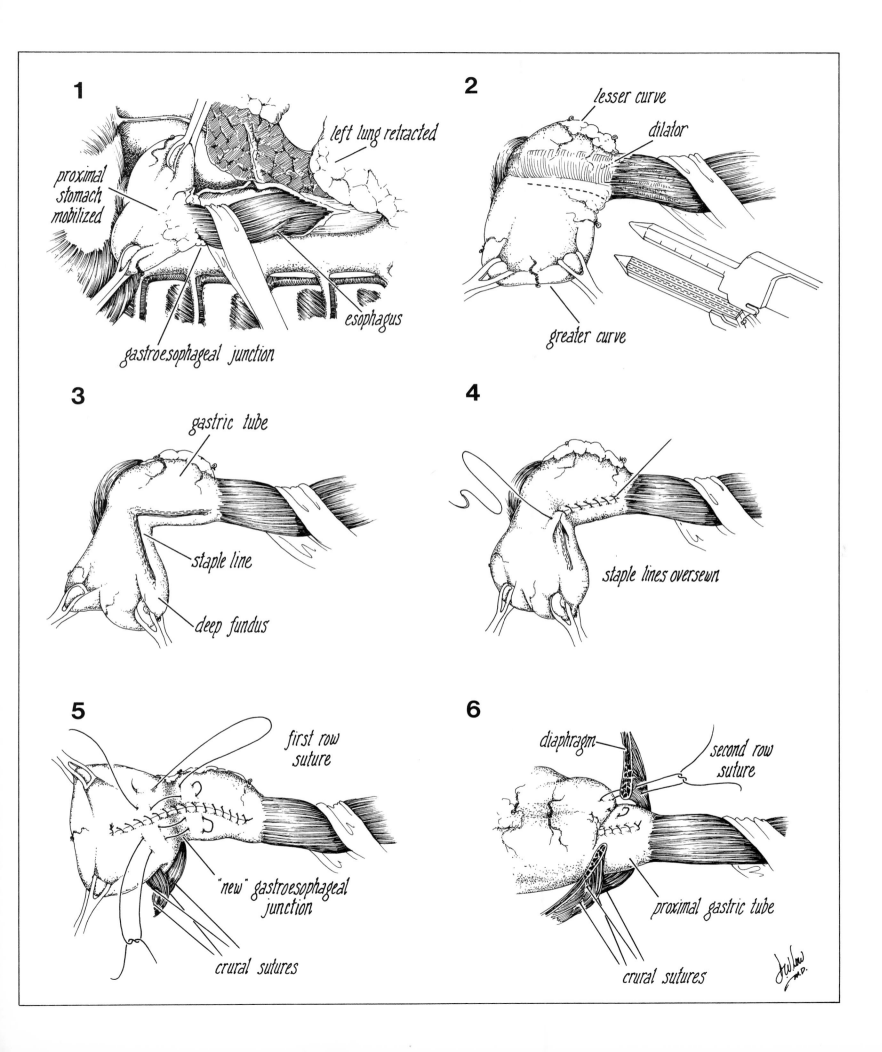

1

left lung retracted

proximal
stomach
mobilized

gastroesophageal junction

esophagus

2

lesser curve

dilator

greater curve

3

gastric tube

staple line

deep fundus

4

staple lines oversewn

5

first row
suture

"new" gastroesophageal
junction

crural sutures

6

diaphragm

second row
suture

proximal gastric tube

crural sutures

Paraesophageal Hernia

The gastroesophageal junction remains anchored in its normal subdiaphragmatic location by posterior attachments in patients with paraesophageal hiatal hernia. The condition is rare and should be differentiated from large sliding hiatal hernias that may compress the lower portion of the esophagus and allow other abdominal viscera to herniate into the chest. Unlike the sliding hiatal hernia, the stomach and a sac of peritoneum rotate through the diaphragmatic hiatus into the left pleural cavity. The lesion may be repaired from the abdomen or by means of a left posterolateral thoracotomy (sixth or seventh rib).

① The stomach and other abdominal viscera are within a peritoneal hernia sac. This sac typically develops adhesions to adjacent mediastinal and thoracic structures.

② The hernia sac is dissected away from adjacent thoracic structures by sharp and blunt dissection. The dissection is carried down to the diaphragmatic hiatus. Usually the stomach can be gently squeezed back into the abdomen once the herniated tissues have been mobilized (nasogastric tube decompression before or during reduction of the hernia is mandatory and a cuffed endotracheal tube should be used to protect against aspiration).

③ The peritoneal sac may be opened to facilitate restoration of abdominal viscera to the abdomen. If necessary, the diaphragmatic hiatus can be incised to facilitate reduction of the hernia.

④ Once the stomach, omentum, and other abdominal viscera are returned to the abdomen, the peritoneal sac is amputated and oversewn at the diaphragmatic hiatus. Three-zero (3-0) absorbable suture is used.

⑤ The defect in the diaphragm is closed with a single row of interrupted 2-0 polyester sutures. The edges of the opening are usually thickened and fibrous; thus closure is not difficult. Space for one finger and the esophagus must remain after the diaphragmatic defect is closed. The distal esophagus should not be mobilized.

⑥ Usually the diaphragmatic defect consists of an enlarged hiatus; occasionally a few muscle bands may be present between the esophageal hiatus and diaphragmatic opening of the hernia.

It is important not to disturb the gastroesophageal junction in patients with paraesophageal hernia because both the location and function of this important mechanism are not affected by the disease.

If a sliding hiatus hernia is associated with herniation of all or most of the stomach and mimics a paraesophageal hernia, the herniated abdominal contents should be first restored to the abdomen. Then a Nissen fundoplication or a Belsey repair should be carried out to restore gastroesophageal function and anatomic location.

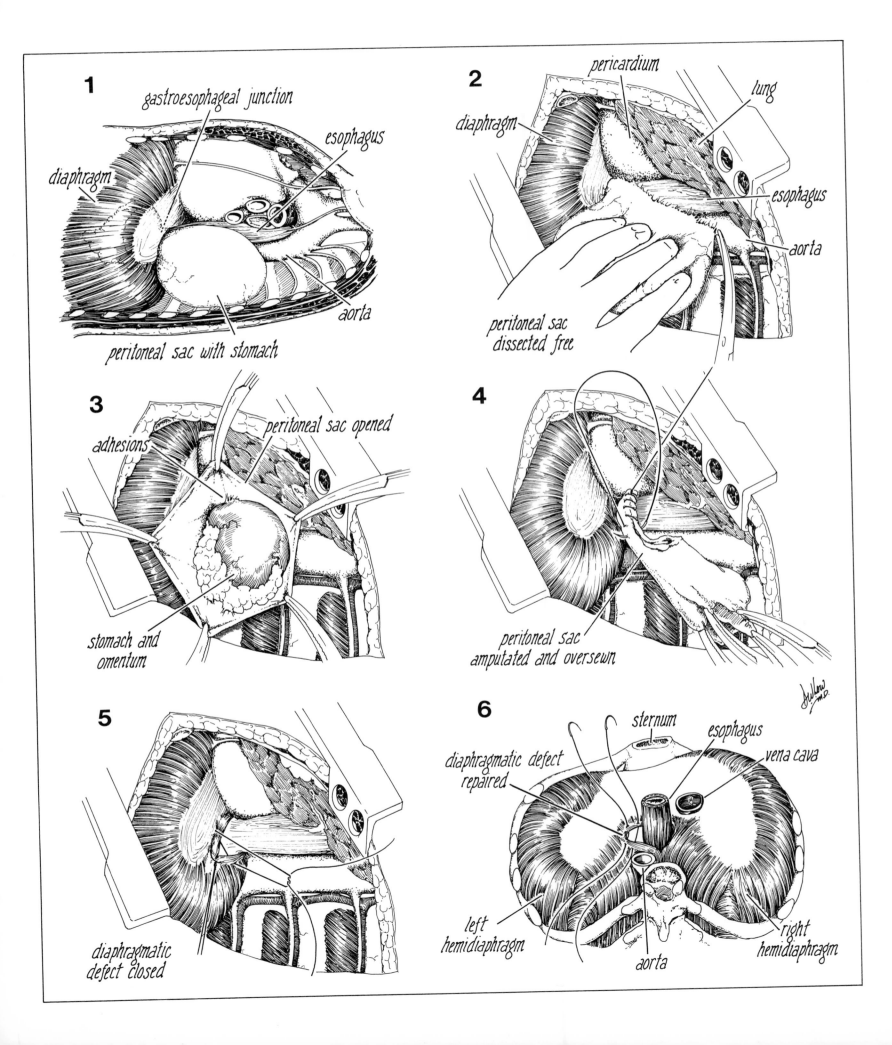

1
gastroesophageal junction
esophagus
diaphragm
aorta
peritoneal sac with stomach

2
pericardium
lung
diaphragm
esophagus
aorta
peritoneal sac dissected free

3
adhesions
peritoneal sac opened
stomach and omentum

4
peritoneal sac amputated and oversewn

5
diaphragmatic defect closed

6
sternum
esophagus
vena cava
diaphragmatic defect repaired
left hemidiaphragm
aorta
right hemidiaphragm

Excision Leiomyoma and Esophageal Cyst

Benign, encapsulated leiomyomas may be removed by enucleation. The tumors may be approached from the right or left side as indicated by the location of the tumor in the esophagus. A posterolateral thoracotomy incision is used and a segmental rib is usually removed.

(1) A lower third esophageal leiomyoma is illustrated. The mediastinal pleura is incised longitudinally.

(2) The esophagus is sharply and bluntly dissected out above and usually below the lesion. Penrose drains are passed around the esophagus to stabilize the organ and improve exposure.

(3) Attenuated esophageal muscle fibers over the tumor are carefully incised in a longitudinal direction until the wall of the tumor is reached. Invariably, this plane is readily apparent if the overlying fibers are incised slowly and carefully.

(4) Using blunt or sharp dissection and with upward pressure against the tumor, the lesion is separated from the surrounding esophageal muscle fibers. A traction suture can be placed in the tumor to facilitate separation from the esophageal mucosa. The tumor is removed as the underlying mucosa and overlying muscle fibers are dissected away.

(5) After removal of the tumor, the mucosa is carefully inspected for small tears or leaks. If found, these are carefully closed with 5-0 monofilament sutures. The separated muscle fibers are reapproximated with 4-0 or 5-0 interrupted nonabsorbable sutures. The mediastinal pleura is closed over the esophagus with a running suture.

ESOPHAGEAL CYST

Esophageal cysts are uncommon but not rare congenital lesions that may be classified as extramural or intramural and as communicating (that is, diverticulum) or noncommunicating. Cysts may vary in size and may present in the mediastinum but communicate with the intestinal tract below the diaphragm. An esophagogram and upper gastrointestinal series may indicate the ostial opening of a communicating cyst or diverticulum.

Either a right or left posterolateral thoracotomy is used. The approach is determined by the location of the cyst. Excision of a small intramural communicating cyst is illustrated.

(6) After incision in the mediastinal pleura, the cyst is located and overlying muscle fibers are incised longitudinally. The cyst may be separated by blunt and sharp dissection as is done for leiomyoma or may be opened to reveal the site of communication. The entire mucosal lining of the cyst is excised. The site of communication (neck) is sutured closed with interrupted 4-0 monofilament sutures. Overlying muscle fibers are also closed over the mucosal suture line with interrupted sutures.

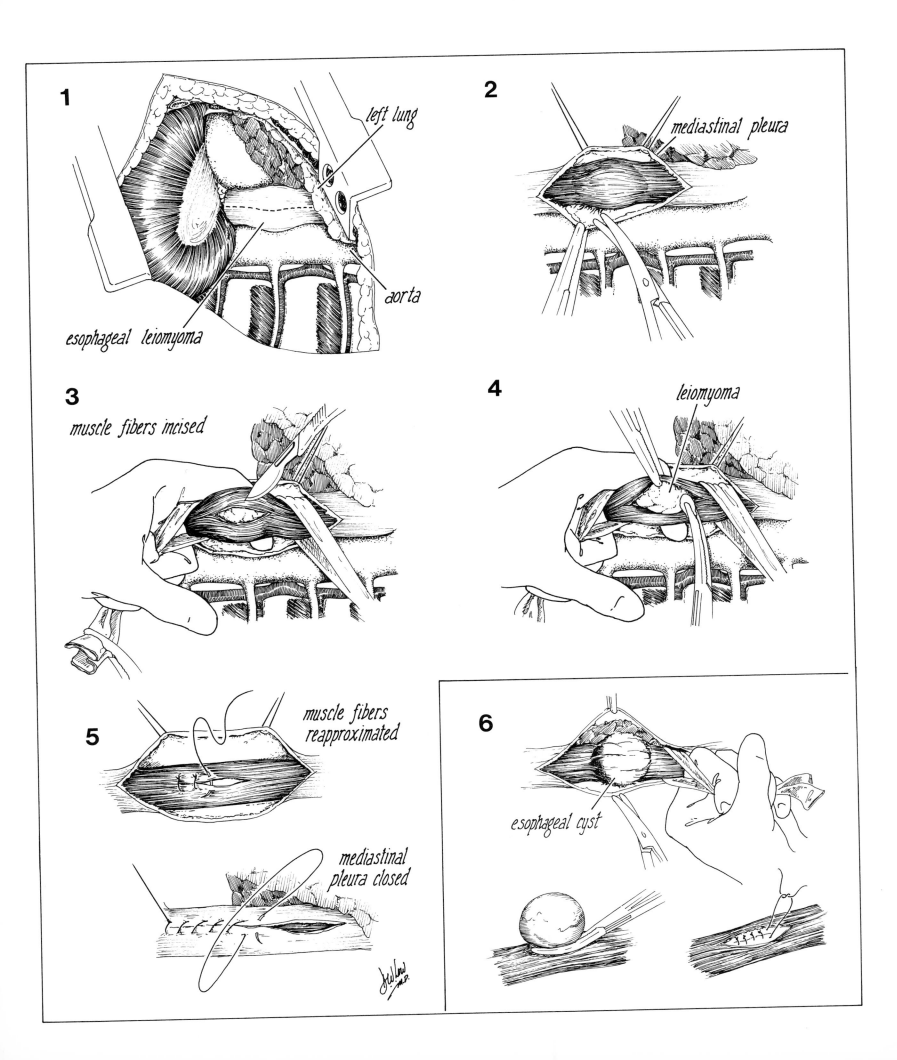

1

left lung

aorta

esophageal leiomyoma

2

mediastinal pleura

3

muscle fibers incised

4

leiomyoma

5

muscle fibers reapproximated

mediastinal pleura closed

6

esophageal cyst

Esophageal Perforation

A variety of causes, which include instrumentation, foreign body, blunt and penetrating trauma, retching, surgical tears, and benign and malignant tumors, may perforate the esophagus. Perforation of the esophagus requires immediate treatment, usually surgery, because the entrance of mouth organisms into the mediastinum causes a rapid, fulminating life-threatening infection.

CERVICAL ESOPHAGUS

Traumatic perforation of the cervical esophagus, usually caused by instrumentation or a foreign body, occurs just above or near the cricopharyngeus muscle. Small tears may be treated by antibiotics, intravenous fluids, and stopping of feedings, but we recommend early operative closure and drainage of most cervical tears.

1. An incision is made along the anterior border of the left sternocleidomastoid muscle. The esophagus is exposed by dividing the omohyoid muscle, inferior thyroid artery, and veins and by retracting the thyroid gland, anterior strap muscles and trachea anteriorly and the carotid artery and jugular vein laterally.

2. Once exposed, the lacerated mucosa is closed with interrupted 4-0 absorbable sutures and the esophageal musculature with interrupted 4-0 polyester sutures. A Penrose drain should be left near the laceration and brought out through the wound.

3. If the injury is recognized late and infection and inflammation have occurred, the retrovisceral space at the site of the lacerated esophagus must be drained. If no distal obstruction is present, the lacerated esophagus will heal without suture. The same incision to suture the esophagus is used; a sump drain is left near the upper esophagus and cricopharyngeus muscle.

THORACIC ESOPHAGUS

Rupture of the intrathoracic and intraabdominal esophagus should be treated by immediate thoracotomy (usually left) as soon as the lesion and its location are recognized. The perforation is most accurately located by radio-opaque swallows and fluoroscopy. The lower esophagus is the most common site of laceration. A left thoracotomy is usually used, but higher perforations may be exposed through a right posterolateral thoracotomy. Prompt recognition of the lesion and operation within 12 hours usually allows closure before tissues become inflamed and friable.

4. The esophagus is exposed through a left posterolateral thoracotomy with excision of a segment of the sixth or seventh rib. The edematous mediastinal pleura over the distal esophagus is incised to expose the lacerated esophagus. Sometimes location of the laceration is difficult and requires dissection and mobilization of the esophagus and careful inspection.

5. Once located, the mucosa and esophageal musculature are closed with two layers of 4-0 interrupted sutures (absorbable suture for the mucosa; polyester for the muscle). If contamination and inflammation are minimal, indicated elective procedures such as Heller myotomy or hiatal hernia repair may be safely carried out. A chest tube should be left near the site of the lacerated esophagus and the mediastinal pleura should be opened wide before the chest is closed.

6. Late recognition of intrathoracic esophageal lacerations (12 hours) threatens life. These are more difficult to treat effectively. As soon as the lesion is recognized and located, but after the patient is prepared by appropriate fluids and antibiotics, the laceration is exposed by thoracotomy. The mediastinal pleura is opened wide and any pockets of serum or pus are drained. The esophagus is dissected and mobilized to locate the site of the laceration. Often the edges of the lacerated esophagus are too swollen and friable to accept sutures. If the edges can be approximated without enlarging the tear, this is done.

To prevent further leakage and contamination, the site of the laceration is covered by a pleural flap. The pleura is often thickened by the local inflammation, but can be mobilized and used to cover the laceration. The pleural flap is hinged on the aorta and is made wide enough to extend at least 1 cm beyond each end of the laceration. The flap should be long enough to easily reach and partially or, if necessary, completely surround the esophagus.

7. Tacking sutures are placed on either side of the laceration to fix the thickened pleura firmly over the site of injury. In addition, edges of the pleura are sutured to the adjacent healthy esophagus with interrupted 4-0 polyester sutures to completely seal the laceration. The area must be drained by one or more chest tubes, including one in the right hemithorax if the right pleura has been opened. Often a gastrostomy is added (separate abdominal incision) to decompress the stomach and lower esophagus.

8. A preference for palliative laser resection instead of placement of a Celestin tube in patients with obstructing, inoperable carcinoma may increase the incidence of perforated carcinomas. If perforation occurs, palliative resection and immediate replacement of the esophagus are the preferred treatment if the patient is eligible. The operation should be done within a few hours of the perforation and does not differ from elective resection. The area of contamination should be drained.

If the patient cannot tolerate total esophagectomy and replacement at one operation, reconstruction of the esophagus can be deferred. A cervical esophagostomy is made first; the distal end of the esophagus is stapled closed; the thoracic esophagus is excised; the mediastinum is drained; the stomach is transected just below the gastroesophageal junction and a feeding gastrostomy is placed.

9. To make the cervical esophagostomy, the cervical esophagus is exposed by means of an incision over the anterior border of either the right or left sternocleidomastoid muscles. Division of the omohyoid and retraction of the thyroid gland and trachea medially and the carotid and jugular vessels laterally exposes the esophagus. The esophagus is mobilized for 4 to 5 cm below the cricopharyngeal muscle. Two traction sutures are placed opposite each other and the distal esophagus is stapled shut with a closing stapler. The staple line is inverted with interrupted 4-0 polyester sutures. The proximal esophagus is brought out the incision. The wound is closed around the esophageal stoma. The edges of the esophagus are sutured to the skin edges with interrupted 4-0 monofilament sutures. Should survival dictate reconstruction, the esophagostomy can be taken down and anastomosed to any esophageal substitute.

Perforation of a carcinoma that is recognized late in a debilitated patient or a patient with an inoperable unresectable carcinoma precludes removal of the thoracic esophagus. This tragedy has a high mortality, particularly if the perforated carcinoma cannot be resected. Surgical management requires division of the cervical esophagus with both ends brought out to the skin, placement of a large gastrostomy tube, and ligation or stapled closure of the gastroesophageal junction and drainage of the perforated carcinoma and contaminated mediastinum by placement of multiple chest tubes by means of a localized posterlateral thoracotomy. Intravenous feeding is required until feeding can be established by means of the gastrostomy. The vagi should not be included in the ligature or staple line at the gastroesophageal junction.

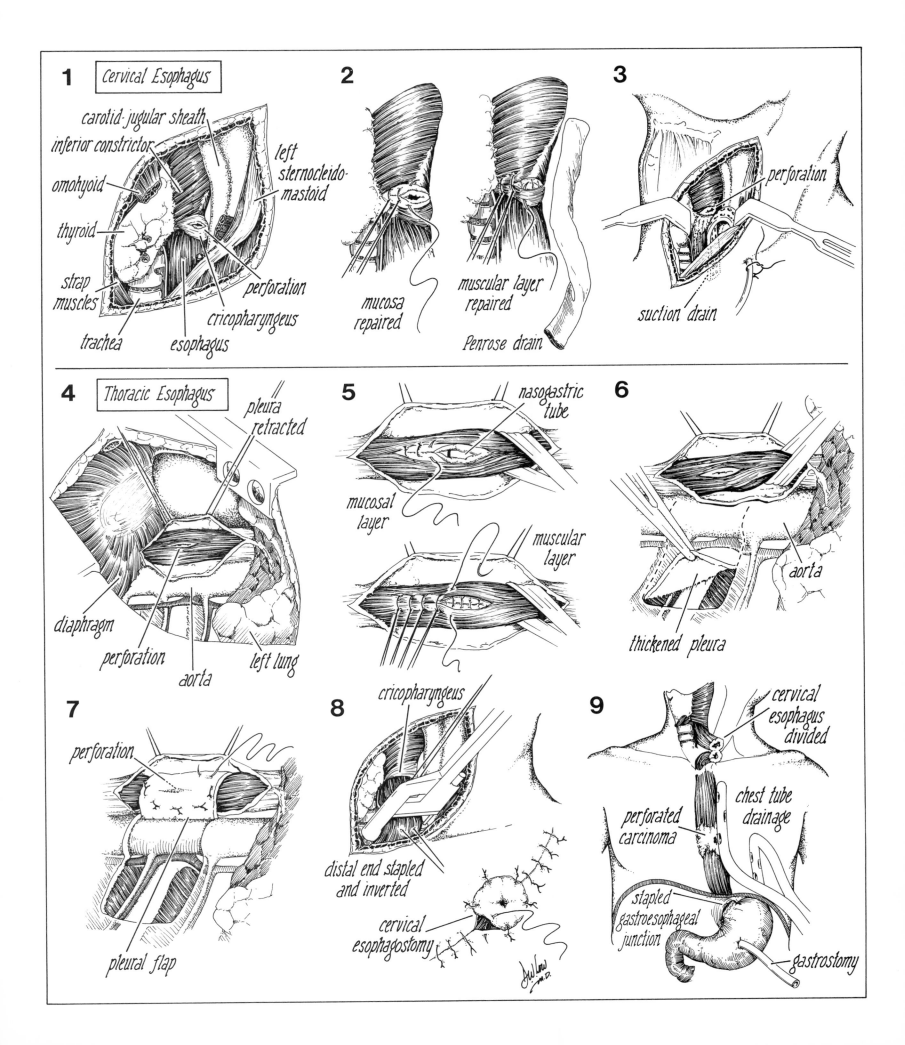

1 Cervical Esophagus

carotid-jugular sheath
inferior constrictor
omohyoid
thyroid
strap muscles
trachea
esophagus
cricopharyngeus
perforation
left sternocleido-mastoid

2

mucosa repaired
muscular layer repaired
Penrose drain

3

perforation
suction drain

4 Thoracic Esophagus

pleura retracted
diaphragm
perforation
aorta
left lung

5

nasogastric tube
mucosal layer
muscular layer

6

aorta
thickened pleura

7

perforation
pleural flap

8

cricopharyngeus
distal end stapled and inverted
cervical esophagostomy

9

cervical esophagus divided
chest tube drainage
perforated carcinoma
stapled gastroesophageal junction
gastrostomy

Esophageal Resection: Gastric Bypass Through Right Thoracotomy

The stomach, colon, or jejunum may be used to substitute for the resected esophagus. The stomach, the most common conduit, has many advantages but exposes the residual esophagus to acid reflux. The colon usually provides the greatest length but requires more extensive mobilization and more anastomoses. The jejunum provides an excellent substitute for the lower and middle thirds of the esophagus, but has a less robust and secure vascular supply as compared to the stomach. The blood supply of all esophageal substitutes remains within the abdomen; thus each conduit is a pedicle graft that replaces or bypasses the esophagus distal to the proximal anastomosis. The use of a free jejunal interposition graft wherein the trunk artery and vein of the pedicle are anastomosed to cervical vessels using microvascular techniques is a new and perhaps experimental procedure with limited indications.

Partial esophagectomy with esophagogastrostomy through a right thoracotomy, sometimes called the Ivor Lewis procedure, is a good operation for resection of middle and lower third esophageal lesions when an intrathoracic anastomosis is desired. In recent years, cervical anastomoses with subtotal esophagectomy are often preferred to intrathoracic anastomoses, even for lower third tumors. Separate laparotomy and right thoracotomy incisions are used. These incisions provide excellent exposure and are versatile and generally well tolerated. Mobilization and advancement of the stomach reduce the anastomoses required, and in most patients provide an acceptable conduit. For middle third lesions, the right thoracotomy incision avoids making the esophagogastric anastomosis at or near the aortic arch.

The patient can be placed supine for the initial laparotomy, and turned and redraped for the thoracotomy incision. It is preferable, however, to position the patient with a sandbag under the right hip, and with the right shoulder and arm pulled anteriorly so that both incisions can be made in the same operative field. A Robertshaw endotracheal tube permits the anesthetist to collapse the right lung during the esophagogastric anastomosis.

(1) An upper abdominal midline or right paramedian vertical laparotomy incision is made. The abdomen and liver are carefully explored for metastasis. The lesser sac is opened to palpate the celiac and splenic nodes. The extent and mobility of the tumor at the gastroesophageal junction are assessed. Fixation of the tumor or invasion of the esophageal hiatus obviates resection for cure. If indicated, resection begins by mobilizing the stomach. A Kocher maneuver is performed. The right gastroepiploic artery along the greater curvature is identified. This vessel is carefully preserved along the greater curvature of the stomach as the omentum and transverse mesocolon are separated from the stomach from the origin of the right gastroepiploic artery medial to the duodenum to the short gastric arteries.

(2) The short gastric vessels are divided and clipped or ligated. If splenic nodes are involved, the spleen can be taken with the upper stomach and included in the specimen.

(3) The gastroesophageal junction is now mobilized. The peritoneum around the junction is excised, and the diaphragm surrounding the esophageal hiatus is separated from the specimen by blunt and sharp dissection. Usually an operable tumor does not break through the esophageal wall to invade the diaphragm and mediastinum at the hiatus. The dissection is carried through the esophageal hiatus to sweep paraesophageal nodes toward the distal esophagus to be included in the resected specimen. The anterior and posterior vagal trunks are divided and clipped. The esophageal hiatus is necessarily enlarged by this dissection so that the stomach can be easily brought up later through the hiatus into the chest.

(4) The left gastric artery is exposed at its origin from the celiac axis and doubly ligated and divided. The gastrohepatic ligament is divided from the celiac axis to the esophageal hiatus. A line of resection across the upper stomach is then determined well below the caudal extent of the tumor. Individual branches of the left gastric artery are separately ligated and dissected away so that a cutting stapler can be placed across the proximal stomach.

(5) The stomach is divided and the distal staple line is turned in and reinforced by a row of interrupted 3-0 polyester sutures. It is often wise to oversew the proximal staple line with a running monofilament suture to reduce the chance of contamination from discharge of esophageal contents into the operative field.

(6) A pyloromyotomy is performed. The serosa and muscle layers of the pylorus and proximal duodenum are carefully incised for a distance of 4 to 5 cm and separated. Incision into the mucosa, particularly the duodenal mucosa, is assiduously avoided. If the mucosa is perforated, a Heinke-Miculitz pyloroplasty is performed by completing the incision through the layers and closing the longitudinal incision transversely by a running 3-0 absorbable suture in the mucosa and interrupted nonabsorbable sutures in the serosa and muscular layers. The proximal stomach, tagged by a long suture, is gently pushed through the esophageal hiatus into the mediastinum. A moist pack or towel is placed over the abdominal incision and contents.

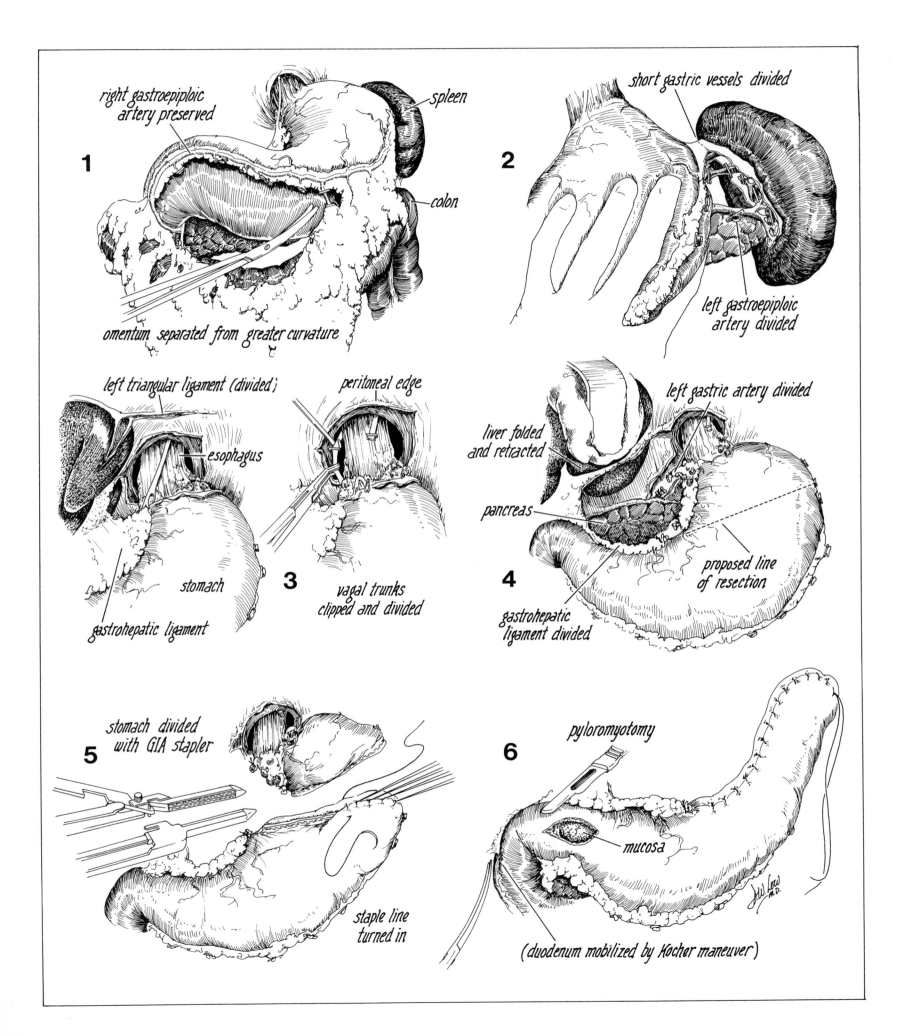

1
right gastroepiploic artery preserved
spleen
colon
omentum separated from greater curvature

2
short gastric vessels divided
left gastroepiploic artery divided

3
left triangular ligament (divided)
esophagus
stomach
gastrohepatic ligament
peritoneal edge
vagal trunks clipped and divided

4
liver folded and retracted
pancreas
gastrohepatic ligament divided
left gastric artery divided
proposed line of resection

5
stomach divided with GIA stapler
staple line turned in

6
pyloromyotomy
mucosa
(duodenum mobilized by Kocher maneuver)

J.W. Low M.D.

(7) The right chest is entered through a lateral thoracotomy after resection of the fifth (for a high anastomosis) or sixth rib. The right lung is allowed to collapse, the pulmonary ligament is divided, and the lung is packed away anteriorly and superiorly. The mediastinal pleura over the distal esophagus is incised. The distal esophagus and all paraesophageal nodes are dissected out. The nodes are swept toward the esophagus as the dissection proceeds. The right medial and anterior wall of the descending thoracic aorta is dissected clean; however, the left pleural cavity is not entered.

(8) After completion of this dissection, the distal esophagus and transected proximal stomach are delivered into the thoracic field. The site for transection of the esophagus is selected. This should be well proximal (cephalad) to the tumor (approximately 10 cm) because of the proclivity of these tumors to spread in the submucosal plane. The distal stomach is gently pulled up with care not to twist or distort the stomach. This brings the pylorus near the esophageal hiatus and the proximal stomach to the proposed site of the anastomosis.

(9) The gastric incision is made several centimeters away from the stapled turn-in and usually caudad to the fundus. A circular incision, approximately 1 cm in diameter, is made at a spot that appears to be well vascularized. Gastric contents are aspirated; bleeding vessels are carefully cauterized.

(10) The distal esophagus is held out of the thoracotomy incision by an assistant or clamp. Either a single all-layer or a two-layer anastomosis may be used. A two-layer anastomosis is illustrated. The gastroesophageal anastomosis is begun by a row of interrupted 4-0 polyester sutures between gastric serosa and muscles, and the muscle layers of the posterior esophageal wall.

(11) The esophageal and gastric mucosa are approximated with a continuous 4-0 adsorbable suture. After the posterior mucosal walls are joined, the anterior wall of the esophagus is transected and the specimen is removed. A nasogastric tube is now passed through the open anastomosis into the stomach. The tube should be firmly fixed to the nose and face (no sutures) to prevent premature dislodgement or removal. The mucosal suture line is continued around the anterior esophageal and gastric walls and tied.

(12) The anterior gastric serosal and muscular layers are sutured to the anterior muscular esophagus with interrupted 4-0 polyester sutures to complete the anastomosis. The surgeon should be able to approximate his thumb and index finger across the anastomosis by invaginating the esophageal and gastric walls.

Additional stomach is "wrapped" over the anastomosis by interrupted 4-0 polyester sutures. The stomach is also sutured to the parietal pleura at three or four sites to prevent tension on the anastomotic suture line.

The laparotomy incision is reopened. Diaphragmatic crura may be approximated behind the stomach to reduce the esophageal hiatus if necessary; usually it is not necessary. At least three fingers should be accommodated within the esophageal hiatus to prevent excessive narrowing. A few interrupted sutures may be placed between the stomach wall and the diaphragmatic hiatus to prevent herniation of abdominal contents. After inspection for bleeding, the abdomen is closed with continuous 2-0 monofilament suture for the peritoneum and fascia, continuous absorbable sutures in the subcutaneous tissue and either skin clips or a subcuticular suture. The thoracotomy incision is closed with interrupted No. 1 absorbable sutures to the intercostal muscles and continuous absorbable sutures in the remaining muscle layers and skin. A single chest tube placed low in the hemithorax is used for drainage.

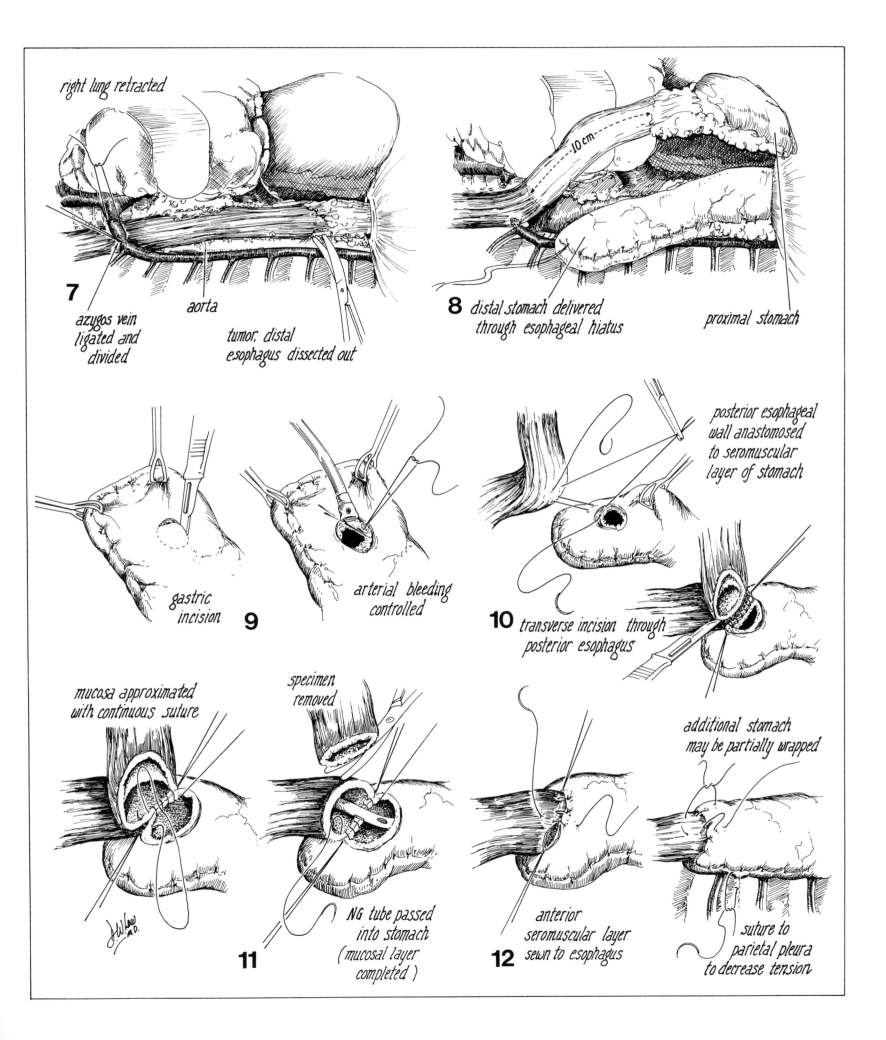

7 right lung retracted

azygos vein ligated and divided

aorta

tumor, distal esophagus dissected out

8 distal stomach delivered through esophageal hiatus

10 cm

proximal stomach

gastric incision

9 arterial bleeding controlled

posterior esophageal wall anastomosed to seromuscular layer of stomach

10 transverse incision through posterior esophagus

mucosa approximated with continuous suture

specimen removed

11 NG tube passed into stomach (mucosal layer completed)

12 anterior seromuscular layer sewn to esophagus

additional stomach may be partially wrapped

suture to parietal pleura to decrease tension

Esophageal Resection: Gastric Bypass Through Left Thoracotomy (Stapled Anastomosis)

1 The patient is positioned right side downward with shoulders perpendicular to the table and hips tilted posteriorly 30 to 40 degrees to provide easy access to the abdomen. A Robertshaw divided endotracheal tube is used. The left chest is entered through a low posterolateral incision over the sixth or seventh rib. The rib is resected, but the costal margin is not divided. The incision allows excellent exposure to the lower esophagus and diaphragm. We no longer use a thoracoabdominal incision carried across the costal margin into the upper abdomen.

The mediastinal pleura over the distal esophagus is incised and the esophagus above the lesion is encircled with a Penrose drain. The pulmonary ligament is divided. A radial incision in the diaphragm is made from the esophageal hiatus to the diaphragmatic attachments to the anteromedial chest wall. This incision denervates the anterolateral portion of the diaphragm, which is a disadvantage. One or more marking stitches on either side of the diaphragmatic incision facilitate later closure of the diaphragm. The diaphragmatic attachments to the esophagus at the gastroesophageal junction are dissected to free the distal esophagus and proximal stomach from the diaphragm.

As an alternative to denervation of part of the diaphragm, the chest wall attachment of the diaphragm may be incised by a curved incision approximately 1.5 cm from the chest wall. The esophagus and proximal stomach are dissected free of the diaphragmatic hiatus, which remains intact.

2 A careful exploration of the abdomen is made to determine the extent of liver or nodal metastasis. The diaphragmatic attachment to the left lobe of the liver is incised to permit rightward retraction of this lobe. If nodes in the hilum of the spleen require removal, the branches of the splenic artery in the hilum of the spleen are ligated and divided and the spleen taken with the proximal stomach in the specimen. With a deep Deaver retractor placed anteriorly through the diaphragmatic incision, the avascular ligaments lateral to the duodenum are incised to perform the Kocher maneuver.

3 The gastroepiploic artery is identified and preserved as the greater curvature of the stomach is separated from the omentum and transverse mesocolon. Either ties or vascular clips are used for the vessels. The short gastric vessels are divided and tied or clipped and the left gastroepiploic artery is taken to complete mobilization of the greater curvature of the stomach.

4 The gastrohepatic ligament is divided to enter the lesser sac. The left gastric artery is identified and distinguished from the splenic and hepatic arteries before double ligation and division. If left gastric nodes require removal with the proximal stomach, these can be dissected toward the proximal stomach and included with the specimen.

The site of transection of the proximal stomach is selected as dictated by the location and extent of the tumor or lesion. Branches of the left gastric artery and short gastric or left gastroepiploic branches are dissected away from the stomach wall and ligated. The proximal stomach is stapled closed and divided using a cutting stapler. The gastric staple line is turned in with a row of interrupted 4-0 nonabsorbable sutures.

5 The distal esophagus and adjacent paraesophageal nodes can now be dissected upward. Node-bearing mediastinal tissues are dissected from the aorta and right pleura and included with the specimen. The dissection continues upward to the level chosen for transection of the proximal esophagus.

The stomach is advanced into the chest. This advancement and the previous mobilization of the stomach brings the pylorus into reasonable view for a pyloroplasty. A careful pyloromyotomy is performed and converted to a Heineke-Mikulicz pyloroplasty only if the mucosa is inadvertently incised.

6 A one- or two-layer esophagogastrostomy is performed at an adequately vascularized site in the anterior wall of the stomach several centimeters away from the gastric turn-in. For a one-layer anastomosis, we use 4-0 monofilament sutures and prefer to tie the knots on the outside against the longitudinal muscle. Suture bites pass through all layers of the esophageal and gastric walls about 4 mm from the edge. The posterior row of sutures is usually placed before any are tied. Anterior sutures are tied as placed. A nasogastric tube is advanced into the stomach after completion of the posterior wall of the anastomosis. If available, some of the redundant stomach wall is tacked to the distal esophagus to reinforce the anastomosis. The gastric pouch is tacked to the chest wall with several sutures to relieve all tension on the anastomosis.

The diaphragm is closed around the stomach with interrupted mattress sutures of heavy nonabsorbable suture. The crura are not approximated, and the reconstructed esophageal hiatus should accommodate two or three of the surgeon's fingers to avoid constriction of the stomach or right gastroepiploic artery. Two or three tacking sutures are placed between the stomach wall and the diaphragmatic hiatus to prevent herniation of abdominal contents.

If a circumferential diaphragmatic incision is used, the edges of the diaphragm are approximated by 0 gauge polyester mattress sutures after the stomach has been brought up into the chest and anastomosed to the esophagus.

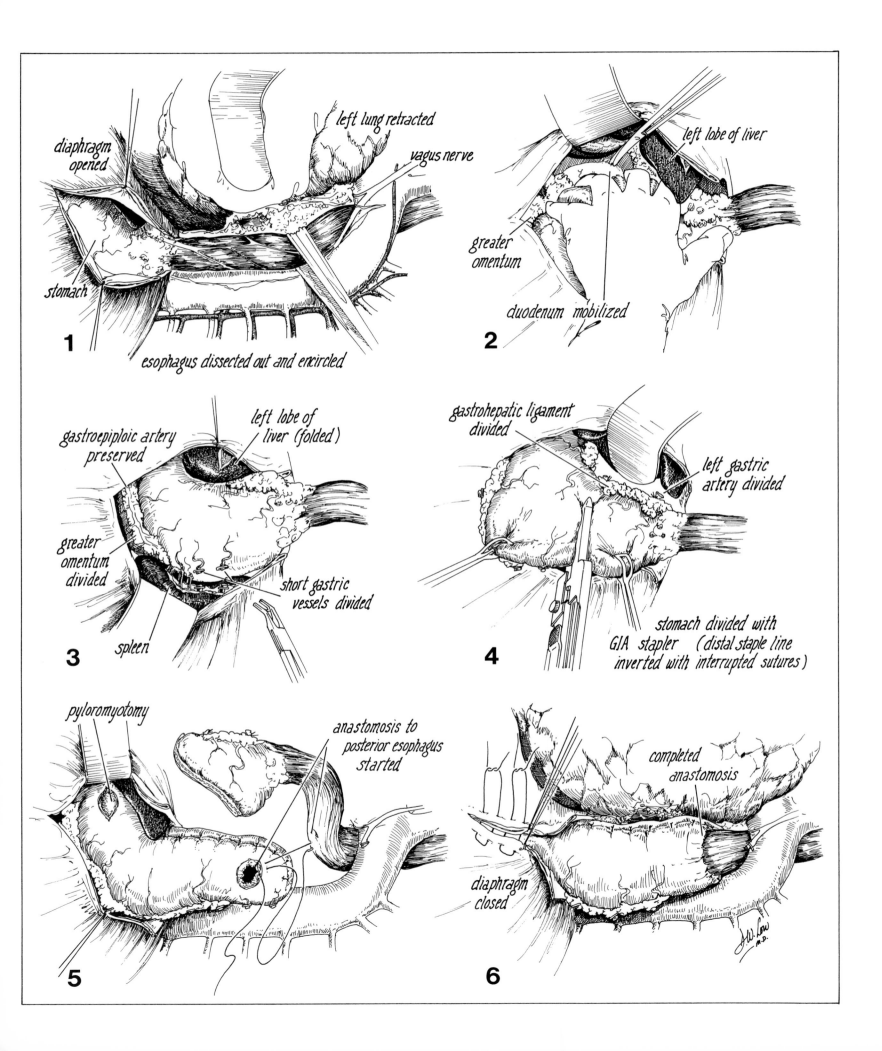

1 diaphragm opened · left lung retracted · vagus nerve · stomach · esophagus dissected out and encircled

2 left lobe of liver · greater omentum · duodenum mobilized

3 gastroepiploic artery preserved · left lobe of liver (folded) · greater omentum divided · short gastric vessels divided · spleen

4 gastrohepatic ligament divided · left gastric artery divided · stomach divided with GIA stapler (distal staple line inverted with interrupted sutures)

5 pyloromyotomy · anastomosis to posterior esophagus started

6 completed anastomosis · diaphragm closed

(7) The esophagogastrostomy anastomosis can also be made with a commercial stapling device (Ethicon Inc., Somerville, NJ). The disposable device is introduced through an incision in the anterior wall of the stomach 8 to 12 cm from the planned gastric anastomotic site. A purse-string suture (3-0 polyester) 2 to 2.5 cm in diameter is placed at the planned site of the gastric anastomosis.

(8) A stab wound is made in the center of the gastric purse-string. The instrument, with or without attached anvil, is introduced into the stomach and passed through the purse-string exit site. The anvil is now attached (if necessary) and the gastric purse-string is drawn up to pull full-thickness gastric wall around the center shaft of the instrument.

(9) A purse-string suture is placed around the esophagus at the planned site of transection. The anterior wall of the esophagus is cut transverse to the longitudinal axis 2 to 3 mm distal to the purse string.

(10) The posterior wall of the esophagus is cut and the anvil is introduced into the esophagus. Allis clamps applied to full-thickness edges of the esophagus facilitate introduction of the anvil.

(11) The esophageal purse-string is drawn up and tied. Both the esophageal and gastric ends are carefully inspected to ensure that full-thickness walls of each organ will be stapled when the instrument is screwed down and fired. When the instrument is fired, staples are driven across the opposing visceral walls and the center tissue (containing the purse-string sutures) is cut away and removed when the instrument is removed. Before firing, the instrument should be adjusted for tissue thickness as recommended by the manufacturer.

(12) The stapled anastomosis is reinforced by a row of interrupted 4-0 polyester sutures in the serosa of the gastric wall and muscular esophagus. The gastrostomy incision is closed in two layers with running sutures.

A single chest tube is placed in the lower hemithorax for drainage and brought out through a stab wound. The thoracotomy incision is closed with interrupted and running absorbable sutures.

7

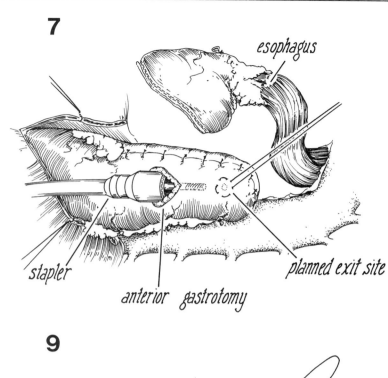

esophagus

stapler

anterior gastrotomy

planned exit site

8

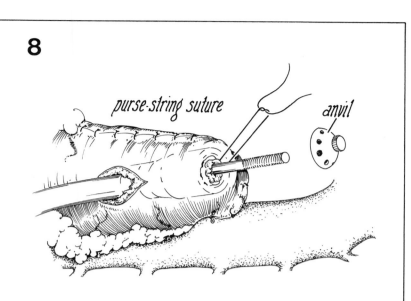

purse-string suture

anvil

9

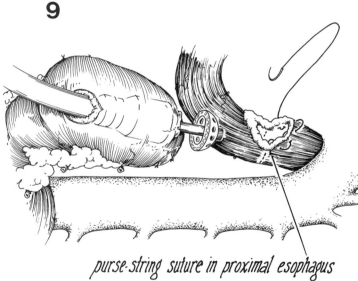

purse-string suture in proximal esophagus

10

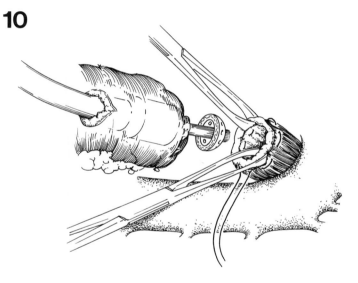

11

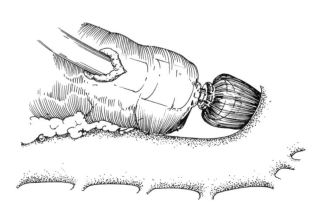

12

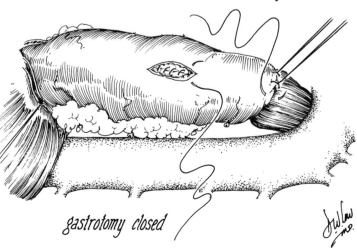

anastomosis reinforced

gastrotomy closed

Subtotal Esophagectomy with Cervical Esophagogastrostomy

This operation brings the stomach into the neck for anastomosis with the proximal cervical esophagus. The operation may be used to bypass the obstructed esophagus or combined with subtotal esophagectomy performed with or without thoracotomy. The stomach may be placed in the posterior mediastinum in the bed of the excised esophagus or in the anterior mediastinum beneath the sternum.

The steps needed to bring the stomach into the neck will be described first, followed by the procedures used to bypass or remove the distal cervical and entire thoracoabdominal esophagus.

The patient is positioned supine with the head turned to the left or right opposite the side of the cervical incision. If simultaneous right thoracotomy is planned, the patient may be turned toward the left with sandbags beneath the right hip and shoulder and the right arm extended overhead to permit access to the right neck. A Robertshaw divided endotracheal tube is used only if thoracotomy is planned.

1 A midline or right paramedian upper abdominal incision is made. After careful exploration and confirmation of operability, the stomach is mobilized by a Kocher maneuver, division of the omentum and separation from the transverse mesocolon, division of the short gastric arteries, division of the gastrohepatic ligament, and ligation and division of the left gastric artery (see Esophageal Resection: Gastric Bypass Through Right Thoracotomy). A pyloroplasty is performed. The peritoneum around the esophageal hiatus is incised, the vagus nerves are divided, and the distal esophagus and paraesophageal nodes are mobilized. The proximal stomach is transected near the gastroesophageal junction with the cutting stapler and the gastric staple line is turned in with interrupted polyester sutures. A heavy traction suture is placed in the proximal stomach to facilitate later advancement of the stomach to the neck.

2 The cervical incision is made parallel to the anterior border of either the right or left sternocleidomastoid muscle. The omohyoid muscle is divided and the cervical esophagus is mobilized medial to the carotid sheath and lateral to the thyroid gland. The recurrent laryngeal nerve is identified and protected.

3 The esophagus is found behind the trachea and mobilized by blunt and sharp dissection for about 3 inches in length. A Penrose tube is passed around the cervical esophagus to facilitate dissection of the cervical esophagus to the thoracic inlet.

Sometimes the thoracic outlet requires enlargement to accommodate the relatively bulky stomach. If indicated, the thoracic inlet is enlarged by dividing the clavicular attachments of the sternocleidomastoid muscle and, as is often necessary, by resecting the head of the clavicle. The clavicular attachments to the sternum and anterior first rib are divided with knife and heavy scissors. A clamp is passed around the clavicle about 4 or 5 cm from the medial end and is used to pass a Gigli saw around the bone. Injury to the subclavian vessels is avoided. The bone is transected. These maneuvers improve visualization of the innominate or carotid arteries, subclavian-jugular venous junction, and distal cervical esophagus, and permit access to the thoracic outlet.

4 Unless the esophagus is removed without thoracotomy, the stomach is brought up into the neck by way of the anterior mediastinum in the parietal space beneath the sternum. From the laparotomy incision, the attachments of the diaphragm to the lower sternum and xiphoid are divided to allow a hand to be passed into the anterior mediastinum. From the neck, the anterior mediastinum is opened by depressing the innominate vein and thymus posteriorly. The heavy traction suture attached to the anterior and cephalad portion of the stomach is passed through the anterior mediastinum into the neck with a large DeBakey or Crafoord clamp. The stomach is then carefully pushed and pulled through the anterior mediastinum into the neck. Great care is taken to prevent tension on the right gastroepiploic artery. Local papaverine may be sprayed on the artery before advancement of the stomach to relieve vasospasm. No sutures are placed between stomach and diaphragm to close the abdominal mediastinal opening.

5 The adequacy of the blood supply of the proximal stomach is carefully assessed after advancement to the neck (as well as before). A spot on the anterior wall several centimeters away from the turn-in is selected for the anastomosis. This spot should easily reach the planned level of the esophageal resection without tension.

The esophagus is prepared for anastomosis as follows. If blind resection is planned (see below), the intrathoracic esophagus is delivered into the neck and held up so that the posterior wall can be sutured to the posterior wall of the stomach opening with interrupted nonabsorbable sutures.

6 If the intrathoracic esophagus is not removed or is to be removed during a subsequent thoracotomy, the esophagus is transected as deep into the thoracic inlet as practical. A closing stapling instrument (RC-60 with long staples, Ethicon Inc., Somerville, NJ) is used to close the distal esophagus. Two traction sutures are placed in the distal segment to hold the distal esophagus after it is transected with a knife. The distal staple line is reinforced with a row of interrupted polyester sutures before it is allowed to descend into the posterior mediastinum. A right-angle clamp is placed across the proximal end of the esophagus. The end is held up out of the wound to expose the posterior esophageal wall. The esophagogastric anastomosis is then made in two layers using an inner running mucosal absorbable suture and an outer interrupted muscular nonabsorbable suture.

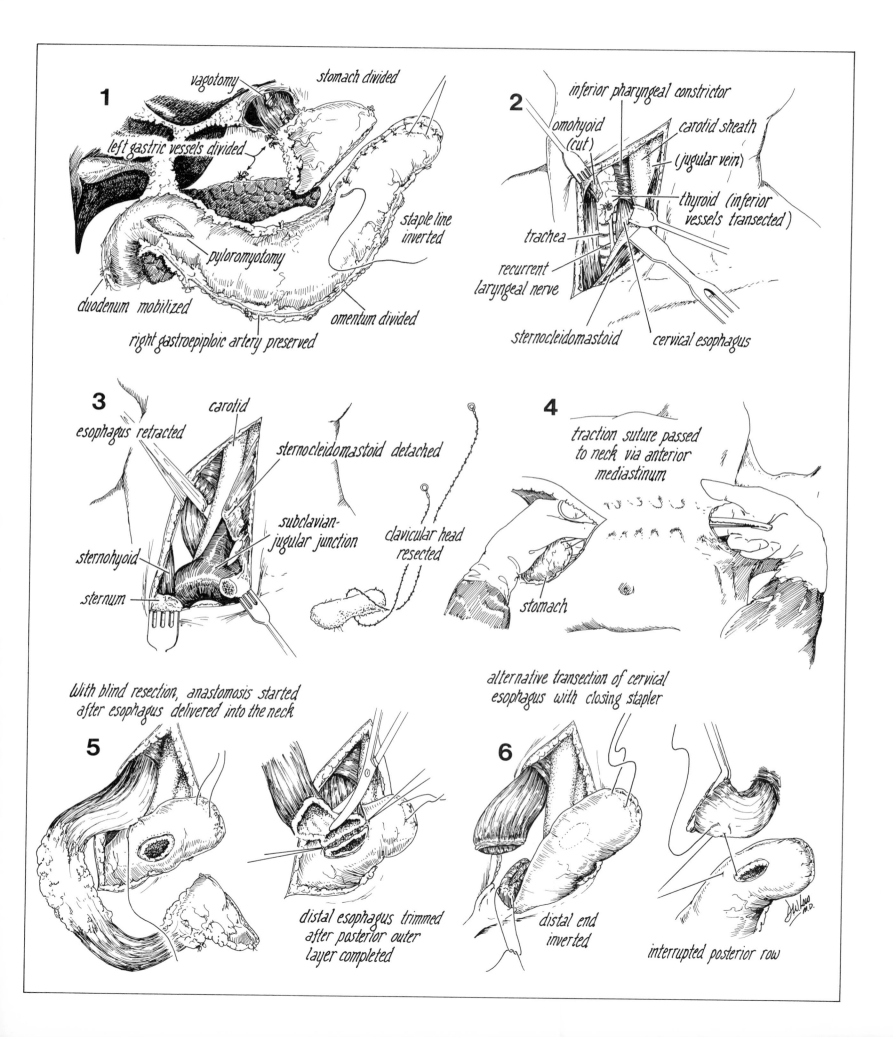

1
vagotomy
stomach divided
left gastric vessels divided
staple line inverted
pyloromyotomy
duodenum mobilized
right gastroepiploic artery preserved
omentum divided

2
inferior pharyngeal constrictor
omohyoid (cut)
carotid sheath
(jugular vein)
thyroid (inferior vessels transected)
trachea
recurrent laryngeal nerve
sternocleidomastoid
cervical esophagus

3
esophagus retracted
carotid
sternocleidomastoid detached
subclavian-jugular junction
clavicular head resected
sternohyoid
sternum

4
traction suture passed to neck via anterior mediastinum
stomach

5
With blind resection, anastomosis started after esophagus delivered into the neck
distal esophagus trimmed after posterior outer layer completed

6
alternative transection of cervical esophagus with closing stapler
distal end inverted
interrupted posterior row

7 A nasogastric tube is advanced into the stomach. The anastomosis is completed with an anterior row of interrupted polyester sutures. After the anastomosis is completed, several traction sutures are used to tack the stomach to cervical structures to relieve tension on the anastomosis. At least one suture in the sternoclavicular ligaments is usually included.

8 If the thoracic esophagus is not being removed, both ends must be turned in. Turn-in of the distal cervical esophagus is illustrated (Panel 6). The distal esophagus is stapled closed and transected just above the esophagogastric junction. A closing stapler with long staples is used. After the distal esophageal-gastric stump is transected, the staple line is reinforced by interrupted 4-0 polyester sutures. This creates a blind tube of esophagus which contains the obstructing lesion and which produces mucus. This closed, mucus-filled segment is generally well tolerated and does not expand to cause symptoms. If it does, it can be removed through a right thoracotomy at a later date.

9 The distal cervical and entire thoracoabdominal esophagus may be removed during the same operation with or without thoracotomy. In our experience, the addition of a simultaneous right thoracotomy to the laparotomy and cervical excisions increases postoperative pain and sometimes causes respiratory complications, and therefore is not recommended for older or malnourished patients. Removal of the diseased esophagus through a thoracotomy incision, however, does permit more complete removal of mediastinal nodes, particularly in the superior mediatinum.

When a simultaneous right thoracotomy is planned, the patient is positioned with sandbags beneath the right shoulder and hip, and with the right arm elevated and supported above the head. A Robertshaw divided endotracheal tube is inserted. The right chest is entered through a lateral thoracotomy incision with resection of the fifth rib.

The pulmonary ligament is divided and the collapsed lung is retracted anteriorly. The mediastinal pleura over the entire thoracic esophagus is divided. The azygos vein is ligated and divided. Superior mediastinal nodes, surrounding the esophagus and trachea, are dissected toward the esophageal specimen as the dissection begins in the thoracic inlet. The turned-in cervical esophagus, with previously dissected adjacent cervical nodes, is delivered into the chest. The dissection proceeds distally using clips and cautery to control esophageal branches from the aorta and bronchial vessels. Subcarinal nodes are usually included in the dissection. After removal of the specimen and control of all bleeding, the thoracotomy is closed with one lower tube to drain fluid collections.

ESOPHAGECTOMY WITHOUT THORACOTOMY

10 The distal cervical and thoracoabdominal esophagus can also be removed without thoracotomy, and it is often possible to perform a fairly complete lymph node dissection of the lower half of the esophagus. The distal esophagus is exposed through the laparotomy incision, which has been carried up to the base of the xiphoid. A large Deaver or (preferably) a "four-in-hand" retractor is placed through the esophageal hiatus after the peritoneum and esophageal-diaphragmatic attachments have been cut. The retractor partially elevates the heart; therefore, careful cardiac monitoring is required during this exposure and dissection (electrocardiogram and arterial and Swan–Ganz pulmonary arterial catheters). Working through this tunnel, the surgeon can visually dissect out the distal esophagus and paraesophageal tissues and nodes up to the tracheal bifurcation and sometimes the aortic arch.

11 The superior segment of the thoracic esophagus is dissected out as far as possible from the cervical incision. Usually it is not possible to carry this dissection more than a few centimeters beyond the thoracic inlet, but lower cervical and a few superior mediastinal nodes can be visually dissected toward the specimen.

12 The remaining esophagus is then blindly extracted from the thoracic inlet, tearing the remaining attached nodes and vessels of the undissected proximal thoracic esophagus. Bleeding is usually minimal and adequately controlled by temporary packing.

The cervical incision is closed with continuous suture and without drainage. The laparotomy incision is also closed without drainage.

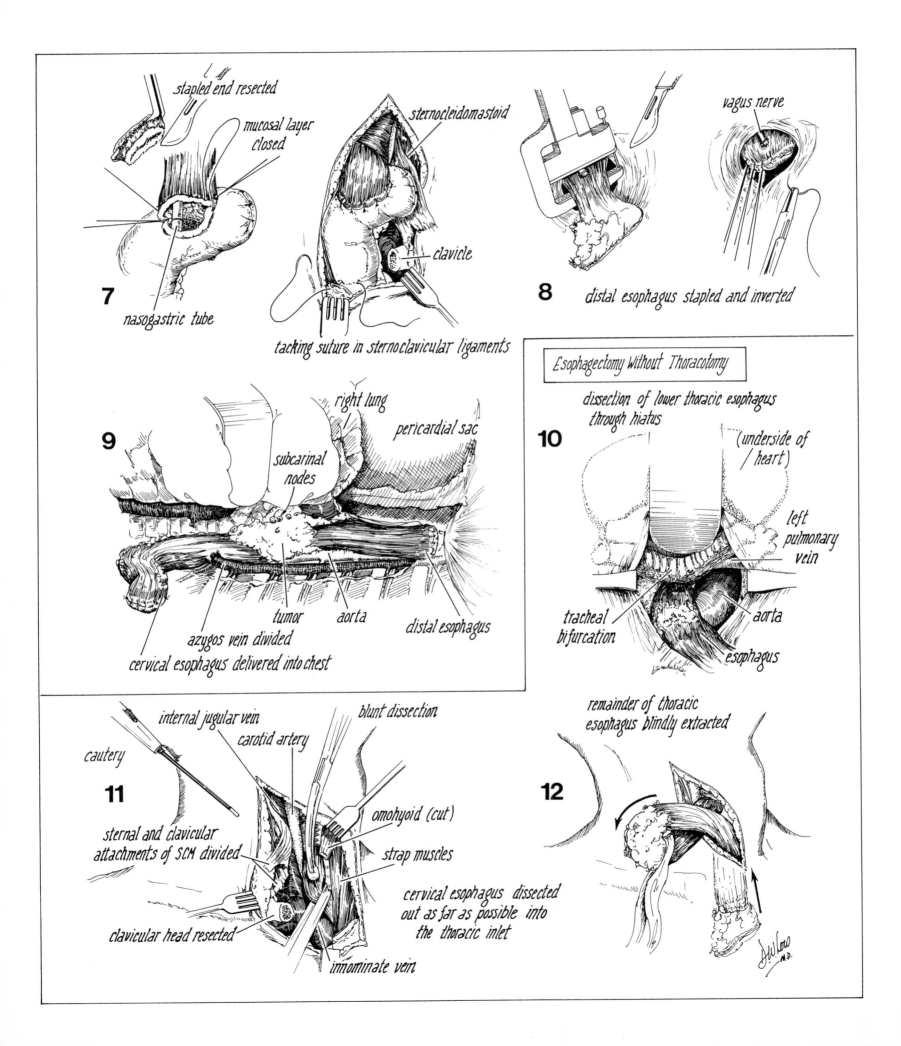

7 stapled end resected

mucosal layer closed

nasogastric tube

sternocleidomastoid

clavicle

tacking suture in sternoclavicular ligaments

8 distal esophagus stapled and inverted

vagus nerve

9 right lung

pericardial sac

subcarinal nodes

azygos vein divided

cervical esophagus delivered into chest

tumor   aorta

distal esophagus

Esophagectomy Without Thoracotomy

10 dissection of lower thoracic esophagus through hiatus

(underside of heart)

left pulmonary vein

tracheal bifurcation

aorta

esophagus

11 internal jugular vein

carotid artery

cautery

blunt dissection

sternal and clavicular attachments of SCM divided

omohyoid (cut)

strap muscles

clavicular head resected

cervical esophagus dissected out as far as possible into the thoracic inlet

innominate vein

12 remainder of thoracic esophagus blindly extracted

Reversed Gastric Tube

The reversed gastric tube can reach the neck, requires only one anastomosis, preserves the gastroesophageal junction, and does not require transection of the vagi and pyloromyotomy or pyloroplasty. Because the conduit depends upon the left gastroepiploic artery, however, the spleen is vulnerable to injury during dissection and construction of the tube. Some surgeons intentionally remove the spleen by an intracapsular dissection of the splenic arterial branches to increase blood flow to the short gastric and left gastroepiploic vessels. A reversed gastric tube is inappropriate for lower esophageal lesions because the proximal stomach and left gastric artery are preserved and the celiac nodes cannot be removed en bloc. Because the vagi and gastroesophageal junction are preserved, the reversed gastric tube has an advantage in the management of patients with benign distal esophageal stricture or patients with malignant tracheoesophageal fistula, particularly those who have been treated by radiation. The operation provides an alternative to bypass in the thoracic esophagus with colon or the entire stomach. The conduit is usually placed substernally, but can be placed subcutaneously or in the posterior mediastinum.

1 The abdomen is explored through a midline or left paramedian incision. The gastrocolic omentum is transected several centimeters away from the gastroepiploic artery. A Kocher maneuver is usually done to mobilize the antrum and duodenum. The left gastroepiploic artery is located and inspected to determine if it can support the conduit. The *right* gastroepiploic artery is divided and ligated near the pylorus. The spleen, splenic hilum, and tail of the pancreas are carefully elevated from the posterior abdomen.

2 A stab wound is made in the anterior stomach wall approximately 5 to 6 cm proximal to the pylorus and 2.5 to 3.0 cm from the greater curvature. A similar stab wound is made in the posterior stomach wall. The linear cutting stapler is placed across both walls of the stomach to the opposed stab wounds and angled toward the pylorus along the greater curvature. After the stapler is fired, it is reloaded and placed parallel to the greater curvature to fashion the gastric tube by stapling the anterior and posterior walls together and dividing the stomach between the two staple lines. To ensure an adequate lumen within the tube, some of the staples at the end of the tube can be removed and a large bougie (60 Fr) inserted along the greater curvature to the fundus. The linear cutting stapler is snugged against the bougie as the tube is cut from the body of the stomach. Usually five to seven stapler firings are required to split the stomach longitudinally from a point proximal to the pylorus to a point 5 to 6 cm from the apex of the fundus. The left gastroepiploic and short gastric arteries are carefully preserved and occasionally sprayed with papaverine to relieve vasospasm.

3 The staple line of the residual stomach is inverted with a running 3-0 monofilament suture to invert the staples and coapt the anterior and posterior seromuscular layers. Ample room should remain between the residual stomach and pylorus so that narrowing of the food channel does not occur just proximal to the pylorus. Interrupted 3-0 or 4-0 polyester sutures placed in the gastric seromuscular layers are used to invert the staple line of the gastric tube, to avoid shortening the tube. Fine bites are taken to ensure that the internal diameter of the final conduit is approximately 2 cm in diameter.

4 Usually, when reversed gastric tube is chosen as a conduit, the esophagus is not transected at the gastroesophageal junction. The gastric tube bypasses the lower esophagus, which becomes a blind pouch when the proximal esophagogastric anastomosis is made. If the esophagus is to be removed or completely bypassed, however, the gastroesophageal junction is carefully dissected free. Every effort is made to preserve as many branches of the left gastric artery as possible. The esophagus is transected at the lesser curvature with the linear cutting stapler. The anterior and posterior vagal trunks are dissected free and preserved before the esophagus is transected. Both staple lines are inverted with running or interrupted polyester sutures.

5 The long gastric tube is now rotated cephalad and, with the aid of traction sutures, passed through a substernal tunnel into the cervical wound for anastomosis in the neck. Because the gastric tube has less bulk than the entire stomach, it is usually not necessary to enlarge the thoracic inlet by resecting the medial head of the clavicle. Usually the reversed gastric tube provides sufficient length to reach the hypopharynx if necessary. There should be no tension on the left gastroepiploic vessel.

6 A cervical esophagogastric anastomosis is made with two layers of sutures. The closed end of the gastric tube is amputated and bleeding blood vessels are checked for adequacy. The anastomosis should not be made if the blood supply to the tube is precarious as documented by the lack of arterialized blood oozing or spurting from the amputated tube stump. The anastomosis is made end-to-end in two layers as described previously for gastroesophageal anastomoses. Nonabsorbable interrupted "tacking" sutures are used to anchor the gastric tube in the neck and to prevent tension on the anastomosis. A nasogastric tube does not have to be used, because the vagi are not cut.

7 The thoracic esophagus may be turned in and left in situ to drain into the proximal stomach, removed by "blind excision" (in which case the vagi may be injured and a pyloromyotomy necessary), or removed by means of a right thoracotomy immediately or at a later date. The cervical wound is usually closed without drainage; however, a Penrose drain is occasionally placed near the anastomosis and brought out through the incision.

Because of the long suture lines, a gastrostomy tube is placed in the anterior wall of the residual stomach. A stab wound is made between two concentric purse-string sutures of 0 absorbable sutures. A large (22 to 24 Fr) mushroom catheter is inserted and the two purse-string sutures are pulled up and tied. The outermost suture is used to tack the anterior stomach to the peritoneum wall at the site of the stab wound made in the abdominal wall for the gastrostomy tube.

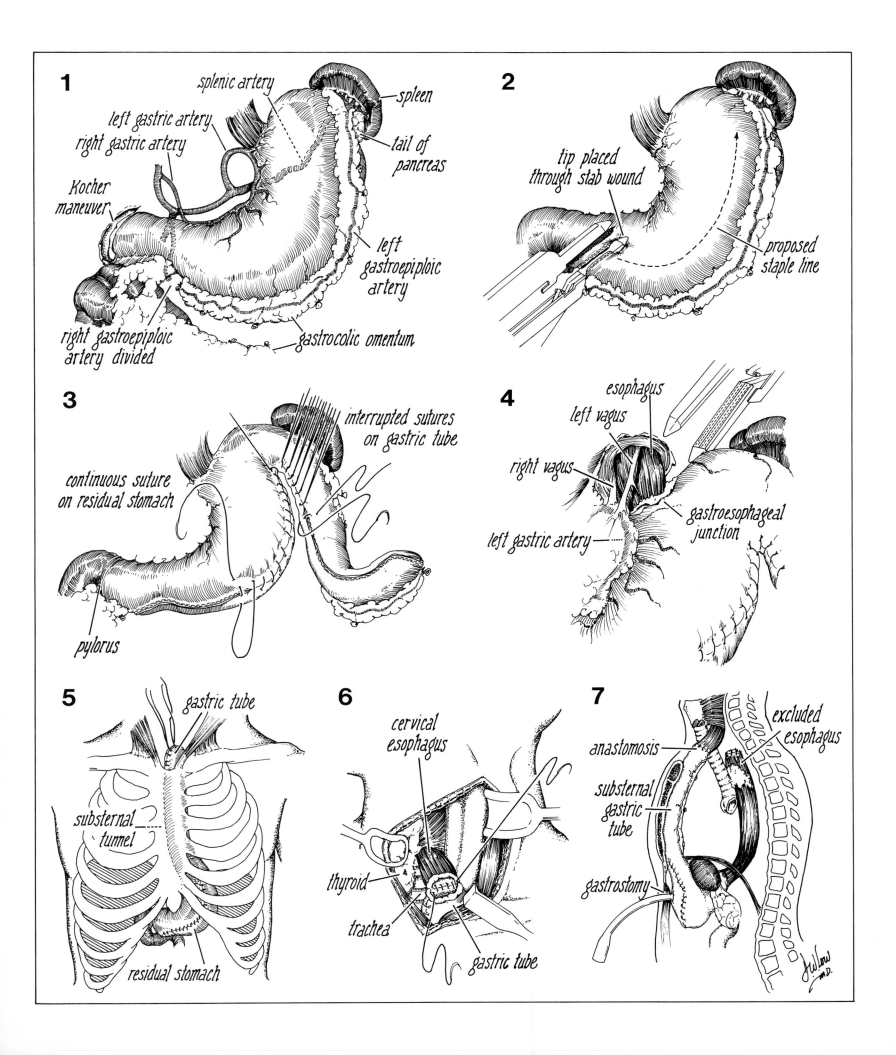

1

splenic artery

spleen

left gastric artery

right gastric artery

tail of pancreas

Kocher maneuver

left gastroepiploic artery

right gastroepiploic artery divided

gastrocolic omentum

2

tip placed through stab wound

proposed staple line

3

continuous suture on residual stomach

interrupted sutures on gastric tube

pylorus

4

esophagus

left vagus

right vagus

gastroesophageal junction

left gastric artery

5

gastric tube

substernal tunnel

residual stomach

6

cervical esophagus

thyroid

trachea

gastric tube

7

anastomosis

excluded esophagus

substernal gastric tube

gastrostomy

Colon Interposition

The right, left, or transverse colon can be used to substitute for the esophagus after partial or subtotal resection. Colonic anastomoses are usually made in the neck; the colon is uncommonly used for intrathoracic anastomoses. Isoperistaltic colon segments are strongly preferred. The colon is prepared for operation by 3 days of low-residue diet, mechanical cleansing, and poorly absorbed oral antibiotics for 12 to 24 hours. The colon is frequently placed in the anterior mediastinum but may be used in the posterior mediastinum, pleural space or beneath the skin and subcutaneous tissue anterior to the sternum.

Although a left thoracoabdominal incision provides excellent exposure, this incision is painful and poorly tolerated by many patients. In thin patients, a left thoracotomy (with resection of the sixth or seventh rib) may be combined with a circumferential diaphragmatic incision to expose the left colon and intrathoracic esophagus. We prefer laparotomy and separate thoracotomy or deferred or no thoracotomy for colon interposition operations. Laparotomy provides better visualization of the colonic mesentery, permits use of the right or transverse colon if the left colon is diseased, and adds little morbidity. In elderly or debilitated patients, esophagectomy is deferred or the esophagus is dissected out from below and removed blindly as previously described.

1 The patient is positioned supine with the face turned opposite to the proposed cervical incision. A midline or paramedian laparotomy incision is made and careful abdominal exploration is carried out to detect metastases. The omentum is dissected from the colon. The hepatic and splenic flexure is mobilized. The superior and inferior mesenteric arteries and colic branches are identified. The selected segment of colon must be long enough to reach the neck easily and must have a series of interconnected vascular arcades that can nourish the selected colon segment from one major colic vessel after one or two other colic vessels are divided. In the illustration, the right colon has been selected and the right colic and ileocolic arteries have been ligated and divided. As illustrated, the left colon and distal half of the transverse colon can also be used. If the left colon, which is preferred by many surgeons, is used, the left colic artery is preserved and the colon is divided proximal to the splenic flexure and at the sigmoid.

Before any colic vessels are cut, bulldog clamps are placed on the designated vessels for 15 minutes. The arcade vessels may be sprayed with papaverine. During this period, a pyloromyotomy may be performed and the cervical incision or the route for the transplanted colon prepared. If the arcades are adequate, the clamped arcade feeder vessels are ligated and divided.

2 The colon segment, which is now supplied by a major colic branch and a series of interconnecting arcades, is stapled closed and divided at each end. The stapled ends are covered with rubber domes to reduce contamination. The illustration shows the prepared right colon based on the middle colic artery.

Intestinal continuity is restored by anastomosis of the two ends of divided bowel. We prefer a two-layer anastomosis.

3 The colon segment is passed behind the stomach. Either the substernal or posterior mediastinal route to the neck is prepared. If simultaneous esophagectomy is planned, the stomach is divided and turned in. If the esophagus is to be resected without thoracotomy, this dissection is done before the colon is advanced into the neck.

4 The regional anatomy of the left neck and cervical esophagus is illustrated. The neck is incised along the anterior border of the sternocleidomastoid muscle, and the omohyoid muscle is divided. The plane between the carotid sheath laterally and the thyroid gland, recurrent laryngeal nerve, and trachea medially is opened to reach the cervical esophagus.

5 A Penrose tube is passed around the esophagus to produce a three-inch loop which is gently pulled into the wound. The ligamentous attachments of the sternocleidomastoid muscle to the sternum and clavicle are divided, and if necessary, the head of the clavicle may be resected to enlarge the thoracic inlet. The superior portion of the anterior mediastinum is bluntly dissected so that the colonic segment can be gently advanced through the anterior or posterior mediastinum to the neck.

6 A heavy traction suture facilitates passage of the colon segment to the neck. Tension on the vascular pedicle, injuries to the delicate arcades, and torsion of the colon segment must be avoided. Adequacy of the blood supply of the cervical colon and absence of venous congestion are confirmed. If blood supply is not clearly adequate, the questionable segment is amputated at a level with a secure blood supply.

7 The esophagocolic anastomosis is made end-to-end or to the side of the turned-in colon several centimeters away. Either the cervical esophagus is divided in the neck and the distal end turned in as previously described, or the transected intrathoracic esophagus is blindly removed.

8 The posterior esophageal wall is sewn to the serosa and muscular layers of the colon with interrupted nonabsorbable sutures.

9 After completing these rows, the esophagus is transected 6 to 8 mm from the suture line. The mucosal layers are sutured together with a running absorbable suture 360 degrees around the circumference. A nasogastric tube may be passed into the stomach or a gastrostomy in the gastric fundus may be used for decompression.

10 The esophagocolic anastomosis is completed with an anterior row of interrupted nonabsorbable sutures. The colon is anchored into the neck by several sutures to cervical structures and ligaments to relieve all possibility of tension.

11 The opposite end of the colon segment is trimmed and anastomosed end-to-side to the anterior or posterior wall of the stomach at approximately its midpoint. Running sutures of 3-0 absorbable material are used for the mucosa; running sutures of monofilament nonabsorbable suture are used for the outer seromuscular layer.

A Stamm gastrostomy using two concentric purse-string sutures may be placed in the fundus of the stomach for decompression. A pyloroplasty or pyloromyotomy is not needed unless the vagus nerves have been divided (which is done if the esophagus is removed, but not if the esophagus is only bypassed).

The neck and abdominal wounds are closed in layers, usually without drainage. A small Penrose drain placed near the esophagocolic anastomosis may be used if the surgeon is insecure about the viability of the anastomosis.

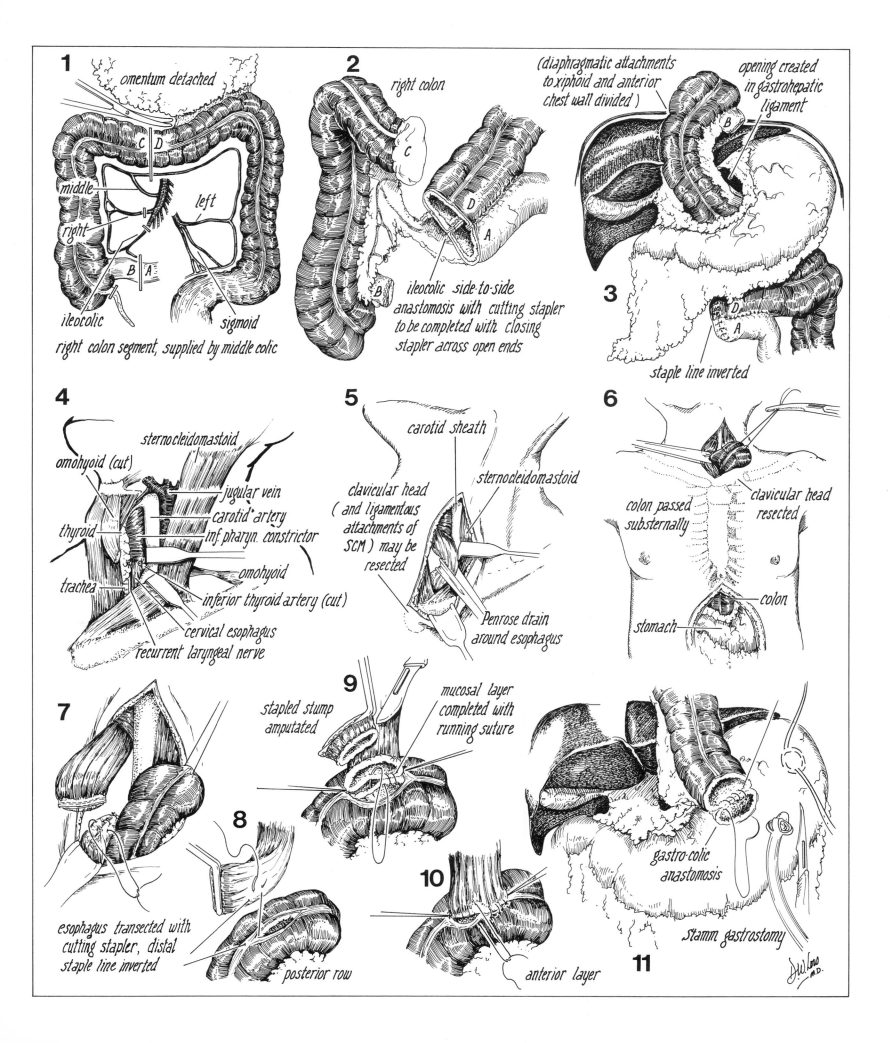

Jejunal Interposition

A segment of jejunum can be used to replace or bypass the middle and lower esophagus. Sometimes the jejunum can be used to replace the entire thoracic esophagus; however, usually the jejunal vascular arcades limit the length of the interposed jejunal segment to an anastomosis within the chest.

The operation can be done through a left thoracotomy and circumferential diaphragmatic incision in thin individuals, but because of the importance of the mesenteric blood supply, separate laparotomy and right thoracotomy incisions (Ivor Lewis technique) are preferred. Thoracoabdominal incision is avoided, although it provides good exposure.

1 After laparotomy and abdominal exploration, the proximal jejunum is isolated and the mesenteric vessels inspected. The first 6 to 10 inches beyond the ligament of Treitz are rarely used because the vascular pattern usually limits the length of the interposed segment. Beyond this proximal segment, however, the vascular arcades are usually sufficient to support a 12- to 14-inch segment pedicled on one of the major branches of the superior mesenteric vessels. The success of a jejunal interposition depends on the adequacy of the blood supply to the selected segment. The mesenteric vessels should be well illuminated and studied before test clamping. Sometimes a segment of proximal jejunum is intentionally removed at the edge of the mesentery to enhance blood flow to the adjacent distal segment. Papaverine is sprayed on mesenteric vessels to alleviate vasospasm. Bulldog clamps are placed on trunk vessels selected for division for 10 minutes before these vessels are ligated and divided. The selected vessels are ligated and divided and the mesentery is carefully divided to the bowel. The jejunum is transected at each end of the selected segment with the linear cutting stapler.

2 Intestinal continuity is restored by anastomosis of the proximal and distal jejunum. A stapled anastomosis is illustrated. Stapled lines are inverted with interrupted 3-0 or 4-0 polyester sutures. The jejunal mesentery is closed with a running suture. The jejunal pedicle is brought through a hole made in the transverse mesocolon behind the stomach.

3 The esophageal hiatus and proximal stomach are dissected to mobilize the distal esophagus and proximal stomach. If the lesion is malignant and near the gastroesophageal junction, the left gastric artery is doubly ligated and divided at its origin for the celiac axis. The lymph nodes in the gastrohepatic omentum can be swept upward toward the proximal stomach to be included in the resected specimen. Likewise, the spleen and its hilar lymph nodes can be included in the specimen by ligating the splenic artery and vein at the upper border of the tail of the pancreas. If the lesion is a benign structure that requires replacement of the lower esophagus, a node dissection is not necessary, and the stomach can be transected just below the esophagogastric junction beyond any squamous cell mucosa.

The stomach is transected at the appropriate level (between the upper and the middle third in the illustration). The distal gastric staple line is inverted with interrupted 3-0 polyester sutures. Any remnants of gastrohepatic omentum or diaphragmatic attachments to the esophageal hiatus are divided. The esophageal hiatus in the diaphragm is enlarged and lymph nodes and fat are resected toward the specimen if the lesion is malignant. A pyloromyotomy or Heineke-Mikulicz pyloroplasty is done. A Kocher maneuver is optional.

4 The right chest is entered through a lateral thoracotomy incision with resection of the fifth or sixth rib. After incision of the pulmonary ligament, the lower esophagus with paraesophageal nodes is dissected free and the distal esophagus and proximal stomach (with or without attached spleen) is delivered into the chest. The jejunal segment is carefully passed into the chest through the esophageal hiatus. The vascular pedicle is checked for pulsations and the proximal pedicle is inspected through the laparotomy incision to ensure that it is not twisted or under tension.

5 The jejunal staple line is amputated and bleeding from the open end of the bowel is inspected. A two-layer end-to-end esophagojejunal anastomosis is carried out with interrupted nonabsorbable outer wall sutures and a continuous mucosal suture. A nasogastric tube is not usually passed through the anastomosis; the bowel is decompressed by either a gastrostomy or by feeding and draining jejunostomies.

6 If curvature of the jejunal loop caused by the vascular arcade tends to kink the esophagojejunal anastomosis, the stapled end of the jejunum, may be turned in with interrupted sutures. The end of the proximal esophagus is anastomosed to the antimesenteric side of the jejunum using a two-layer anastomosis. The jejunal segment is sutured to the parietal pleura in several places to prevent tension on the suture line.

7 The opposite end of the jejunum is amputated at the level necessary for anastomosis to the stomach. Redundant proximal jejunum should be removed without compromising the blood supply to the remaining segment before the gastric anastomosis is made. The anastomosis can be made at the cardia if a benign stricture has been resected. It can also be made on either the anterior or posterior gastric wall. After a 1.5 cm hole is made in the stomach away from the gastric turn-in, the anastomosis is made with either the one-layer full thickness technique or the two-layer method, which we prefer.

The hole in the transverse mesocolon around the jejunal pedicle is carefully closed around the pedicle to prevent an internal hernia. The jejunum is tacked to the diaphragmatic esophageal hiatus with two or three sutures.

The chest incision is closed, with one chest tube left for drainage. The laparotomy incision is closed without damage.

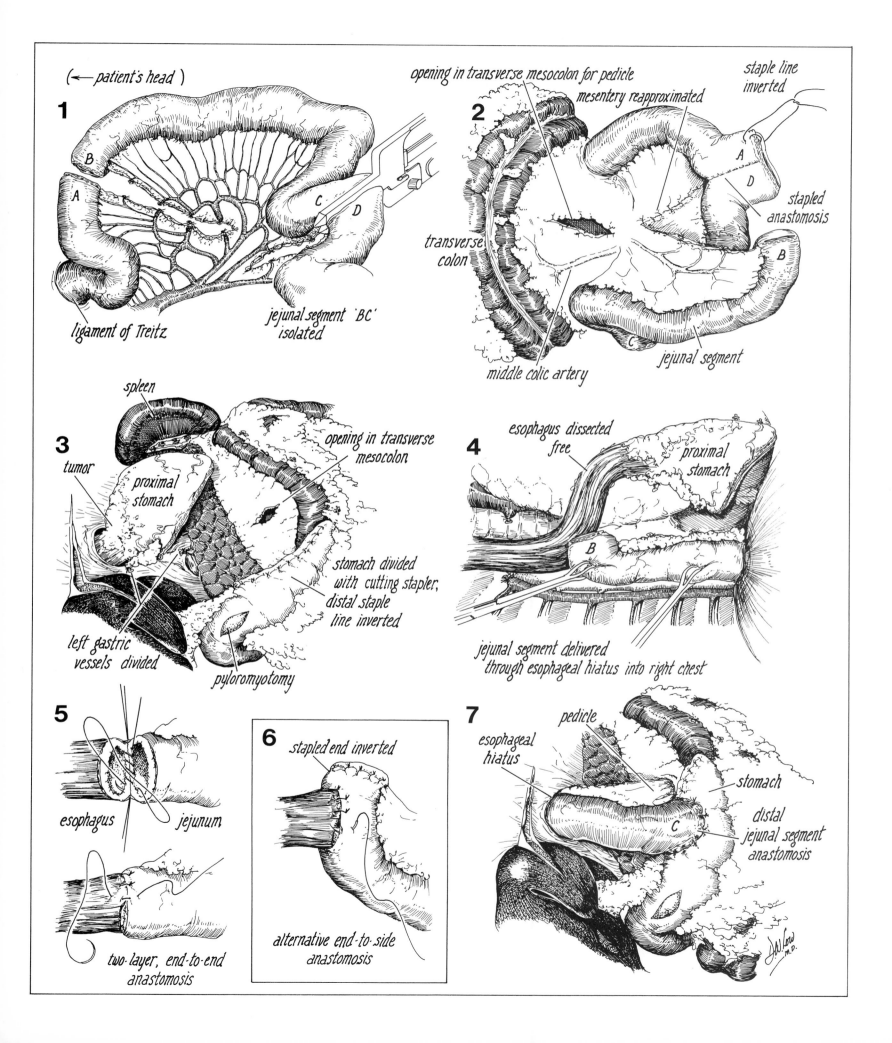

1 (← patient's head)

B

A

C

D

ligament of Treitz

jejunal segment 'BC' isolated

2 opening in transverse mesocolon for pedicle

mesentery reapproximated

staple line inverted

A

D

stapled anastomosis

B

transverse colon

C

jejunal segment

middle colic artery

3 spleen

opening in transverse mesocolon

tumor

proximal stomach

stomach divided with cutting stapler, distal staple line inverted

left gastric vessels divided

pyloromyotomy

4 esophagus dissected free

proximal stomach

B

jejunal segment delivered through esophageal hiatus into right chest

5

esophagus   jejunum

two-layer, end-to-end anastomosis

6 stapled end inverted

alternative end-to-side anastomosis

7 pedicle

esophageal hiatus

stomach

C

distal jejunal segment anastomosis

Index